Using Dental Materials

Eleanor D. Vanable, CDA, RDH, EdD
Professor of Dental Health
Community College of Rhode Island
Lincoln, Rhode Island

Laurence R. LoPresti, DMD
General Dental Practice
Lincoln, Rhode Island
Adjunct Professor of Chemistry
Dean College
Franklin, Massachusetts

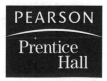

PEARSON

Prentice
Hall

Upper Saddle River, New Jersey 07458

Library of Congress Cataloging-in-Publication Data

Vanable, Eleanor D.
   Using dental materials / Eleanor D. Vanable, Laurence R. LoPresti.
      p. ; cm.
   Includes index.
   ISBN 0-8385-1576-2
   1. Dental materials.
   [DNLM: 1. Dental Materials. 2. Dentistry, Operative—methods. WU
190 V217u 2004] I. LoPresti, Laurence R. II. Title.
RK652.5 .V36 2004
617.6'95—dc21

                                                    2003013208

Publisher: Julie Levin Alexander
Assistant to Publisher: Regina Bruno
Acquisitions Editor: Mark Cohen
Assistant Editor: Melissa Kerian
Editorial Assistant: Mary Ellen Ruitenberg
Marketing Manager: Nicole Benson
Channel Marketing Manager: Rachele Strober
Director of Production and Manufacturing: Bruce Johnson
Managing Production Editor: Patrick Walsh
Production Liaison: Alexander Ivchenko
Production Editor: Jessica Balch, Pine Tree Composition

Manufacturing Manager: Ilene Sanford
Manufacturing Buyer: Pat Brown
Design Director: Cheryl Asherman
Design Coordinator: Maria Guglielmo-Walsh
Cover and Interior Designer: Janice Bielawa
Composition: Pine Tree Composition, Inc.
Manager of Media Production: Amy Peltier
New Media Project Manager: Stephen Hartner
Printing and Binding: Banta Book Group
Cover Printer: Phoenix Color Corp.

Pearson Prentice Hall™ is a trademark of Pearson Education, Inc.
Pearson® is a registered trademark of Pearson plc.
Prentice Hall® is a registered trademark of Pearson Education, Inc.

Pearson Education, Ltd., London
Pearson Education Australia Pty. Limited, Sydney
Pearson Education Singapore Pte. Ltd.
Pearson Education North Asia Ltd., Hong Kong
Pearson Education Canada, Ltd., Toronto
Pearson Educación de Mexico, S.A. de C.V.
Pearson Education—Japan, Tokyo
Pearson Education Malaysia, Pte. Ltd.
Pearson Education, Upper Saddle River, New Jersey

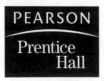

10 9 8 7 6 5 4 3 2 1
ISBN 0-8385-1576-2

TABLE OF CONTENTS

PREFACE

This book is intended for allied dental personnel who want to understand the clinical use of dental materials. Our aim is to answer the "why" questions students have as they begin learning the basics of materials preparation and use. Students tell us understanding is easier when theory can be related to a "story," that is, a real-world experience to which they can attach their new knowledge. Over the years we have developed a framework for teaching materials in which dental procedures are the story. We begin with the basics, such as what items are made with materials, provide routine terminology so each class member can understand what the others are saying, then proceed to the stories: prevention, diagnosis, cosmetic improvement, tooth restoration, and replacement. Better student and graduate understanding has in turn led to more meaningful patient education, plus more conscientious materials preparation and use. We hope you also find this framework useful.

For all teachers, how to teach to many different types of learners is a major consideration. In this text, we have attempted to provide several different learning avenues: the written word, pictures of procedures that may be unfamiliar to the beginning student, traditional self-tests, crossword puzzles, and case studies. It is unlikely that each student will want to complete all of the learning exercises, but we hope that each will find more than one learning method that is helpful. We welcome your comments and suggestions.

ACKNOWLEDGMENTS

As John Donne has said, "no man is an island, entire of itself." A book is completed only with the generous help of many people. We are sincerely grateful to Bob Ready of Cerami-Tech Dental Lab for the porcelain pictures, John Asciolla of Asciolla and Sons Dental Lab, Inc., for the denture pictures, Jan Asciolla and Kathleen Mangan for their unfailing encouragement and good humor, and Rich Lake and Donna Albanese of Patterson Dental for help obtaining pictures. Pamela Coletti, Maria Costa, Theresa Gagne, Debbie Libucha, Melissa Makowski, Gretchen Pratt, Lori Sylvia and Michelle Vincent set up, posed for, and cleaned after numerous pictures. Diane Bourque, Gene Grande, Norm Grant, Donna Medas Patton, and Linda Richard arranged for use of suitable photographic facilities and equipment, and provided helpful demonstrations and advice. Pamela Wood, Linda Pettine and Pamela Coletti read and commented sagely on portions of the manuscript.

Patients, as always, were extremely helpful. On request, they willingly posed and allowed pictures of their restorations to be used. Confidentiality prohibits our naming them but they know who they are and that we are appreciative. Mark Cohen and Melissa Kerian, our editors at Prentice Hall, provided helpful direction and the patience we needed when the demands of work, family and book collided.

Thank you to Michelle, Eric and Julia LoPresti for yielding the computer as needed, and to Dave and Andy Vanable for providing publishing experience plus that ever-valuable commodity, moral support.

Eleanor Vanable
Laurence LoPresti

REVIEWERS

Kathleen H. Alvarez, RDH, BS
Instructor
Department of Dental Hygiene
Cypress College
Cypress, California

Karmen Aplanalp, RDH, BS, MEd
Director and Clinic Coordinator
Dental Hygiene Program
Dixie State College
St. George, Utah

Esther Andrews, CDA, RDA, RDH, MA
Former Chairman
Dental Hygiene Program
Minnesota State University
Mankato, Minnesota

Kathy Gibson, CDA, MS Ed
Coordinator for Dental Assisting
John A. Logan College
Carterville, Illinois

Joan E. Miranda, CDA, RDH, MEd
Professor and Coordinator
Dental Assisting Program
Professor
Dental Hygiene Program
Rose State College
Midwest City, Oklahoma

Robert Patterson, DDS
Director
Dental Hygiene Program
Howard College
Big Spring, Texas

Betty Scott
Instructor
Dental Assisting Program
East Central College
Union, Missouri

Carol Wesley Wright, RDH, BS, MEd
Adjunct Associate Professor
Dental Hygiene Program
Northern Virginia Community College
Annandale, Virginia

SECTION

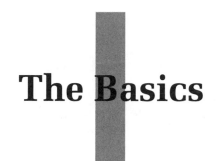

The Basics

Like all fields of study dental materials has its own terminology and a set of basic facts that all students of that subject must understand. These are presented in the next four chapters. Special attention must be paid to this section as this material must be mastered in order to understand the remaining chapters.

For the student, the world of clinical dentistry lies beyond this book. Dental materials technology advances over time and materials in the future may be very different than the ones we use today. However, the principles of use and the evaluation of the materials properties will not change because the laws of chemistry and the biology of the human body control them. By knowing the basics of material science any future material can be assessed properly using the information in this section.

WHY DENTAL MATERIALS?

OBJECTIVES

After studying this chapter, you should be able to:

1. Understand the differences between direct and indirect restorations.
2. Understand the differences between fixed and removable restorations.
3. Identify different types of impressions and the materials needed to make them.
4. Describe the various uses for models.
5. Explain the function of and be able to identify implants, mouthguards, splints, and sealants.
6. Explain what abrasives are used for.
7. Have a basic understanding of the uses of waxes in dentistry.

Almost any procedure performed in a dental office or clinic requires the use of some material. Choosing the right material for any procedure is a bit like choosing a dress or shirt. It has to meet a number of requirements—color, cost, fit, comfort—and have the ability to take the wear and tear of use and cleaning. This book is about understanding materials—making sure the right one is selected, used properly and cared for properly. An introductory knowledge of materials will go a long way toward developing proficiency in their use, and by so doing, improving your patients' satisfaction with the procedures you complete for them.

▼ RESTORATIONS ▼

When teeth are damaged they do not heal nor do new teeth grow once the permanent dentition is complete. Damage may be caused by dental decay, trauma, or various other causes. These damaged teeth and oral tissues need the services of a dental professional to restore their original shape and size to allow for proper chewing, speech and appearance. Tooth repairs are termed *restorations*. They are divided into two basic categories depending on where they are formed.

Direct Restorations

Restorations formed in the patient's mouth are termed *direct restorations.* They are commonly called fillings. A direct restoration is chosen when the need is to restore the tooth as close to original condition as easily, quickly and inexpensively as possible, and enough tooth structure remains to retain the restoration in the tooth. Direct restorations are pictured in Figure 1-1.

Direct restorations are made of different materials, some of which are similar to natural teeth and one of which is not. Materials that appear natural are termed *esthetic materials*. It would be wonderful if we had esthetic materials that could be used for every restoration. Unfortunately, for some situations esthetic materials may not be the best choice. They tend to be more expensive, technique sensitive and some are not particularly strong, so some restorations are made of nonesthetic materials.

Indirect Restorations

An *indirect restoration* restores to good condition a tooth that has been damaged, similar to a direct restoration, but is *not* made in the tooth. An indirect restoration is made outside the mouth and held to the tooth by cement or a bonding agent. Cements and bonding agents are

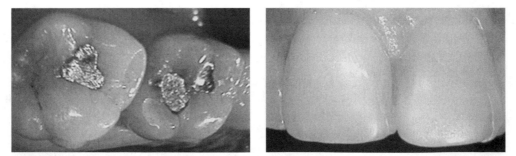

FIGURE 1-1 Direct restorations. The left side shows two old amalgam restorations. The right side shows two composite restorations. Both of the front teeth are missing their corners. One side is several years old and the other is only 1 year old. Can you tell which is which?

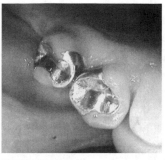

FIGURE 1-2 Inlays. This shows two inlays that are older than the restorations in Figure 1-1. Note how new they still look.

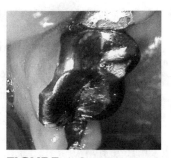

FIGURE 1-3 Onlay. This shows an onlay on an upper molar. Note how this restoration covers the entire chewing surface of the tooth but not the entire side.

adhesives. They attach two solid materials together by interlocking them, joining them chemically or both mechanisms.

An indirect restoration is placed when access is particularly difficult or the restorative material requires some type of processing that cannot take place in the mouth. For example, porcelain, the most natural-looking material in dentistry, may require processing at over 1500° Fahrenheit.

Single Tooth Restorations

There are several types of indirect restorations, differentiated by how much of the natural tooth is being restored. A *veneer* covers only the facial surface, to improve its appearance. A veneer may be placed when the enamel of a tooth is discolored, improperly formed, chipped or the tooth itself is not correctly aligned.

An *inlay* (Figure 1-2) restores one or more tooth surfaces, just as a direct restoration does. The dentist makes an inlay when enough of the original tooth structure is present to hold the inlay in position without difficulty.

An *onlay* (Figure 1-3) also restores one or more tooth surfaces, but specifically includes the edge of a biting surface or the cusp(s) of a chewing surface in the restoration. An onlay is made when a biting edge or cusp is too badly broken down to restore, or is missing.

A *crown* (Figure 1-4) replaces all the surfaces of the natural crown of a tooth. An artificial crown may be made when the natural crown is badly broken down but enough tooth structure is present to provide adequate support for an artificial replacement. A crown may also be made to improve a patient's appearance.

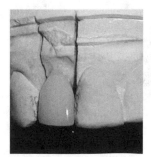

FIGURE 1-4 Crown. This shows a porcelain fused to metal crown on the die used to make it.

▼ REPLACEMENTS FOR MISSING TEETH ▼

Replacements That Are Fixed in Position

A *bridge,* or *fixed partial denture,* is a single restoration that replaces one or more missing teeth and is permanently attached to teeth next to the spaces where the missing teeth were located. Each replacement tooth is termed a *pontic,* and each attachment tooth is an *abutment tooth.* Each restoration used as a connector to an abutment tooth is an *abutment.* Each pontic and each abutment is also termed a *unit.* Dental personnel frequently refer to a bridge by the number of units it contains. So a bridge with two pontics and three abutments would be considered a five-unit bridge.

There are several types of bridges. A *conventional bridge* (Figure 1-5) has crowns over the abutment teeth and is cemented into place. A *bonded bridge* (Figure 1-6) has metal, wing-like plates that conform to the abutment tooth or teeth and are bonded in place. This requires less tooth preparation than a conventional bridge. A bonded bridge may also be called a *Maryland bridge.*

A bridge that has a pontic at either or both ends rather than an abutment is called a *cantilevered bridge.*

Replacements That Are Removable

Dentures are removable tooth replacements. They are used when there is not enough support for a fixed restoration, there is great damage to the oral structures that requires rebuilding or the patient chooses not to have a fixed restoration. They are divided into two major categories: a *full denture* (Figure 1-7) replaces all the teeth and associated tissue in one dental arch; a removable *partial denture* (Figure 1-8) replaces some of them. Patients often speak of a full or partial denture as a plate or partial plate. An *overdenture* (Figure 1-9) is a removable denture (either full or partial) that is held in place by implants or a few remaining natural tooth roots. It has special attachments in the denture that fit over restorations in the mouth. Removable partial dentures have a frame made of metal or plastic, a place to put the replacement teeth termed the *saddle* and usually clasps that attach to the remaining teeth in order to keep the partial denture in the mouth.

Full dentures are held in place by the patient's muscles and the adhesion between the denture and the gums. The adhesion works like two plates of glass with water between them. Although the plates of glass can be very hard to pull apart this type of retention requires a very close fit between the gums and the denture. Try sticking something bumpy to a glass plate. As the space between the objects gets larger the adhesion disappears.

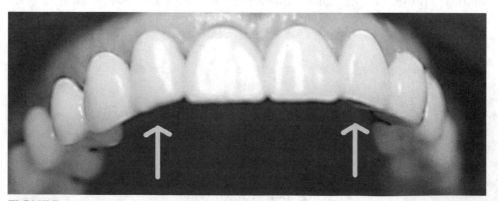

FIGURE 1-5 Fixed partial denture. The arrows point to prosthetic teeth that have no natural root underneath them. They are supported by the crowns on the adjacent teeth.

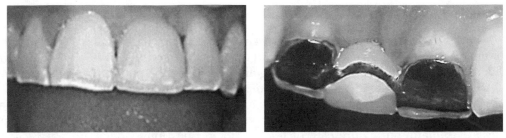

FIGURE 1-6 Maryland bridge. This is the front and the back of the same bridge. The natural teeth are intact on either side of the pontic. On the palatal aspect one can see the two metal retainers that are bonded to the teeth.

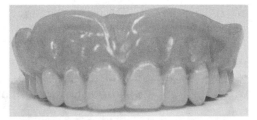

FIGURE 1-7 Full denture. Note that it not only has teeth but also recreates the gingival contours that are lost.

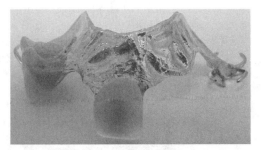

FIGURE 1-8 Removable partial denture. Note that the frame is metal and has clasps on the side that grab the teeth to hold the partial in place.

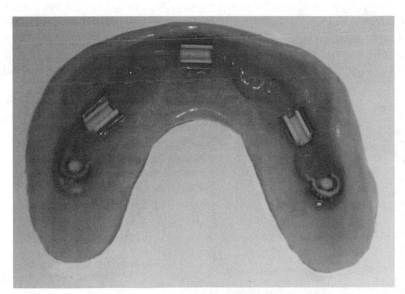

FIGURE 1-9 Overdenture. This has two types of attachments; the long ones go over a bar and the round ones fit into a special keeper. This upper denture is completely stable in the patient's mouth without covering the whole palate.

▼ MODELS ▼

A *model,* or *cast,* may be made of a patient's teeth. It duplicates the patient's teeth in dental stone. A model can be used to study and diagnose the conditions in a patient's mouth when he or she is not present or as a teaching aid to educate the patient. Models used for study or patient education are termed *study models* (Figure 1-10).

Casts are also used to make a restoration or appliance to fit a particular patient. Because each patient's mouth is different, whatever is being made may not fit adequately unless it is made on a duplicate of the mouth in question. Models on which something is made are termed *working casts.* A working cast of only one tooth is termed a *die* (Figure 1-11).

Dental personnel often do not differentiate between study models and working casts; generally calling them all models. Dies, however, are usually referred to as dies.

▼ IMPRESSIONS ▼

A mold of the patient's mouth must first be made if a duplicate is to be created. That mold is termed an *impression.* To make an impression, dental personnel put a soft material in a small mouth-shaped tray (Figure 1-12), place it over the patient's teeth and surrounding tissue, and let it set. The material is then removed from the mouth and used as a mold for making a duplicate.

There are many different types of impressions to meet specific needs: study model impressions, preliminary impressions, counter (or opposing) impressions, secondary (or final or mucostatic) impressions, occlusal registrations (or bites), triple tray (or dual) impressions, and check impressions.

A *study model impression* is used to make a model for study, diagnosis or teaching.

A *preliminary impression* is a fairly, but not highly, accurate impression used to pour a model on which an item that will not place stringent accuracy or processing demands will be made.

A *counter,* or *opposing, impression* is an impression of the arch opposite the one of interest. This and an accurate *occlusal registration,* or *bite* (a record of how the patient's teeth fit together) allows the laboratory technician to fabricate a restoration that will fit the patient well.

A *final* (or *secondary* or *mucostatic) impression* (Figure 1-13) is a very accurate one. The model or die made from it will be used for fabrication of an indirect restoration. Indirect restorations must fit the patient precisely.

A *triple tray impression* is so called because it does three jobs at once. It is made with only one tray, not three as the name implies. Impression material is placed on both sides of

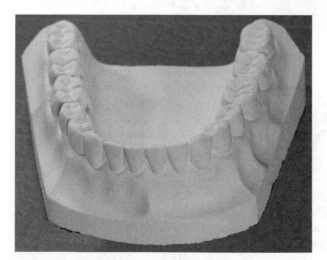

FIGURE 1-10 Study model. This model is used to study a patient's teeth in detail.

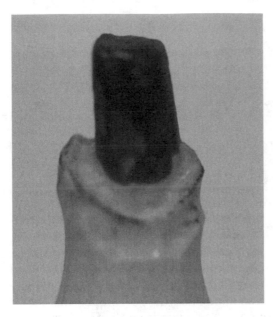

FIGURE 1-11   Die. This will be used to make a crown for this tooth in the laboratory. The tooth is only a stump because it has been cut down to receive the crown.

the tray, the tray is positioned between the teeth and the patient is asked to close gently. When the material is set and the tray has been removed, the impression material has recorded the anatomy of both arches as well as how the teeth close together; the tray has taken a final impression, an opposing impression and a bite all at once. A triple tray impression may also be termed a *dual impression* because what it is actually doing is taking an impression of both arches at once.

A *check impression* is a quick impression to assess the progress of a tooth preparation. Although dentists become near wizards at visualizing the structure of holes cut in teeth to prepare them for receiving restorations, occasionally it is advisable to visualize a preparation more concretely. This is done by pushing a small piece of soft wax into the preparation, then withdrawing it and looking at and often measuring the result.

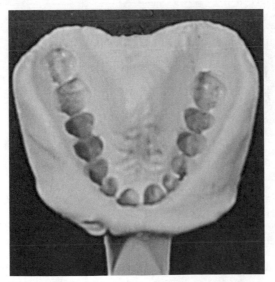

FIGURE 1-12   Alginate impression. This is a full mouth impression for a study model.

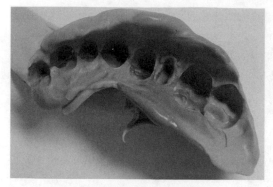

FIGURE 1-13 Polyvinylsiloxane impression. This is a quadrant impression showing the indentations of the teeth, which will be filled to make a model (Figure 1-10) or die (Figure 1-11).

▼ CUSTOM TRAYS ▼

Many impressions are made with stock trays, that is, trays designed to fit many people "pretty well." Stock trays come in a limited number of sizes. When a really good fit is necessary, the "pretty good" fit of a stock tray may not be adequate. A tray that fits only one person, but fits him very well, is constructed for those times. To construct a custom tray, a preliminary impression is taken, a working cast is made from the impression, and a tray is made on the cast (Figure 1-14). This tray is then used to make a second, much more accurate impression. Do you remember what this second, more accurate impression is termed?

▼ IMPLANTS ▼

An *implant* is a replacement for the root of a tooth that has been lost. It is anchored onto the jaw bone or more commonly anchored within the bone. There are two basic types: subperiosteal and endosseous. A *subperiosteal implant* consists of a replacement tooth or teeth attached to a supporting framework that fits between the bone and its covering periosteum. While these were very popular in the 1980s, they have largely been supplanted by *endosseous implants* (Figure 1-15). These consist of a support that is anchored in the jawbone. The supporting substructure may be shaped like a blade, a screw, or, most commonly, a cylinder. The cylindrical ones are often called *root form implants* as they replace

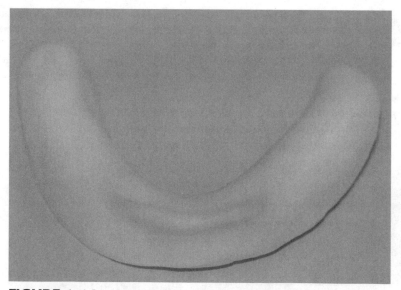

FIGURE 1-14 Custom tray. This particular one is made for a denture impression. They can also be done for impressions of the teeth as in Figure 1-13.

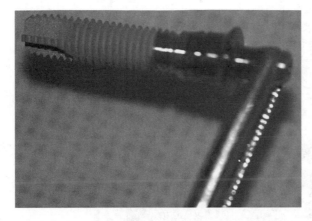

FIGURE 1-15 Endosseous implant. The actual implant is on the left ready to be inserted. The driving cap and driver will be removed after it is placed.

a single root. Subperiosteal implants, then, are placed on the bone and endosteal implants are anchored within it. Fixed or removable restorations can be placed on the implants.

▼ MOUTHGUARDS ▼

Athletes are sometimes hit with balls, bats, elbows or other things in the course of play. The result can be devastating to the teeth and jaws. Mouthguards are worn to protect against such injury. A *mouthguard* (Figure 1-16) is a protective flexible plastic cover that fits over the teeth and absorbs and distributes traumatic forces to a limited degree. Studies show that properly made athletic mouthguards can dramatically reduce the number and severity of oral, facial and head injuries suffered during athletic competition.

▼ SPLINTS ▼

Splints are also used to redistribute forces. There are two basic types: occlusal splints and periodontal splints. An *occlusal splint* (Figure 1-17) is a protective layer of hard plastic placed over the grinding surfaces of the upper teeth. It repositions the lower jaw so as to reduce stress on the muscles of the jaw and the joint between the lower jaw and the skull, the temporomandibular joint. It also serves as a layer through which grinding forces can be distributed around the arch, and which the patient can grind away rather than grinding down the teeth. When the protective layer, or splint, is worn through, it can be replaced. This type of splint, often called a *nightguard,* is usually worn at night and may be prescribed for patients experiencing pain in the jaw area.

Periodontal splints are used to transfer some of the chewing forces on a tooth to adjacent teeth, thus relieving the bone and soft tissue surrounding a weakened tooth of some of

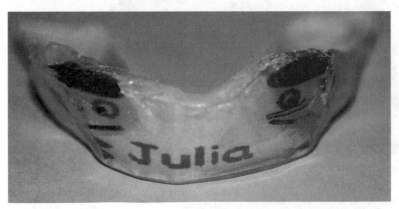

FIGURE 1-16 Athletic mouthguard. Mouthguards made in the dental office fit better and can be customized.

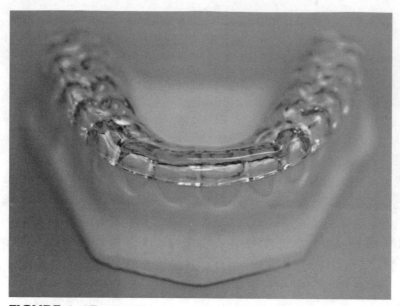

FIGURE 1-17   Occlusal guard. This allows a patient who grinds his teeth to make plastic dust rather than tooth dust.

their burden of support. A periodontal splint (Figure 1-18) may be a piece of wire, cloth, metal or plastic that is bonded to the weakened tooth plus adjacent ones, or it may consist of one or more connected restorations. Periodontal splinting helps to hold the compromised tooth in position and is done to provide a period of time during which that tooth can develop stronger natural support.

▼ SEALANTS ▼

A *sealant* (Figure 1-19) is a thin plastic coating placed on the deep grooves and pits of a tooth to prevent caries. A sealant works by preventing decay-causing microorganisms and the acids they form from contacting the enamel surface. This in turn prevents the microorganisms from entering, and the acid from dissolving out, the mineral crystals that form the enamel structure of the tooth.

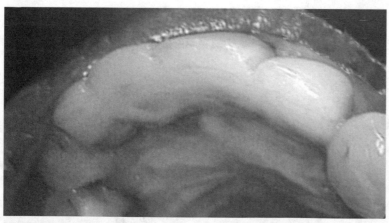

FIGURE 1-18   Periodontal splint. A wire behind the tooth is covered with composite material to hold mobile teeth in a more rigid position. It is, however, impossible to floss between them unless the floss is slipped under the splint between each pair of teeth.

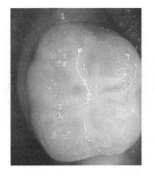

FIGURE 1-19 Sealants. Teeth have narrow fissures on the biting surfaces that can be a starting place for decay. By filling those grooves with sealant material the chance of decay disappears.

▼ PROCESSING MATERIALS ▼

Some materials are used to help complete another process rather than to make something on their own.

Abrasives

Cutting, shaping and polishing natural teeth and restorations are done with abrasives. *Abrasives* are hard particles that are used to remove stains from, smooth, shape and cut tooth structure and the materials that replace it. There are several types of abrasives, each most useful for specific procedures. Abrasives can have a different hardness or particle size and take different forms but they all work by friction, wearing away at the substance. The harder and larger the particle the faster the wear will be. As friction always produces heat as a by-product it is important not to let excessive heat build up when using abrasives. Dental personnel routinely select and use polishing agents that contain mild abrasives. Since patients are keenly interested in beautiful teeth, this is a group of frequently used materials!

Processing Waxes

Waxes are sometimes used to help complete a task. For example, sticky wax holds broken pieces of a denture in correct position temporarily so they may be permanently rejoined in that position. Utility wax may be used to change the fit of an impression tray or make it more comfortable for the patient. Base plate wax is used in the fabrication of dentures. A number of waxes are illustrated in Figure 1-20.

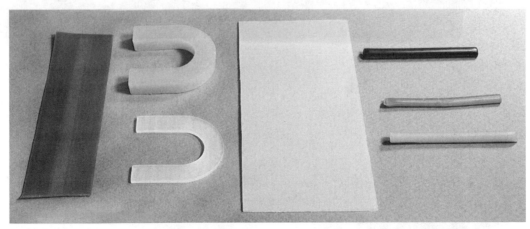

FIGURE 1-20 Waxes. Each of these waxes is used for a different purpose. They not only vary in color but hardness and melting temperature also. The dark-colored stick is so hard it will fracture if dropped, while the stick next to it is completely soft at room temperature.

▼ MATERIALS USED ▼

Although a wide variety of items are made with dental materials, surprisingly few types of materials are used. Most are metal, glass, plastic, or natural material such as resin or ground rock. You already know much about these types of materials from your experience with them in everyday life. Through study and practice you can build on the knowledge you already have to develop valuable skill in using dental materials.

KEY POINTS

✓ Materials are used in almost every dental procedure
✓ Materials are used to make items that will
   • Prevent oral disease or injury
   • Restore tooth form and function
   • Replace lost teeth
   • Be used temporarily to help make something else
✓ Many types of items are made but few types of materials are used
   • Metal
   • Glass
   • Plastic
   • Adhesives
   • Natural materials

SELF TEST

Questions 1–5: Identify the pictured item and indicate why it is used.

1.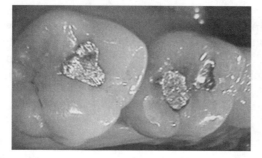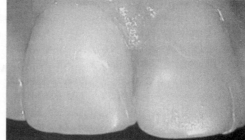

2.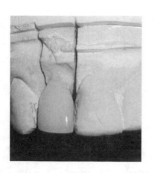

3.

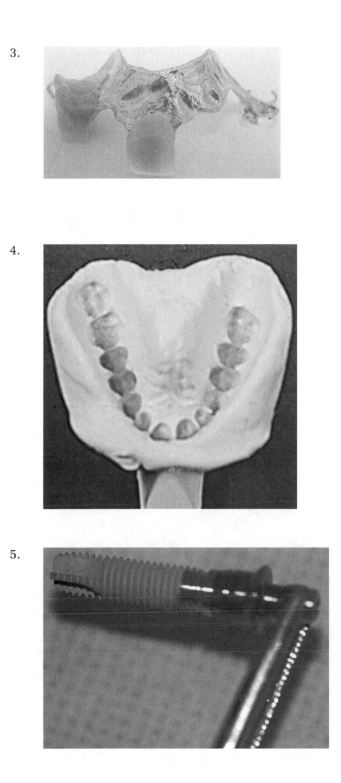

4.

5.

Questions 6–10: Assume the dentist has asked you to include patient education as a routine part of your seating procedures before the appointment begins. About which option would you educate each patient described below?

6. A 12-year-old girl who is very excited that she will be able to play field hockey on a team this year now that she is in junior high school
   a. Sealant
   b. Direct restoration
   c. Periodontal splint
   d. Mouthguard

7. A frail 83-year-old woman who lost her mandibular right central incisor in an automobile accident several weeks ago
   a. Bonded bridge
   b. Implant
   c. Partial denture
   d. Both *a* and *c*
   e. All of the above

8. A 6-year-old boy whose father has accompanied him to a routine examination appointment
   a. Impressions
   b. Sealants
   c. Direct restorations
   d. Nightguard

9. A 43-year-old man with extensive internal stains on all of his maxillary incisors
   a. Conventional bridge
   b. Esthetic veneers
   c. Study models
   d. Full denture

10. A 36-year-old woman who has a badly decayed crown on a mandibular left first premolar that has a sound root
    a. Occlusal splint
    b. Direct restorations
    c. Indirect restorations
    d. Sealants

THE VOCABULARY OF MATERIALS USE

OBJECTIVES

After studying this chapter you should be able to:

1. Define biocompatibility.
2. Define microleakage, and explain why it happens and why it is undesirable.
3. Explain what color is and how it is perceived.
4. Understand the differences between opaque, translucent, and transparent.
5. Explain the differences between the three states of matter and how matter can be converted from one state to another.
6. Define and explain the different mechanical forces that are found in the mouth.
7. Explain how materials fail.
8. Discuss the effect of water on polar and non-polar materials and why these are important.
9. Choose the proper material type for various dental procedures.

Every field has its own vocabulary; the study of dental materials is no exception. Such terminology enables precision in oral and written communication. Dental personnel are interested in the characteristics of materials themselves as well as how materials interact with conditions in the mouth and the patient's general health, for these are the factors that determine which materials will be chosen for use in a particular situation. Understanding the terminology presented in this chapter will help you to discuss items made of dental materials with your professional colleagues, read the directions for how to use a specific material that are inserted in its product package, decipher a product label or material safety data sheet, and educate yourself about the rapidly changing materials field as you read dental articles throughout your working life.

▼ BIOCOMPATIBILITY ▼

Biocompatibility is essentially tissue kindness. Biocompatible materials do not cause undesirable effects to cells, tissues, or body systems. Undesirable effects include such processes as irritation, toxicity and sensitivity.

Irritation is an exaggerated local response of the skin or mucous membrane to a material. Typical responses include soreness, redness, inflammation and sometimes formation of small blisters. *Sensitivity* is an allergy-type response to a foreign substance, in this case a dental material, and *toxicity* is poisoning. Ideally, a material will not cause any of these reactions. These reactions will be discussed in more detail in the next chapter.

Toxicity is normally not a problem, because all dental materials must undergo rigorous testing and obtain federal approval before being cleared for use in patient care. However, sometimes irritation and sensitivity do occur. Dental personnel will not choose to use a material to which a patient is known to be allergic and will remove a material that was placed but to which the patient now exhibits sensitivity. On the other hand, the causes of irritation include more than simply reaction to a material. If a patient experiences irritation, nearby materials will be one factor that will be evaluated for possible contribution to the problem.

▼ MICROLEAKAGE ▼

Microleakage (Figure 2-1) is the entrance of fluids into the microscopic space that exists between the tooth and some restorations. Although extremely small, the space is large enough to permit fluids from the oral cavity to enter and travel beside and under the restoration.

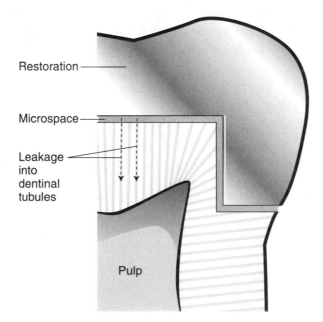

Restoration

Microspace

Leakage into dentinal tubules

Pulp

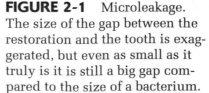

FIGURE 2-1 Microleakage. The size of the gap between the restoration and the tooth is exaggerated, but even as small as it truly is it is still a big gap compared to the size of a bacterium.

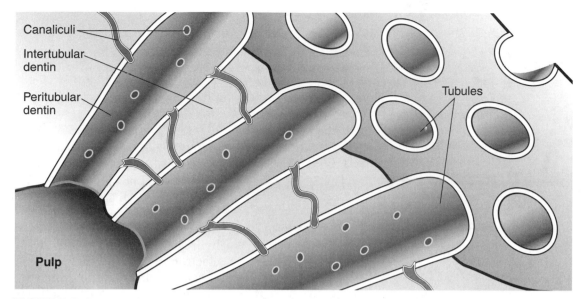

Canaliculi

Intertubular dentin

Peritubular dentin

Tubules

Pulp

FIGURE 2-2 Dentin. You can see that dentin is not a solid mass microscopically but has channels in it.

These fluids may carry microorganisms, chemical ions and colored pigments. Because the tiny tubes (tubules) that form dentin (Figure 2-2) were cut to prepare the tooth for the restoration, they are open to entrance of fluids and dissolved substances. Fluids, microorganisms and dissolved substances entering a tubule can merge with and diffuse through the fluid normally present in the tubule and affect the pulp. This may result in pulp irritation or sensitivity, decay around the restoration or discoloration of tooth structure.

Two types of materials have been used to block this process: varnish and bonding agents. *Varnish* was conventionally painted on the exposed end of the cut tubules to seal them. This was believed to prevent unwanted fluids and dissolved substances from entering, but in recent years this technique has been largely abandoned in favor of bonding. *Bonding* is a method of attaching a material to the tooth surface so the restoration and tooth are continuous with one another, thereby eliminating microleakage.

Two types of bonding, mechanical and chemical, can be used to attach a restoration to a tooth, or two restorative materials to each other. *Mechanical bonding* (Figure 2-3) requires treating the tooth or restorative surface in such a way that many small depressions are made. A thin liquid is flowed into these depressions and hardened. This creates a series of very tiny interlocked fingers that hold the two solids together securely.

Chemical bonding is attraction between contacting atoms of two solid materials. The attraction may be created through sharing surface electrons (Figure 2-4) or by developing

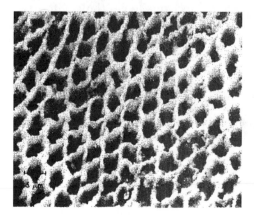

FIGURE 2-3 Etched enamel. This is the tooth surface after treatment to dissolve some of the surface material. You can see how rough and intricate the surface is and how a material flowed onto the surface would fill all the indentations and get locked into place. (Photo micrograph reprinted from Daniel S. Harfst: *Mosby's Dental Hygiene: Concepts, Cases, & Competencies,* p. 441, 2002, by permission of the publisher, Mosby Elsevier Science.

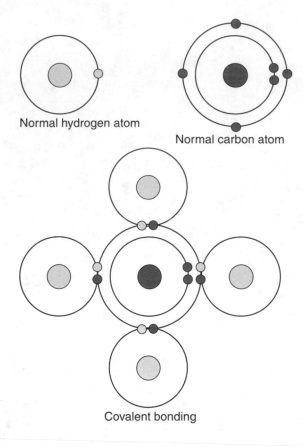

Normal hydrogen atom

Normal carbon atom

Covalent bonding

FIGURE 2-4 Making methane. In this example each hydrogen atom shares one electron with a carbon atom. All atoms like to have full electron shells. The inner shell fits two electrons so hydrogen, which only had one electron in the shell, now has access to another electron from the carbon atom and now has a filled shell. The second shell can hold eight electrons. Carbon starts with four in that shell and by sharing one with each hydrogen atom, it also fills its shell. This type of bond is often called *covalent bonding*.

weak electric currents between adjacent ones (Figure 2-5). Depending on the type of bond, the atoms involved and the amount of surface affected, this type of bond can be very strong or fairly weak. One of the goals of learning about dental materials is to maximize the strength of bonds between the tooth and restoration. This bonding is very sensitive to handling variation, so dental professionals must be knowledgeable about the handling characteristics of each material in order to effect the best possible outcome.

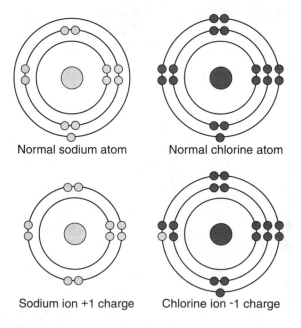

Normal sodium atom

Normal chlorine atom

Sodium ion +1 charge

Chlorine ion -1 charge

FIGURE 2-5 Making table salt. Some atoms prefer to take or give up electrons to get their outer shells filled. In this example sodium has just one electron in its outer shell, which it gives away to the chlorine atom, which had seven in its outer shell. Since electrons carry a negative charge, the sodium atom becomes positively charged and the chlorine atom negatively charged in this exchange. The two atoms will then stay close to each other because their charges attract.

Color

Dental personnel and patients alike are concerned that whenever treatment is done the result is pleasing to look at. Accordingly, color is a major consideration. Color is created when light is reflected from an object and the reflections are visible. There are many ways to look at color. The most useful way for dentistry is to look at color as a combination of three attributes: hue, value, and chroma. To create a perfectly natural appearance, all aspects of a material's color need to match the patient's own tooth structure.

Hue is what is normally considered the color name (red, for example). Light travels in waves. Each wave has a section that goes up and a section that goes down. Measuring from the peak height of one wave to the peak of an adjacent one is a measure of the *wavelength* of that wave. Human eyes and brains are capable of perceiving different wavelengths as different colors. The hue, then, is a measure of the wavelength of the light but is generally known by the name of the color with which it corresponds.

Value refers to the lightness or darkness of the hue. It is equivalent to changing the brightness on your television. The hue stays the same but as the brightness goes up the color has more white added to it and as the brightness goes down it will have more black. Since white and black together are gray, we call the blending of the two the gray value.

Chroma refers to the vividness, or strength, of a hue. This is a measure of how much of the color there is. It is the difference between one thin coat of paint or many thick ones. Vividness is created by saturation of the reflected light with wavelengths of that hue. It is the measure of the height of the wave.

Shade Selection

A *shade guide* (Figure 2-6) is used when an esthetic restorative material is selected. The guide is a series of samples of the same material in different shades and strengths, enabling selection of the one most closely resembling the patient's own.

Shades should be selected in natural light. Sunlight is composed of light of all wavelengths. An artificial light does not emit wavelengths of all colors. Since humans depend on the reflected light's wavelengths to perceive the color, in artificial light we might misjudge the actual color. Shades should also be selected when the tooth is moist, as moisture

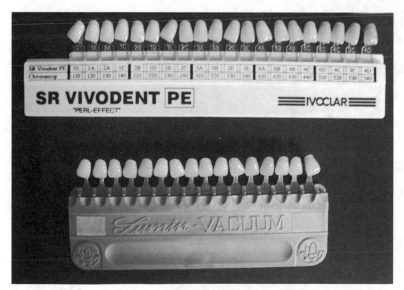

FIGURE 2-6 Shade guides. Shade guides contain tabs of different shades to match esthetic material to the patient's teeth.

changes light reflection slightly. Since teeth are normally moist with saliva and the tooth is dried during the restorative procedure, a restoration will match more precisely when its color is chosen in a moist environment. Additionally, shades should be selected prior to the placement of dental dam, a thin "raincoat" placed to isolate a tooth from its surroundings (Figure 2-7). The dam reflects its own color onto adjacent tooth structure, slightly changing the tooth's shade. The shade selected prior to dam placement will not be adulterated by reflected light from the dam. All of these considerations suggest that shades should be selected prior to the beginning of a dental procedure. At that time the dental light is not yet needed, the tooth is still moist, and dam has not yet been placed.

Penetration of a Material by Light

Materials interact differently with light. Some permit light to pass through; these materials are *transparent*. Others absorb all or part of the light as it attempts to pass through. *Opaque* materials absorb all light and *translucent* materials absorb only part of it. These differences are easily seen on a daily basis. Clear water lets light pass through; it is transparent. A white lampshade will absorb some light but not all; it is translucent. A wooden fencepost does not permit light to pass through; it is opaque.

Everyday experience also teaches us that whether light passes through an object or is absorbed by it is not dependent solely on the type of material of which the object is made. Although wood is certainly expected to absorb more light than water, material thickness and light wavelength also play a part. Shorter wavelengths penetrate more easily. Thicker objects absorb more light. Consider a sheet of white paper, the type normally used for copying everyday letters and school tests. If two sheets of this paper, the top one blank and the bottom one a printed letter, are held up to light, the printing on the bottom page will show through the top page well enough to be read. If several sheets are placed on top of the letter, the printing on the bottom sheet will no longer be visible. Each sheet along the way is translucent; it absorbs part of the light. Eventually, the overlying paper is thick enough to absorb all of the light.

Tooth enamel is translucent but the underlying dentin is opaque. Materials which replace enamel appear more natural if they are translucent and those which replace dentin appear more natural if they are opaque. Enamel and dentin are also of different thicknesses in different areas of a tooth. For restorations to appear natural, they must combine area-

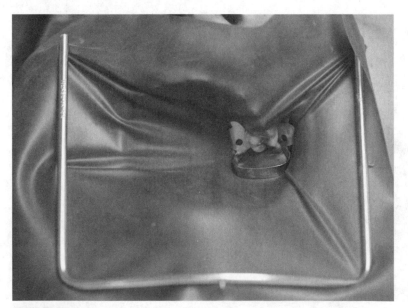

FIGURE 2-7   Dental dam. Notice how only the tooth to be worked on is exposed so the tongue and the rest of the oral structures are held out of the way.

appropriate thickness of an opaque deeper layer simulating dentin with a translucent top layer simulating enamel.

Emission of Light by a Material

Some materials absorb light, then emit it at a different wavelength. This is termed *fluorescence.* This effect is best seen in ultraviolet light (black light) where some objects will show up clearly and some will not. Ultraviolet light has a longer wavelength than visible light and those objects that seem to glow are emitting light at a shorter wavelength than the light hitting them.

Teeth are fluorescent. When looking at other people in natural light one is not normally conscious of dental light emission, but may be subliminally aware of sparkle. That subtle sparkle is fluorescence. A restorative material will look more natural if it fluoresces slightly and emits at the same wavelengths as natural teeth.

▼ MATERIAL PHYSICAL PROPERTIES ▼

State of the Material

Some dental materials are solids and some are liquids. A *solid* has a definite shape. The atoms, or building blocks, of which it is composed are relatively still and the material appears firm. A *liquid* does not have a definite shape; it conforms to the shape of its container. Its molecules are moving smoothly and easily to assume the container shape.

Solids

There are three types of solid materials: molecular solids, metallic solids and nonmetallic solids. Molecular solids (Figure 2-8) have regular arrangements of their internal atoms or molecules but they are not bound together tightly. Think of bowling pins as aligned for play. The regular, rhythmic spacing of the pins is similar to the spacing of one layer of a molecular solid. Regular arrangements of soccer balls or marbles would provide the same type of structure: similar items with equidistant spacing but not bound to one another. Molecular solids are predictable. They have regular structures, melting and solidifying temperature ranges, and tend not to flow when solid. Paraffin wax is an example of a molecular solid.

Metallic solids (Figure 2-9) also have regular arrangements of their internal atoms but they have bonds between atoms formed by charged particles called electrons. Like molecular solids they have regular structures, melting and solidifying temperature ranges, and

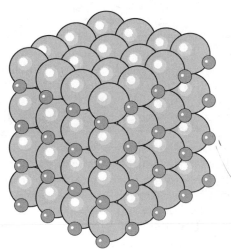

FIGURE 2-8 Molecular solids. Note the very regular arrangement of the atoms in this structure but remember they are all just stacked, not tightly bonded.

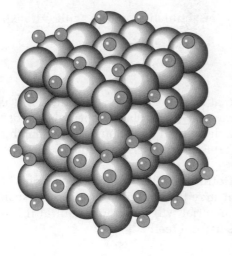

FIGURE 2-9 Metallic solids. Note that this also has a regular arrangement of atoms, but in this case the electrons are not bound as tightly so the edges betwen molecules are less distinct. Since these loosely held electrons can move easily, and electricity is just moving electrons, these solids are good electrical conductors.

tend not to flow when solid. The electrons that form the bonds can move through the solid however. This makes metallic solids good conductors of heat and electricity.

Non-metallic solids are in actuality a very large molecule formed by all the atoms in the solid. This group does not conduct electricity well and tends to have high melting points. Porcelain is a non-metallic solid.

Another important group of chemical compounds, polymers, also needs to be discussed. *Polymers* are long strings of identical chemical units that are connected together by chemical bonds. They are like paper chains. Each link of the chain in a polymer is called a *monomer.* Plastics are composed of a collection of very strong polymer chains that are loosely bound to one another. To picture this, think of lots of paper chains all mixed up on the floor at random. You can pull one chain out of the collection because it is not connected to the others but doing so may be difficult because the chains could be tangled together. Some polymers are cross-linked, meaning that the chains of polymers have chemical bonds between them; think about looping links between two of the long chains. This makes it very much more difficult to remove a single chain since it is bonded to many others.

Solids can also be categorized as *regular* or *amorphous* solids. Regular ones have consistent units in their structure. This means that they will arrange themselves into a regular structure, which will give consistent melting and solidifying temperatures.

Amorphous solids have a mixture of many different atoms and thus cannot assemble into a regular structure. Their melting and solidifying temperature ranges are less regular and the material may flow after solidifying.

Flow

The ability to move in a smooth, uninterrupted manner to conform to the shape of a container is termed *flow.* Some materials flow well; others do not. The measurement of the resistance to flow for a material is known as *viscosity.* Water has arbitrarily been given a viscosity of 1. Materials that flow more easily than water have viscosities of less than 1 and those that have more resistance to flow than water are greater than 1. Think of water and molasses. Water flows easily when poured but molasses, with a high viscosity, flows very much more slowly. Some materials flow slightly after they are set (hardened). Flow after set is *creep.* Dental amalgam, the material used to make silver fillings, creeps.

Some materials have a viscosity that changes depending on the pressure placed on them. Those materials that flow more easily in response to pushing are *thixotropic* materials. Some soft dental impression materials, dental bleaches and fluoride gel preventive materials are thixotropic. This allows the operator to turn the tray they are carried in upside down to place it into the mouth in the proper orientation but allows the material to flow easily into the spaces around the teeth when pressure is applied.

Set

Materials which set when cooled have a *thermoplastic* set. *Plastic* means able to be shaped, and *thermo-* refers to temperature. Each time thermoplastic materials are heated they become liquid, and are able to be shaped again, thus thermoplastic set is reversible. Candle wax is a familiar thermoplastic material that sets when cooled but can be liquefied again by heating. In fact, waxes are thermoplastic materials commonly used in dentistry. Any thermoplastic material used in the mouth must soften at a temperature enough above mouth temperature that its set doesn't begin to reverse until it is in the mouth but it must not soften at such a high temperature the patient will be burned by the material.

Thermoplastic material setting is the only type of setting that is reversible because it is a change of physical state, not a chemical change. Materials which set by changing their chemical structure rather than by just changing their state from liquid to solid are said to have an *irreversible set.* An irreversible set cannot be undone without damaging the material; once set, the material stays set. For example, a material such as an egg or cake, which sets when heated, is exhibiting a *chemical* change and proceeds only in one direction. Neither the egg nor the cake can be returned to their initial state.

A material that sets when exposed to light is *light cured.* Dental polymers for direct restorations often set in response to light. Setting of polymers occurs because monomers in the material join to form polymer chains. For this reason we often refer to the setting of polymers as *polymerization.* Thus, a polymer with a set which begins on exposure to light is a *light cured* or *light polymerized* material. Other polymers set when heated and are termed *heat cured* or *heat polymerized.*

Materials which set when mixed with another material have a *chemical set* because a chemical reaction starts when the two components are mixed. Polymers that are mixed and then set from a chemical reaction are termed *self-cured* or *cold cured.* Self-cured means the material cures itself once mixed, and cold cured indicates application of heat is not required for set, although much heat is given off in the chemical reaction.

Dual set materials cure from exposure to light or heat and through a chemical reaction. The material is mixed, then placed and exposed to light. Light exposure creates a rapid, but not always complete, set. The chemical set which occurs from mixing two materials occurs more slowly, but more completely. Dual set materials garner the advantages and offset the disadvantages of both light and chemical curing. Additionally, whenever light is used to cure a material, the light itself generates heat as it is used. Some dual set materials also factor in this heat as a curing agent.

Response to Mechanical Forces

Load

A *load* is a force placed on a material. That load may be pushing, termed *compression;* pulling, termed *tension;* cutting (both pushing and pulling), termed *shearing;* or twisting, termed *torsion* (Figure 2-10).

Load on a material changes it. The material resists the force, rearranging its internal structure and perhaps changing its shape in an attempt to preserve its integrity. When the load is removed the internal arrangement will return to its original state, if possible. However, if the force is sufficiently strong, or occurs frequently enough or for a long enough period of time, regaining the original state may be impossible. Permanent shape change and material weakening or breakage may occur.

Dental personnel use specific terms to describe the interaction of a material with force. *Stress* refers to the amount of force applied to a specified area of the object. *Strength* refers to resistance to stress. *Strain* refers to the internal rearrangement of atoms to adjust to the stress. While you can't see strain it does change the position of the atoms and molecules in the material. *Deformation* is a change in shape that results from combined effect of the strain. *Relaxation* is the attempt by a material to return to its original state before the stress was applied. *Elasticity* refers to temporary deformation followed by a return to original

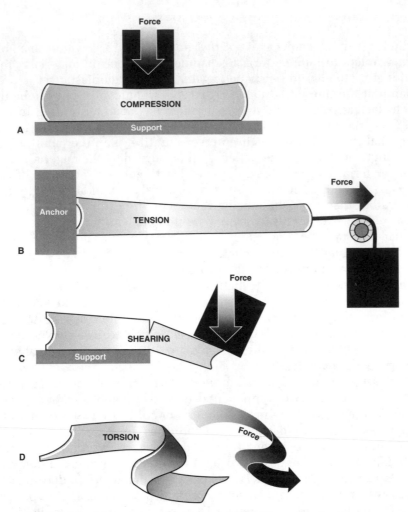

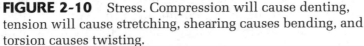

FIGURE 2-10 Stress. Compression will cause denting, tension will cause stretching, shearing causes bending, and torsion causes twisting.

state. When the *elastic limit* is passed, the material cannot completely regain its original size and shape, and permanent deformation occurs (Figure 2-11). When the ultimate, or greatest, strength is passed, the material breaks. Breakage is termed *fracture.* Using this terminology, we can rewrite the paragraph above as follows:

> A material may be strained by compressive, tensile or shearing stress; or by torsion. If the force applied to the material is below the elastic limit of that material it relaxes on removal of the stress. If the stress surpasses the elastic limit of the material, it yields, and deformation or fracture occurs.

Now let us look at an example. Think of a rubber band. It can be pulled to be made larger, slipped over items you want to keep together and then released. When released, it will try to return to its original size and shape, but sometimes has been enlarged too much and remains a bit big. If it has been very much enlarged, it sometimes breaks. In materials terms, a tensile stress was placed on the rubber band. The stress caused sufficient strain that the yield strength of the band was surpassed and the band enlarged to fit over the items. Release of the band removed the stress, ending the resulting strain and triggering band relaxation. The band is usually sufficiently elastic to relax completely and return to its original state. Sometimes, though, deformation remains. Occasionally, stress and the resulting strain on the band surpass its ultimate strength, and the band breaks.

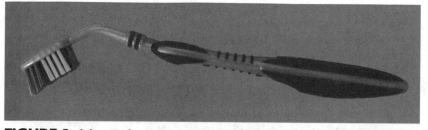

FIGURE 2-11 Deformation. The handle of this toothbrush has been permanently deformed to help the patient reach the lingual surface of the lower incisors more easily. What kind of stress was applied?

Strength

As noted, strength is the ability to resist stress. It comes from material type and thickness. Wood, for example, is more resistant to indentation from poking it with a finger (compressive stress) than jelly is.

Types of strength are used to indicate different points in the resistance process. *Yield strength* is the point just before a material must give in and begin to change shape, that is, the point of greatest resistance before it begins to yield to the load. *Ultimate strength* is the point just prior to fracture. It is the greatest, or ultimate, resistance before the material is overwhelmed by the stress and breaks. Types of strength are also used to indicate resistance to particular types of loads. *Compressive, tensile* and *shearing strength* are the resistance of a material to those stresses.

Some materials have the ability to yield to compressive forces without fracturing; this allows them to be hammered into a shape. The measure of the ability of a metal to be flattened in this way is *malleability. Ductility* is the ability of a metal to be drawn into a fine wire; it is the resistance of a metal to tensile stresses.

Thermal Expansion and Contraction

If a material is heated, it expands; if cooled, it shrinks. This is termed *thermal expansion* and *contraction*. Tooth structure also expands and contracts when heated or cooled. Different materials respond to temperature changes at different rates. The measure of the rate of change in volume of a material to change in temperature is termed the *coefficient of thermal expansion*. Heating and cooling of teeth occurs in everyone's mouth every day. All kinds of foods, from hot drinks to iced desserts, are eaten and temporarily change the mouth temperature. When the teeth are temporarily expanding or contracting in response to these temperature changes, the materials in the mouth are too. If the material in a restoration expands faster than the tooth, it will push against the tooth surface. If it contracts faster, it will shrink away from the tooth.

These differences in expansion and contraction rates cause compressive and tensile forces on the teeth and restorations that can lead to fracture. If the material is bonded to the tooth and shrinks faster than the tooth surface, the shrinking material will pull on the bonding material, which will in turn pull on the tooth. Repeated pulling on the bond weakens it and may cause it to break. A broken bond no longer seals the tooth–restoration interface against microleakage. Repeated, frequent pulling on the tooth as a material shrinks, alternated with the pushing that occurs when it expands faster, hastens tooth weakening and fracture.

Materials that undergo thermal expansion and contraction at a rate similar to tooth structure are less likely to contribute to bonding agent or tooth fracture. The coefficient of thermal expansion of a material is thus clinically very significant and dental personnel can compare the numbers for different materials to learn those which have rates similar to natural teeth. Dental personnel can also learn the resistance to tensile stresses of a particular bonding agent; different agents have different abilities to resist the tensile stresses they experience as restorative materials and teeth expand and contract.

Abrasion Resistance

Abrasion resistance is resistance to wear. *Wear* is friction caused by rubbing. Think about using a loofah sponge to rub callused skin from your heels and elbows. The rubbing dislodges the outer skin cells because the skin has very little resistance to the sponge. On the other hand, if you were to scrub a badly burned pot with the loofah sponge, chances are that it would take a lot longer to remove the unwanted burned material. The burned material in the pot has better abrasion resistance than skin.

Summary of Forces

Loading and resistance interactions take place every day between materials and teeth. During chewing, compressive, tensile, shearing and abrasive forces are placed on the teeth and supporting tissues. Hot and cold foods cause materials and teeth to expand and contract. The result of these processes may be wear, weakening, deformation or fracture of tooth or material.

Response to Electrochemical Forces

Fluids in the mouth are at different times acid, basic and neutral. Most people understand that acids in the mouth attack teeth, contributing to formation of caries. Acids also attack whatever materials are present, and may break their chemical bonds, actively eroding and weakening the material.

Electricity is a flow of electrons along a conducting medium. Because electrons have a negative charge they always flow toward the positive pole. Saliva and dental materials contain chemical ions, some with a positive electrical charge and some with a negative one. An electrical current can be generated in the mouth from a negative to a positive pole using saliva as the conducting medium. Electrical current can shift electrical attraction forces within materials, resulting in ion loss, material dissolution and weakening. Restoration edges are particularly vulnerable to this process.

Metal materials may discolor when attacked by electrochemical forces. This is termed *tarnish* (Figure 2-12). Tarnish is a surface layer that can be removed by polishing.

Metal restorations may also become pitted and break apart from electrochemical assault. Most people are familiar with this process in the form of rust on metal fences or car parts. Disintegration of this type is deeper than tarnish and results in a change in the material itself. It is termed *corrosion* (Figure 2-13).

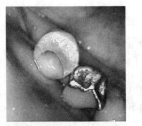

FIGURE 2-12 Tarnish. Note how the surface of the older restoration on the right is discolored compared to the new restoration.

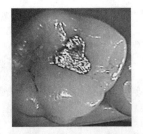

FIGURE 2-13 Pitting. Note how rough the surface of the restoration has become due to the pitting.

▼ RELATIONSHIP BETWEEN SET MATERIAL AND MOISTURE ▼

The mouth is a wet place. The interaction between any material used in the mouth and oral fluids will partly determine how accurately the item made with the material fits, how well it stays where it is put, and how long it serves the patient. The importance of this relationship has given rise to a number of terms describing its aspects.

Wetting refers to how well a liquid covers the surface of a solid. Think water and a dining table. Assume half of the table has been waxed and half remains to be done. If the water is spilled on both halves of the table, it will cover, or wet, a larger area on the un-waxed half. Try it on a piece of wood with wax on one half. The water will cover less area on the waxed half. The water has a higher contact angle with the waxed portion of the wood. A higher contact angle of a liquid with a solid means less wetting has occurred; lower ones, more wetting (Figure 2-14). Wetting is important in dentistry when a liquid material must be flowed over a solid surface, such as when impression material must cover the teeth and gingiva or a bonding agent must flow over a cavity preparation.

Since most of the time the oral cavity is coated with moisture, it is important to know how materials act when in contact with water. Some materials have low contact angles on water-covered surfaces and others do not. Materials that cover those surfaces easily with low contact angles are *hydrophilic,* that is, water loving. In other words, hydrophilic materials tend to wet the tooth, soft tissue or impression surface well. Materials that do not combine well with water are *hydrophobic,* water fearing. Hydrophobic liquids tend to bead up on the surface unless it has been dried or a wetting agent was applied to it to help wetting occur. Surfaces of the teeth and soft tissue are wet, so materials placed on the tooth surface can be joined to it more easily if they are hydrophilic. Similarly, impression materials used for making a mold of hard or soft tissue anatomy will record much better detail and can be poured with a liquid model material more easily if they are hydrophilic.

Sorption, termed *absorption* in everyday discourse, is the drawing of fluid into a solid. When a paper towel is used to mop up spilled orange juice, the towel is absorbing the juice. A material that absorbs fluid will swell. Sometimes this is an advantage, sometimes a disadvantage. If the enlarged material fills an oral space more completely, fit against the tissues may be improved or leakage into the microspace between a tooth and restoration decreased. If the material enlarges too much, pain may result from pressure of the overly large item against tissue. Additionally, oral fluids can carry dissolved pigments from food, medicine, etc. These coloring agents can be absorbed into items made with dental materials and stain them.

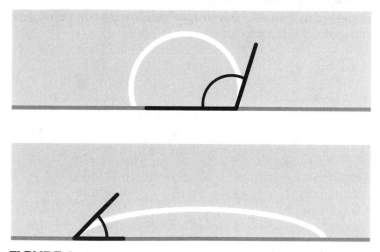

FIGURE 2-14   Wetting of surfaces. Note how a large contact angle results in less of the surface being covered than a small contact angle.

Solubility is the ability of a substance to dissolve in a liquid. Something that dissolves in a particular liquid is said to be *soluble* in it; one that does not is *insoluble.* The liquid in which a substance dissolves is a *solvent* for that material. Instant coffee dissolves in water stirred with a spoon. Water is the solvent; coffee is soluble in it; the spoon is insoluble.

Solubility is liquid- and material-specific. Water dissolves soap but not hair. Cocoa dissolves quickly in milk, the marshmallows very slowly and the spoon not at all. Solubility is similar to sorption in that it is sometimes helpful and at other times detrimental. It is useful for a medication to dissolve in a pleasant-tasting solvent, for example, but not at all helpful for the cement that holds a restoration on a tooth to dissolve. Since the mouth is a wet area, undesirable dissolution of material can and does occur.

Disintegration is the breaking up of a solid. It is the end process of a number of processes to which fluid and material interactions contribute. Since dental materials are solids placed in a fluid environment, the thin edges of restorations are vulnerable to disintegration. When edges disintegrate, a visible open area, or *ditch* appears, and dental personnel speak of ditching around the restoration.

▼ CHOOSING A MATERIAL ▼

Most oral conditions are predictable but each patient combines them in unique ways. Dental personnel choose to use a certain material for a particular patient because it will not harm the patient's health, is easy enough to use and they believe it will be able to withstand that patient's oral conditions. When choosing materials to use, take what you know about the characteristics of a material, evaluate them in relation to your patient's conditions, and select the best available fit. There is no perfect material, but there are some truly excellent ones.

KEY POINTS

✓ Dental personnel use specific words to describe the characteristics of a material.
✓ Such words enable concise precision in communication.
✓ Words may describe
  • The material itself.
  • Conditions in the mouth.
  • Interactions between a material and the mouth.
✓ Learning the correct words will enable you to speak and write so that other dental professionals understand exactly what you mean.

Questions 1–5: Using professional terminology, how would you describe each item or condition illustrated below?

1.

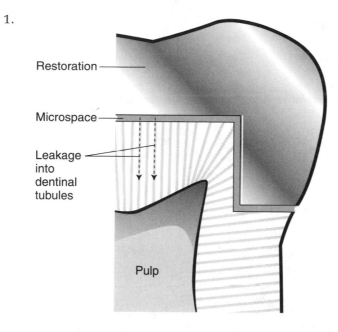

Restoration

Microspace

Leakage into dentinal tubules

Pulp

    a. tarnish
    b. bonding
    c. microleakage
    d. deformation

2.

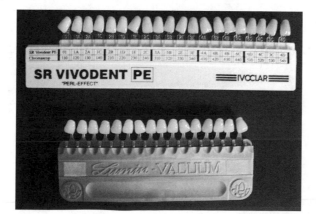

    a. etched surface
    b. thermal expansion
    c. metallic solid
    d. microscopic appearance of dentin

3.

    a. dental dams
    b. shade guides
    c. viscosity gauges
    d. die molds

4.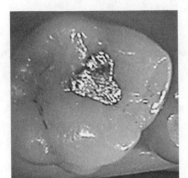
   a. esthetic restoration
   b. implant surface
   c. tarnish
   d. pitted restoration

5.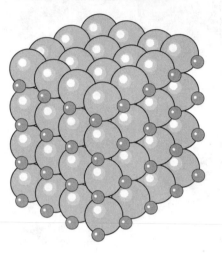
   a. enamel
   b. dentin
   c. polymer
   d. molecular solid

Questions 6–10: Assume you are speaking with the dentist. What term would you use to convey your meaning precisely?

6. The patient's crown needs to be attached to the tooth surface. You would say it needs to be
   a. bonded.
   b. cured.
   c. thermoset.
   d. polymerized.

7. The material you are using does not flow well at all. You would say it has high
   a. loading.
   b. strain.
   c. viscosity.
   d. sorption.

8. The material you are using has to be mixed, then exposed to visible light. You would say the material is
   a. light cured.
   b. dual cured.
   c. thixotropic.
   d. elastic.

9. You are reading and relaying the contents of the informational insert in a new material. It states the material may dissolve in, and must be protected from, oral fluids for the first 24 hours following placement. You would say the material is _____ in oral fluids and must be protected for the first 24 hours following placement.
    a. soluble.
    b. galvanic.
    c. expansile.
    d. toxic.

10. The new material you were using should have hardened when a light was placed on it, but did not. You would say the material did not
    a. flow.
    b. disintegrate.
    c. bond.
    d. cure.

USING MATERIALS SAFELY

OBJECTIVES

After studying this chapter, you should be able to:

1. Describe programs to assure the safety and quality of dental materials.
2. Discuss how chemicals can cause harm.
3. List procedures to maintain the integrity of a chemical.
4. Describe agencies that regulate or guide safe dental practice.
5. List and discuss the elements of the Hazard Communication Standard.

6. Decode hazardous chemical warning labels that use the National Fire Protection Association coding system.
7. Describe procedures for spill and leak clean-up.
8. Discuss the characteristics and clean-up of mercury.
9. Describe approved methods for disposal of regulated and non-regulated waste, including hazardous chemical waste.
10. List basic actions that should be taken to prevent transmission of infection in dental practice.

▼ PATIENT SAFETY ▼

A basic rule of patient care is, "First, do no harm." We do the patient no favor if we treat in a manner that cures one problem but causes another. You know from your reading in Chapter 2 that materials can be toxic and an individual patient may experience irritation or sensitivity from exposure to a specific material. Anything used in the mouth must be safe and of high quality. Two programs are designed expressly to meet this need: the Food and Drug Administration (FDA) approval process and the American Dental Association (ADA) Acceptance Program.

FDA Approval Process

The FDA is a federal agency charged with ensuring the safety of medical and dental drugs, materials and devices. Dental materials and new equipment manufacturers are required to obtain approval from the FDA before placing a material on the market. To request approval, the manufacturer submits extensive information about the product to the agency, which then uses that information to determine product safety and effectiveness. When indicated, additional testing or information may be required. Products determined to be safe are approved and may be marketed under the conditions specified in the approval decision.

Professionals experiencing problems with an FDA-approved product are encouraged, or in some cases required, to notify the agency through its adverse event reporting program. Agency personnel monitor the reports and periodically reevaluate and reclassify approved items if indicated.

ADA Acceptance Program

The ADA acceptance program is voluntary. The manufacturer must pay a fee to participate, so not all manufacturers choose to do so. A manufacturer seeking to participate submits data about a product to the ADA's Council on Scientific Affairs. Members of the Council evaluate the data provided and may arrange for submission of additional information or testing results as well. Products found to be safe and effective are accepted. Accepted products may place the ADA Seal of Acceptance on the product, and may use it with a specified statement in advertisements promoting product purchase. Information about accepted products may be found on the ADA's Web site at *www.ada.org/public/topics/seal.html.*

Dental personnel who experience problems with an accepted product are encouraged to notify the ADA. Such reports provide a valuable service to the manufacturer, who learns what improvements are needed; to the Council, by identifying products for which reevaluation may be indicated; and for clinical dental personnel, who ultimately receive better products to use.

Private Resources

Several private Web sites also offer unbiased information concerning material and device safety and quality. The Dental Advisor provides laboratory and clinical data on dental materials through monthly newsletters and *www.dentaladvisor.com.* Clinical Research Associates is a nonprofit organization that evaluates dental materials and devices for effectiveness and clinical usefulness, then publishes the results in a newsletter and at *www.cranews.com*. Reality is a full-service company that tests and publishes information about esthetic dental materials, techniques and research at *www.realityesthetics.com*.

▼ PERSONNEL SAFETY ▼

Harm from Chemicals

Dental materials are chemical substances and as such may cause harm. They may be toxic to plants, animals and/or people. They may eat other substances away, or damage the air, soil or water. They may catch fire or explode. Additionally, materials may become contaminated with blood or saliva and transfer disease-causing microorganisms from patient to patient, from a patient to a dental health worker or from a worker to a patient. Such results of material use rarely happen in dentistry nowadays because by law everyone who uses materials must be trained to follow procedures to control infection and to store, use, decontaminate and dispose of materials safely. When correct procedures are followed, dental materials are safe to use.

Hazard Control

Whether a chemical will harm you or not depends on several factors: the amount to which you are exposed, the length of time over which the exposure takes place, the strength of the chemical and the route by which it enters the body. Other things being equal, stronger chemicals, received as larger doses in a shorter period of time, cause greater harm. This type of exposure is termed *acute,* and reactions usually appear rather quickly—sometimes within minutes or hours. Typically, dental personnel receive *chronic* rather than acute exposure, from using small amounts of a material many times a day over a long period of time. Chronic exposure may cause harm, but the effects are not seen for months or years.

Chemical Strength

Chemicals may degrade from exposure to heat, cold or light. They also have a *shelf life,* that is, they degrade when stored too long before use. All materials should be protected from light and stored at the temperature recommended by the manufacturer. Any material that has passed its expiration date should not be used.

The FIFO (first in, first out) system has long been used to assure proper rotation of materials during storage. When a new shipment is received, new packages are stored behind those already present. Packages for use are taken from the front.

Material degradation is also of concern during purchasing. Dental supply companies often offer specials—lower prices if a material is purchased by a certain date or in a large amount. These specials may be a great bargain, or not. If a sale is being used to clear material nearing its expiration date from the supply house, or if the amount that must be purchased to obtain the lower rate is too large, the dental practice may not be able to use it all before the expiration date. Ask about and monitor expiration dates; discarding unused material is largely an avoidable expense!

Chemical Exposure

Chemical exposure may occur through normal use, accidental leakage or spill, or improper waste handling. Chemicals can enter the body via inhalation, ingestion or absorption through the skin or conjunctiva of the eye. Most chemicals have a preferred route of entry. Some enter only by that route; others can exploit several means. Most harmful chemicals target specific body organs; some can damage many.

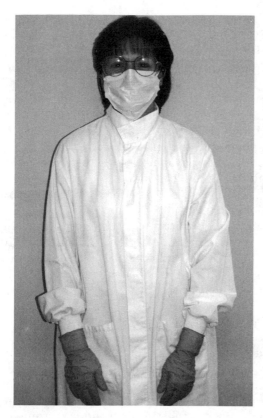

FIGURE 3-1 Personal protective equipment (PPE).

Most dental personnel are not chemists, and are not aware of the method of entry the chemical they are using prefers or of the particular health problems it can cause. Accordingly, we routinely protect ourselves against all methods of entry by wearing what is termed *personal protective equipment* (PPE) whenever we are treating patients or handling chemicals (Figure 3-1). A mask, safety glasses with solid side shields, gloves and laboratory coat protect against chemical entry through the nose, mouth, eye lining, hands or skin.

Some chemicals, particularly disinfectants or methacrylates, can degrade patient care gloves; some emit fumes that pass through the masks we normally wear. When working with disinfectants, we wear thick, more resistant *utility gloves.* Small amounts of methacrylates such as those used at chairside can be safely handled using patient care gloves, but the larger amounts used in the laboratory may require use of heavier, more resistant nitrile or vinyl. Different masks specially designed for filtering fumes may need to be worn when using noxious chemicals.

Regulatory Agencies

How do we know when to exercise special vigilance? Because chemicals can be hazardous, specific laws, regulations and guidelines exist to protect and teach workers to use chemicals safely. Laws are broad policy statements passed by a governmental body that set a government goal—worker education, for example. A law typically delegates responsibility to a specific agency to develop regulations that set forth acceptable means of meeting the goal. Regulations developed by the agency have the force of law and must be followed. Guidelines may be issued by any agency and are suggested means of meeting a goal; their adoption is voluntary. Several agencies have specific roles in the chemical safety regulation process.

The Occupational Safety and Health Administration (*www.osha.gov*) issues regulations designed to protect workers by preventing disease transmission and promoting hazard control in the workplace. The Bloodborne Pathogens Standard and the Hazard Communication Standard codify many of these regulations. Chemical safety impacts dental practice most immediately through the Hazard Communication Standard.

The Centers for Disease Control (*www.cdc.gov*), the National Institute for Occupational Safety and Health (*www.niosh.gov*) and their parent agency, the United States Public Health Service (*www.usphs.gov*), issue guidelines for safe medical and dental practice. Although these guidelines do not have the force of law, many states have adopted laws requiring their implementation. CDC, NIOSH and USPHS guidelines are followed by federal agencies, including the armed services, and are influential in all states.

The Environmental Protection Agency (*www.epa.gov*) issues regulations designed to protect plants, animals, air, water and soil from chemical harm.

The National Transportation Safety Board issues regulations designed to assure safe transportation of chemicals over our nation's highways.

The Organization for Safety and Asepsis Procedures (*www.osap.org*) is a voluntary national organization of dental personnel, manufacturers, infection control professionals and other interested persons that provides information, policy statements and guidelines regarding safe dental procedures and equipment. OSAP has become a respected, influential organization in the short period of time it has been operating.

Requirements of the OSHA Hazard Communication Standard

The basic premise of the Hazard Communication Standard is that an informed worker will be a careful, safe worker. Dental personnel learn what can cause harm, the kinds of harm that can occur and how to protect themselves. Once armed with accurate information, they can independently practice appropriate procedures. Perhaps the simplest way of thinking about hazard control is this: safety is job #1; what is the safest procedure for me to use?

Written Program

Every dental facility must have a written hazard communication program. It should contain a copy of the standard, assign the various safety responsibilities to specific employees, list requirements for labels and other forms of warning, and policies and procedures for employee information and training. Information should be included regarding established procedures to maintain the current program and evaluate its effectiveness. The written program must be available to all employees who have actual or potential exposure to chemical hazards.

Material Safety Data Sheets (MSDS)

A chemical manufacturer or importer must provide the purchaser with an information sheet (MSDS) about a chemical substance before or when it is initially shipped, and on subsequent purchases if the information changes. The MSDS must be dated, in English, and include current information about the identity of the material; describe its physical and chemical characteristics; any health, environmental, flammability or reactivity risks associated with use; procedures for safe storage, handling, clean-up and disposal; and information about how to contact the manufacturing company for answers to any questions the user may have. In actual practice, most suppliers include a current MSDS with every shipment of dental materials.

Chemical Inventory

Any facility that uses chemicals must maintain a comprehensive file of current MSDS sheets, one for each material in use. This file serves as an authoritative resource about the chemicals an employee may encounter and must be available to all workers with actual or potential chemical exposure. Because manufacturers usually include an MSDS with every shipment, it becomes the dental facility's responsibility to check the new MSDS against the one in the file and ensure the most recent information is included.

Training

Chemical safety policies and procedures must be written and accessible to employees. Dental personnel must be trained in safe chemical use policy and procedure on hire and whenever a new physical or health hazard is introduced. Training records should be maintained and available for inspection by OSHA representatives.

Labeling

Chemical containers must be labeled. The label must be legible and cannot be defaced. The label must contain the chemical or common name of the substance, potential hazards from its use, and the manufacturer's name and address. If a chemical is moved to a secondary container and will not be used immediately by the person who transferred it, the secondary container must be labeled with the same information required on the original container.

▼ EYE AND FIRE SAFETY ▼

Although not mentioned in the Hazard Communication Standard, other OSHA regulations require eye and fire safety protection in workplaces. Eyewash stations and fire extinguishers must be available and located near the area where a chemical is used. Personnel must be trained in their use. Fire exits must be clearly marked.

▼ OTHER CHEMICAL LABELING PROGRAMS ▼

Clinical dental personnel are busy people. They need information about chemical hazards that can be rapidly absorbed and understood. Because MSDSs present comprehensive information, their routine use may require more time and chemical expertise than dental personnel ordinarily have. A number of rapid read-out labeling programs have been developed to meet this need; the National Fire Protection Association system is most frequently encountered.

A number from 1 to 4 is placed in each of three diamonds to indicate the risk of fire (red), chemical reactivity (yellow), and biohazard (blue). Letters or picture symbols are placed in a fourth (white) diamond to alert the user to any special precautions required (Figure 3-2). The label provides a capsule version of the MSDS information, allowing appropriate safety precautions to be put into practice quickly.

▼ SPILLS AND LEAKS ▼

Chemical spills and leaks must be cleaned up promptly. If a substantial amount of gas leaks, the office or clinic may need to be evacuated temporarily. Recommendations of the appropriate MSDS are followed for liquid clean-up. A general purpose spill kit (Figure 3-3) should be available for use if needed. Such kits may contain nitrile utility gloves, a neutralizing absorbent powder such as bicarbonate of soda (baking powder), a small disposable dustpan and brush, and a disposal bag. Once collected, the spilled material should be disposed of in accordance with the manufacturer's recommendations.

▼ MERCURY ▼

Mercury is a component of dental amalgam restorations. Mercury itself is highly toxic; the restoration, once set, is not. Mercury can be absorbed through the skin or conjunctiva of the eye and can cause damage to the nervous and gastrointestinal systems, skin and mucous membranes. It is liquid but vaporizes at slightly above room temperature. The vapors are easily inhaled. Accordingly, spilled mercury cannot be cleaned up in a manner that in-

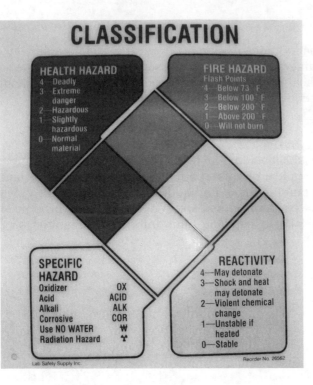

FIGURE 3-2 National Fire Protection Association label. Notice how each color informs about a different type of hazard.

volves touching or motorized vacuuming. Mercury spill kits (Figure 3-4) should contain heavy nitrile gloves, mercury absorb sponges, mercury absorbing powder, a small disposable dustpan and brush, and a disposal bag.

▼ WASTE DISPOSAL ▼

Dental practices generate non-regulated and regulated waste. Regulated waste is either biologically or chemically hazardous. Non-regulated waste is neither and may be discarded in unlabeled, leakproof, closed containers such as polyethylene bags.

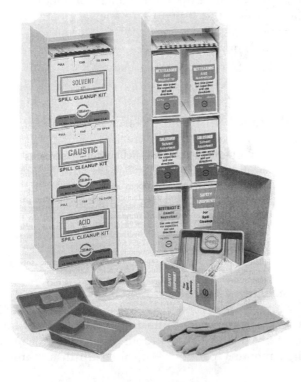

FIGURE 3-3 Chemical spill kit. This kit is complicated but offers protection against a variety of chemical spills. (Photo courtesy of Lab Safety Supply, Inc., Janesville, WI)

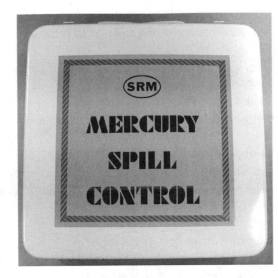

FIGURE 3-4 Mercury spill kit. This kit needs to be available if amalgam is used. If no amalgam is used in an office, then this kit can be dispensed with.

Biohazardous waste is potentially infectious or contains sharps. Potentially infectious waste includes extracted teeth, body tissue, fluid blood, or blood-soaked gauze. It most be placed in a closed, fluid-impervious container, usually red, labeled with a biohazard symbol.

Sharps, including needles and other items as defined by the dental practice, must be disposed of in a dedicated puncture-proof container located as close to the site of use as possible.

Hazardous chemical waste, as defined by the appropriate MSDS, must be labeled *Hazardous* and the MSDS-recommended disposal procedures followed.

Reputable hazardous waste companies should be employed to dispose of all types of hazardous waste. Chemical safety is "cradle-to-grave." Every agency involved in the manufacture or importing, transportation, use or disposal of hazardous material is responsible for its effects on the environment for up to 20 years following its disposal. Improper disposal can lead to extensive fines.

▼ INFECTION CONTROL ▼

As noted, dental materials can become contaminated and transmit infectious microorganisms from the patient to a dental health care worker, from one patient to another, or from a worker to a patient. Rigorous infection control procedures are essential to safe, modern dental practice. Comprehensive information relating to infection control in dentistry is a complex subject that is beyond the scope of this text, however. The information below is presented as a series of basic infection control actions that should be taken by all personnel who provide, or assist in providing, dental treatment. The interested reader is referred to the OSHA Bloodborne Pathogen Standard, the current CDC Guidelines for Infection Control in Dentistry, and clinical texts in dental assisting and dental hygiene for more extensive information.

1. Accept and truly believe in the importance of infection control procedures in dentistry.
2. Educate yourself regarding the best procedures to use, then follow them.
3. Be immunized against diseases of concern in dentistry for which vaccination is available and recommended.
4. Do not participate in patient care procedures when you are ill with a transmissible disease.
5. Screen patients' medical histories carefully for information (hepatitis or tuberculosis, for example) that may require modification in treatment procedures.

6. Keep good records of information patients and their health care providers disclose about chronic transmissible diseases patients have and keep this information *confidential.*

7. Conscientiously follow hand hygiene, gloving and hand lotion use procedures recommended for dental health care workers.

8. Follow standard precautions *every* time you work with a patient.

9. Handle needles and sharp instruments carefully; recap needles using a needle shield or scoop technique.

10. Use sterile water or sterile saline solution during surgical treatment.

11. Reprocess (clean, sterilize, disinfect and barrier protect) instruments, supplies, and work areas as required in the OSHA's Bloodborne Pathogens Standard and recommended in the CDC's Recommended Infection Control Practices for Dentistry.

12. Use heat sterilization for dental handpieces.

13. Monitor sterilization equipment and procedures on a regular basis.

14. Notify your employer if you suffer an exposure to blood or bodily fluids during treatment, operatory clean-up or instrument reprocessing procedures.

15. Follow recommended procedures for postexposure prophylaxis.

16. Clean and disinfect treatment waterlines, and monitor the quality of water in dental units, on a regular basis.

17. Dispose of regulated medical waste, including extracted teeth and biopsy specimens, in accordance with state and local laws and regulations.

KEY POINTS

✓ Dental materials contain hazardous chemicals.

✓ Patient, personnel and environmental safety during material storage, use, transport and disposal are ensured by a network of volunteer standards and federal, state and local regulations.

✓ Protect yourself and your patients when using dental materials by:
   • Wearing appropriate personal protective equipment.
   • Storing and handling materials correctly.
   • Cleaning material spills and disposing of waste materials as recommended by the manufacturer.
   • Following recommended infection control practices.

✓ Correct procedures for storing, handling and disposing of hazardous materials are learned by consulting the appropriate MSDS.

✓ To promote employee health and safety, OSHA requires all dental practices to maintain the following:
   • Written chemical safety program.
   • Chemical inventory.
   • Chemical labeling.
   • MSDS file.
   • Employee training.

✓ OSHA also requires that all employees with actual or potential chemical exposure have access to the employer's written chemical safety program.

Questions 1–4: Explain the purpose of wearing each item of personal protective equipment shown here.

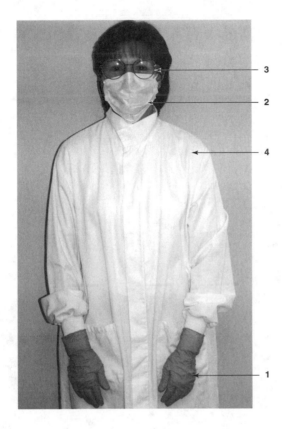

5. If your employer asked you to obtain a copy of the Hazard Communication Standard, where could you get it?

6. You have been delegated responsibility for overseeing the office's chemical safety program. As part of this responsibility, you are training a new employee. How will you explain chronic chemical exposure to her or him?

7. You are cleaning the operatory after a tooth extraction. What should you do with the extracted tooth?

8. One of your colleagues accidentally spilled some bonding agent. How should this spill be cleaned up?

9. When you see the logo below on a material package, what do you know about the material?

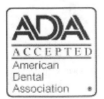

10. Describe the shelf life of a material.

USING MATERIALS SENSIBLY

OBJECTIVES

After studying this chapter, you should be able to:

1. Describe the general properties of metal alloy, glass and plastic.
2. Recognize and state the use of common items used to package and prepare dental materials.
3. Describe the following mixing techniques:
    a. Rotary
    b. Fold and press

c. Stropping
d. Figure 8
e. Stirring
4. Describe how to mix and gather materials packaged as powder and liquid or two tubes of paste.

▼ UNDERSTANDING MATERIAL SELECTION ▼

Common sense goes a long way when working with dental materials. A myriad of products is available but many are made with the same basic ingredients: metal alloy, porcelain, glass, and plastic. You already have experience using these materials in everyday life. If you think about their characteristics in everyday use and compare them to conditions in the mouth, you will understand why a particular material is selected for a given dental use and another is not.

Metal Alloy

An alloy is a mixture of metals. Using a mixture enables the manufacturer to incorporate the desirable characteristics (properties) of each metal and use the others to offset its undesirable properties to a limited degree.

Metals have some properties in common. They are relatively strong; hard; resistant to compressive, tensile and shearing loads; opaque; nonesthetic; and inexpensive. They conduct heat and cold well, tarnish and corrode, can transmit electrical currents, and melt at relatively high temperatures. They are quite smooth and can be polished to a high shine. They are useful in parts of the mouth where strength is needed, appearance is not critical and cost is a consideration.

Because of these properties, metal restorative materials are used for direct restorations in posterior teeth, where biting forces are greater and appearance is less critical; on anterior palatal surfaces, which are not usually seen in daily activities; and to construct crowns, bridges, inlays, onlays, appliance parts, and implants when strength or cost is more important than appearance.

When used in the mouth, metal restorations tend to provide excellent longevity of service. In recent years their popularity has decreased because of poor esthetics and concerns about safety. Available evidence indicates metal dental restorations are safe but appearance remains a problem.

Porcelain and Glass

There are some small differences in the chemistry of porcelain and glass but the terms are used interchangeably in this book since their properties are similar and the applications of both are the same. Both are made from naturally occurring elements—basically sand for glass, and clay and rock for porcelain. Life has taught you that glass is transparent, can be tinted a variety of colors, and is translucent when tinted. Because tooth enamel is translucent, using tinted glass for the outer parts of a restoration can mimic tooth structure beautifully. Glass does not conduct heat, cold or electricity well, nor does it tarnish or corrode. It melts at relatively high temperatures and is quite smooth, but can be eaten away by acid, especially hydrofluoric acid. It may also crack or craze and breaks relatively easily under tensile load. It is, however, very strong in compression. That is why you can stack porcelain dishes in tall stacks without breaking any, but if you hit the edge of one on a countertop you will be cleaning up dish shards.

Some dental porcelains are engineered to expand and contract at approximately the same rate as tooth enamel in response to heating and cooling. Materials with similar expansion and contraction rates do not push and pull at each other in confined spaces as readily as those that expand and contract at different rates. Less pushing and pulling results in less material and tooth structure fatigue, therefore fewer restoration and tooth fractures.

Glass reacts little with body tissues. This means it does not tend to cause tissue irritation or sensitivity, a very important property. The gingival tissue in contact with smooth porcelain will be healthier than with plastic esthetic restorative material.

Glass is made from silica, a principal ingredient of sand, which is a relatively inexpensive material. Obviously, having to be fired at high temperatures means that these restorations are made indirectly. Even though the materials may be inexpensive, the techniques for fabricating porcelain or glass restorations are time-consuming and require an exceptionally high degree of skill and some special equipment. Restorations made with glass materials may require a substantial financial investment.

Porcelain or glass is selected where appearance is critical, biting forces are weaker or tissue reactivity must be kept to a minimum. The patient must also elect to make the investment required. Porcelain is used for veneers, crowns, and inlays, and there are some porcelain materials that are recommended for short span bridges. Crowns made solely with porcelain, termed *jacket crowns,* are generally placed only in the anterior, although that is changing as porcelain materials increase in strength and accuracy. Posterior porcelain crowns are reinforced with metal. This decreases their esthetic value but increases their strength and improves the fit. The fit problem is due to the shrinkage of porcelain during the firing process, which can be as great as 10%.

Plastic

Plastics are polymers. Polymers are long, tumbled chains of very large molecules. As you know from personal experience, plastics tend not to be as strong as metal, but are more flexible then either metal or glass. They can be translucent or opaque and may be tinted a variety of colors. They melt at relatively low temperatures and do not conduct heat, cold or electricity well. The techniques used to place direct plastic restorations in the mouth are more difficult and time-consuming than those used to place amalgam. This and the cost of the materials make plastic direct restorations more expensive than metal ones.

Plastic restorative materials shrink during curing. They also expand and contract at a very different rate from tooth structure, pushing and pulling on the plastic bonds with which they are attached to teeth. Curing shrinkage and pulling on the bonds holding materials to teeth may break them, leading to the microleakage that the bond was designed to eliminate.

Another important property of most polymers is their inability to displace water. They tend to be repelled by water and surfaces that will have polymers applied need to be kept dry. With some newer bonding and impression materials, however, some fancy chemistry has overcome this obstacle. Therefore, it is important to know whether the particular polymer you are using is hydrophobic or hydrophilic.

Plastics used for direct restorations are actually a mixture of polymer and some hard substance like quartz or glass for wear resistance and translucency. This type of mixture is known as a *composite.* The amount and type of the filler used influences the properties of the material and will be discussed in greater detail later in the book.

Polymers have traditionally been used where esthetics are important, strength less so. Veneers, anterior restorations and crowns can be made with composites. Denture teeth and other esthetic appliance parts, mouthguards, nightguards, sealants, custom trays, bleaching trays, periodontal splints and all types of temporary restorations have long been made with plastics.

Improvements in polymer materials in recent years have led to a dramatic expansion in their use. Posterior composite restorations, crowns, bridges and inlays, as well as appliance frameworks and clasps are now placed with increasing frequency. Polymer liners, adhesives and bonding agents are extremely popular. The greatest number and variety of dental fabrication techniques are now completed using polymer chemistry.

▼ ANTICIPATING MATERIAL NEEDS ▼

So many products with minor variations in preparation technique exist it is impossible for one person to know and use them all. The key phrase here, though, is minor variations. A few basic types of equipment are used to complete a limited number of basic material

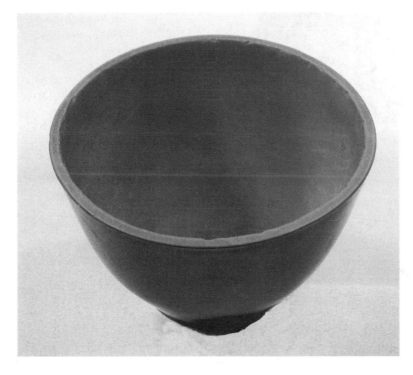

FIGURE 4-1 Rubber bowl. This bowl is made of soft rubber so is quite flexible.

preparation techniques. These techniques make common sense, can be learned relatively quickly and used as the basis for preparing and using the particular brand favored in your office or clinic.

▼ BASIC EQUIPMENT ▼

Bowls

Bowls are used to hold relatively large amounts of material. Two types are in common use: flexible and nonflexible (Figure 4-1). Mixing is done in flexible bowls. Nonflexible bowls are used for auxiliary tasks, such as soaking, transporting or storing materials.

Pads and Slabs

Similar to paper writing pads, dental pads (Figure 4-2) are disposable paper surfaces, held together with an adhesive coating on at least one end. They are used to mix materials on. The paper may have a fluid-resistant coating if the liquid being used will soak through paper. Pads are available in a variety of sizes. Once used, the top paper is detached and thrown out. The majority of mixes are now completed on pads, which are inexpensive and require minimal time for cleanup.

Slabs are reusable mixing surfaces. They are usually glass, but may be plastic. Glass slabs (Figure 4-3) are used for mixing zinc phosphate cement, which generates heat during setting and must be mixed on a surface that dissipates heat. Other materials may be mixed on a slab but this is not popular because of the cleaning necessary before it can be used again. Cleaning any slab is easier if excess material is wiped away with a gauze square immediately after use.

Spatulas

Similar to mixing spoons in a kitchen, spatulas (Figure 4-4) are used to mix two or more materials into one whole. There are several types and each is used to mix specific materials.

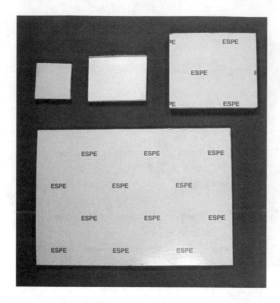
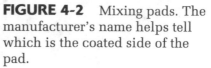

FIGURE 4-2 Mixing pads. The manufacturer's name helps tell which is the coated side of the pad.

Vacuum Formers

Vacuum formers are small machines (Figure 4-5) that soften and adapt plastic materials to working casts. The machines use a heating element to soften the plastic and a vacuum to adapt the material to the model.

Pressure Formers

Pressure formers (Figure 4-6) also soften and adapt plastic materials to models. In this case, a heating element softens and pressurized air adapts the material.

Model Trimmers

Model trimmers (Figure 4-7) cut finished models to esthetic proportions. Cutting is accomplished by pushing the models against a rotating abrasive disk.

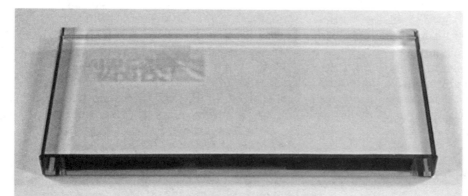

FIGURE 4-3 Glass slab. This is cleaned and reused.

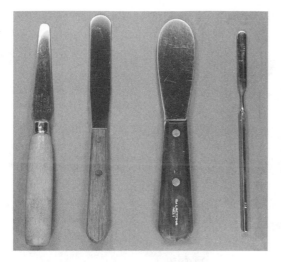

FIGURE 4-4 Spatulas. Different materials demand differently shaped mixing devices. These spatulas are from left to right: impression spatula, plaster spatula, alginate spatula, and cement spatula.

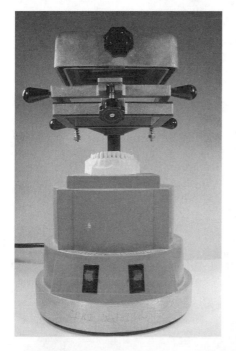

FIGURE 4-5 Vacuum former. The upper section contains a heating element; the middle section holds the plastic to be softened; and the base holds the model and a vacuum pump to suck the softened plastic down tightly over the model.

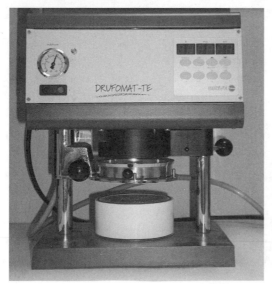

FIGURE 4-6 Pressure former. This time the plastic is again heated by an element above it but a piston presses the softened plastic over the model.

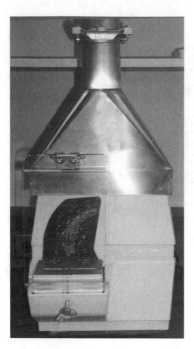

FIGURE 4-7 Model trimmer. Note that there is a shield over the abrasive disk to protect against objects hitting the operator and a dust collector to remove the ground plaster or stone.

Curing Lights and Light Boxes

Lights (Figure 4-8) and light boxes (Figure 4-9) are used to cure polymers. A curing light is placed as near as possible to, but not touching, the uncured light-sensitive material. The light is activated to initiate polymerization. Similarly, an item made of light-sensitive material is placed in a light box. The door is closed, a timer set and the light activated. The cured item is removed from the box at the end of the light cycle.

Amalgamators

Also termed *triturators,* amalgamators (Figure 4-10) are small machines that mix a pre-measured unit dose of a material by shaking it. A container is placed in the machine, speed

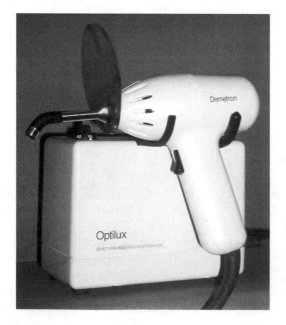

FIGURE 4-8 Curing light. The bulb is in the gun section. The light is emitted by the light guide, which is removable for sterilization. The base contains the timer. Notice the shield to protect the operator's eyes.

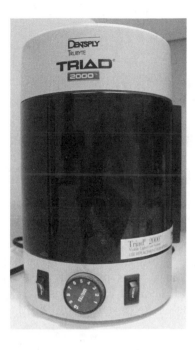

FIGURE 4-9 Light boxes. For materials that can be removed from the mouth, this unit with a rotating base and up to three lights inside gives a more complete cure.

and duration of shaking selected, and the machine activated. These machines were originally designed to mix amalgam, hence the name amalgamator. Amalgam is used less frequently nowadays, but amalgamators are now used to mix a variety of other premeasured materials in addition to amalgam.

▼ COMMON METHODS OF PACKAGING MATERIALS ▼

How a material is packaged informs you how it will be prepared.

Powder and Liquid

Powder and liquid must be measured and mixed. Powders are measured with scoops (Figure 4-11). Large amounts of liquid are measured in marked cylinders or graduates

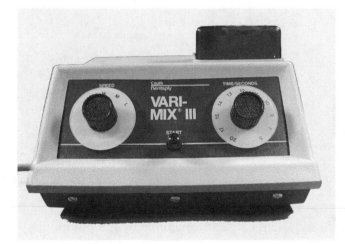

FIGURE 4-10 Amalgamator. The left-hand dial controls the speed of the mixings and the right dial controls the time. The capsule is inserted under the spring-loaded cover on top to protect the operator should the capsule or its contents get loose.

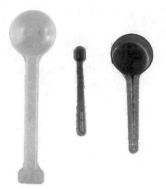

FIGURE 4-11 Scoops. They come in a variety of shapes, sizes, and colors. Just make sure you use the correct one for the powder being used.

(Figure 4-12) and small amounts are measured with fluid droppers (Figure 4-13). Each type of powder requires its own specific scoop and each type of liquid its own specific measure. For this reason, the correct scoop and liquid measure are always kept with powder and liquid materials. Some are even integral parts of the powder and liquid containers themselves.

Large amounts of powder and liquid are mixed in a bowl; small amounts are mixed on a pad or slab. In either case, a suitable spatula will be needed.

Two Tubes of Paste

Equal lengths of two paste materials are squeezed onto a paper pad when the pastes are packaged in two tubes (Figure 4-14). Although the lengths of the materials will be equal, the amounts may not. This is because the size of the openings on the two tubes may be different. One material is a base, the other a catalyst. They will be different colors and are mixed with a spatula to form one blended whole.

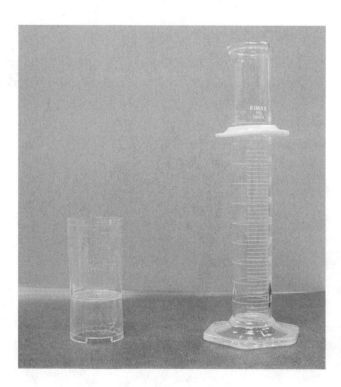

FIGURE 4-12 Cylinders. The graduate on the right can be used for a variety of materials, the one on the left is useful only for one manufacturer's product.

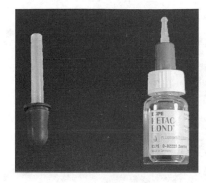

FIGURE 4-13 Droppers. Some droppers are dipped into the liquid and others are built into the bottle.

Sheets

Sheets, or squares, of plastic (Figure 4-15) are softened and adapted to models in vacuum former or pressure former machines. Sheets of wax, which are rectangular, are softened in warm water or over a low flame.

Capsules

Capsules (Figure 4-16) are small cylinders that contain premeasured unit doses of powder and liquid separated by a thin membrane. Some capsules use special tools to mix the two components but in many the action of the trituration breaks the membrane, allowing the two components to mix. The capsule is placed in an amalgamator that is activated to shake the capsule for a specified number of seconds. The capsule is then opened, the capsule re-assembled and discarded, and the mixed material placed with a hand instrument.

Tips

Tips (Figure 4-17), like capsules, are unit doses of powder and liquid separated by a plastic membrane in a closed container. They too are placed in an amalgamator to be shaken until mixed. Unlike capsules, they are designed to fit into a small, hand-held applicator gun. The trigger is activated to squeeze the mixed material out the tip directly onto the area of use.

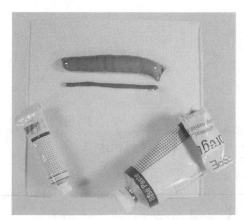

FIGURE 4-14 Pastes. Notice how the paste is proportioned by length, not volume.

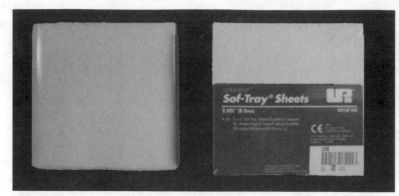

FIGURE 4-15   Sheets. These sheets vary from quite soft to very rigid and come in a variety of colors so that many different appliances can be created.

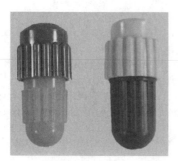

FIGURE 4-16   Capsules. Capsules are color coded for type and for the amount of material contained in the capsule.

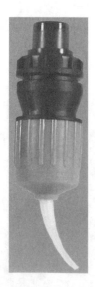

FIGURE 4-17   Tip. Note how it looks like an amalgam capsule but has a tip to extrude the mixed material. The groove near the top is to position it in a gun for injection into the cavity preparation.

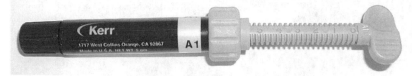

FIGURE 4-18 Syringe. Syringes generally contain light-cured materials. The screw is turned to expel material from the opposite end.

Syringes

Syringes (Figure 4-18) are disposable, single-compartment containers that hold multiple doses of premixed material. A portion of the material is squeezed onto a paper pad and placed in the desired area with a hand instrument.

Cannulas

Similar to syringes, cannulas (Figure 4-19) are disposable, single-compartment containers that hold multiple doses of a premixed material. However, they are fitted with a long, narrow tube through which the material is expelled directly onto the area of interest.

Cartridges

Cartridges are disposable, two-compartment containers that hold multiple doses of unmixed material. They are placed in a large, hand-held applicator gun (Figure 4-20) capable of pushing separate plungers into the two compartments. A disposable, cylinder-shaped tip containing a rotary mixing device is attached to an opening at the front of the cartridge. Squeezing the gun handle pushes the plungers into the compartments, forcing both materials into the tip. The rotary device in the tip mixes the materials as they pass through it. Because the tip does the mixing automatically, this technique is termed *automixing,* and the hand-held gun is termed an *automix syringe.*

▼ COMMON PREPARATION TECHNIQUES ▼

A powder and liquid, or two pastes, will be mixed with one or more of the motions described below.

- Rotary—move flat side of spatula in circles (Figure 4-21).
- Fold and press—with spatula edge, pull powder toward liquid. At liquid, turn spatula to flat side and press (Figure 4-22).

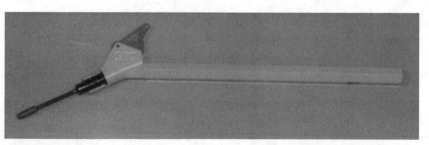

FIGURE 4-19 Cannula. A cannula has a straw-like end that can dispense or draw up material.

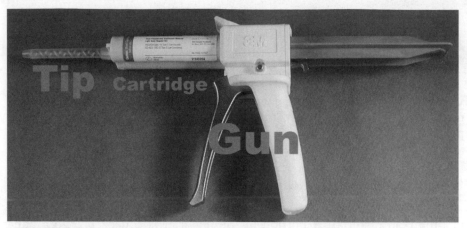

FIGURE 4-20 Automatic syringe and cartridge. The cartridge has two containers. When the trigger is squeezed the material is pushed into the tip, which combines the two parts into a homogeneous mix.

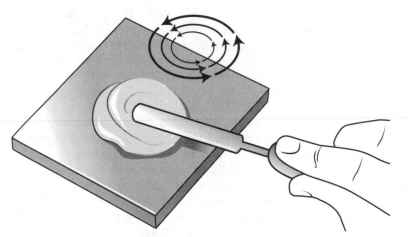

FIGURE 4-21 Rotary mixing. The spatula is kept against the pad and moved in a circular motion.

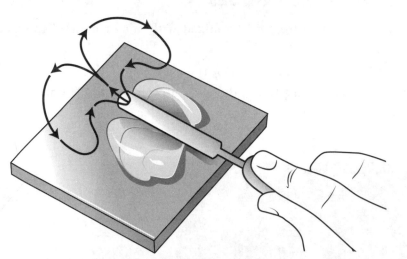

FIGURE 4-22 Fold and press mixing. In this case the material is continually swept into the center of the pad, folded onto itself, pressed firmly, and then the spatula is lifted off the pad and the cycle repeats.

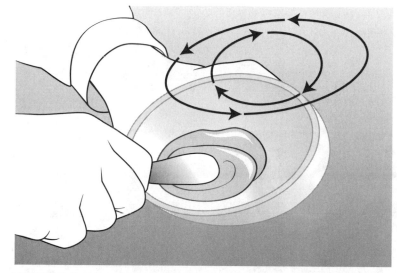

FIGURE 4-23 Stropping. The bowl is tipped toward the mixer and is rotated, and the spatula is swept back and forth across the inside surface. Alternatively, the bowl may be rotated and the material pressed against the side of the bowl in the opposite direction of the bowl movement. The alternative technique is pictured here.

- Strop—using flat side of spatula, sweep back and forth across a surface (Figure 4-23).
- Figure 8—strop, lifting spatula slightly when switching from one direction to the other (Figure 4-24).
- Stir—submerge spatula tip in material and move it in circles (Figure 4-25).
- Gather from a pad—scrape spatula along length of pad to pick up all material. Place back on pad by moving spatula a short way in reverse direction, rotating wrist slightly and pressing. Repeat pickup and replacing process. Pick up again and use (Figure 4-26).

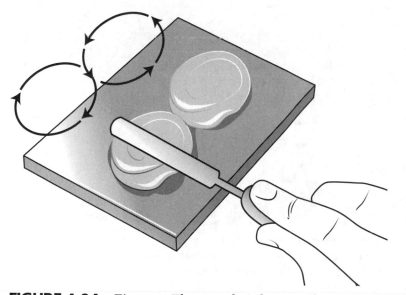

FIGURE 4-24 Figure 8. The spatula is kept on the surface and moved in a figure 8 pattern.

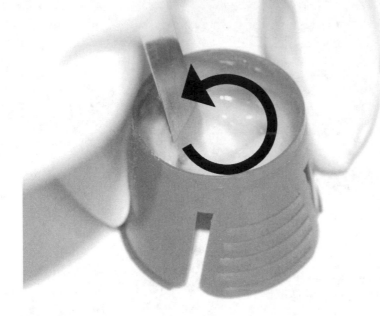

FIGURE 4-25 Stirring. Note the spatula tip is kept submerged to avoid creation of air voids in the mix.

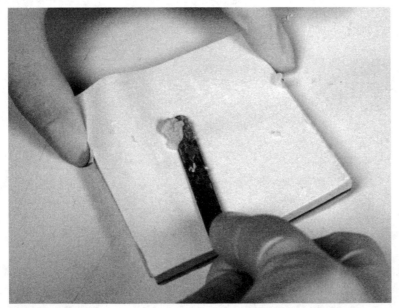

FIGURE 4-26 Gathering from a pad. Using the edge of the spatula, the material is brought to the center from one side, then the wrist is turned away from the body to remove the material from the flat side. The process is repeated on the other side of the pad. The spatula is then forced under the mass of material to pick it all up as one neat whole.

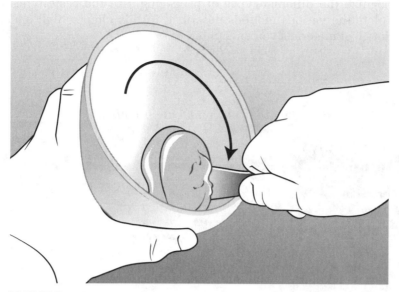

FIGURE 4-27 Gathering from a bowl. The spatula is raked down the side of the bowl in a perpendicular orientation and then after one turnaround flipped horizontally with all the material stuck to it.

- Gather from a bowl—scrape spatula along side of bowl to pick up all material. Scrape both sides of spatula on edge of bowl. Repeat pickup and replacement process (Figure 4-27).

KEY POINTS

✓ There are many different materials but they are prepared using relatively few techniques.
✓ How a material is packaged tells you how it will be prepared.
  - For powder and liquid materials: mix using a bowl or pad and spatula
  - For paste materials in tubes: mix using a pad and spatula
  - For materials in syringes and cannulas: no mixing—place directly where it will be used, or place on pad and carry to mouth with hand instrument
  - For materials in capsules or unit dose tips: mix in amalgamator and carry to mouth in an applicator gun or hand instrument
  - For materials in cartridges: place in an automix syringe, affix tip and squeeze handle
  - For single sheets of wax or plastic: soften with heat
✓ Mixing of powders and liquids, or pastes, will be done with one or more of these motions:
  - Rotary—move flat side of spatula in circles
  - Fold and press—with spatula edge, pull powder toward liquid; at liquid, turn spatula to flat side and press
  - Strop—using flat sides of spatula, sweep back and forth across a surface
  - Figure 8—strop, lifting spatula slightly when switching from one direction to the other
  - Stir—submerge spatula tip in material and move it in circles
  - Gather from a pad—scrape spatula along length of pad to pick up all material. Place back on pad by moving spatula a short way in reverse direction, rotating wrist slightly and pressing. Repeat pickup and replacing process. Pick up again and use.
  - Gather from a bowl—scrape spatula along side of bowl to pick up all material. Scrape both sides of spatula on edge of bowl. Repeat pickup and replacement process.

✓ Learning to recognize the different types of packaging, use the basic types of equipment, and complete the various motions described in this chapter will enable you to prepare the majority of materials you encounter.

SELF TEST

Questions 1–5: Identify and state the use of each item pictured below.

1.

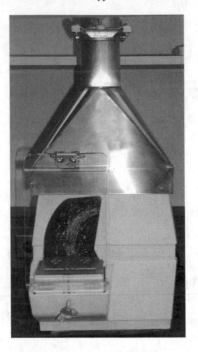

2.

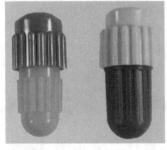

3.

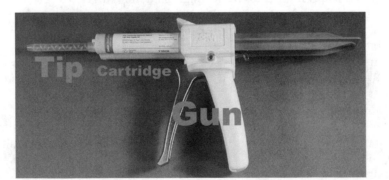

4.

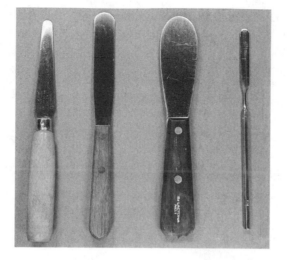

5.

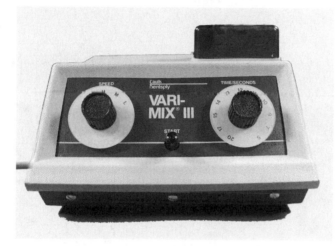

Questions 6–10: Indicate how each task listed below would be accomplished.

6. Mix powder and liquid that are packaged in a unit dose tip
   a. Place in flexible bowl and strop with spatula
   b. Place on a paper pad and combine with a rotary motion
   c. Soften in warm water or over a low flame
   d. Place in an amalgamator, select time and speed of shaking, activate timer

7. Mix two pastes that are packaged in a cartridge
   a. Measure with correct scoops, knead with fingers
   b. Place equal lengths on a paper pad, blend with spatula
   c. Place in automix syringe, affix tip, squeeze handle
   d. Soften and adapt with heat in a vacuum former

8. Place material packaged in a tube with a cannula
   a. Eject directly onto area of interest
   b. Place in automix syringe, affix tip, squeeze handle
   c. Place in flexible bowl, stir with spatula
   d. Mix in amalgamator, eject onto paper pad, carry to mouth on hand instrument

9. Proportion two pastes packaged in tubes: place
   a. Equal amounts of the materials on a slab
   b. Equal lengths of the materials on a pad
   c. An equal number of scoops of the materials in a bowl
   d. The tubes in a syringe, add mixing tip, push handle

10. Prepare items needed to mix a large amount of powder and liquid: obtain correct
    a. Scoop, liquid measure, spatula and flexible bowl
    b. Syringe, tip and mixing machine
    c. Slab, spatula, and measures for powder and liquid
    d. Capsule, amalgamator and measures for powder and liquid

Preventive, Diagnostic, and Cosmetic Materials

This section contains primarily information about materials used to help the patient avoid dental problems. These materials are used to prevent problems from occurring, finding problems that are in their early stages when they are easy to repair, or to make the smile look better. An attractive smile is often an incentive for the patient to maintain his or her mouth even more conscientiously. The rest of the sections in this book deal with materials that restore tooth form and function after damage. This section strives to make the procedures discussed in the other sections unnecessary.

ABRASIVES

OBJECTIVES

After studying this chapter, you should be able to:

1. Define the term *abrasive*.
2. Describe abrasion.
3. Indicate how particle size, speed, smoothness, hardness and application pressure affect abrasion.
4. List means of avoiding tissue damage, retaining an abrasive on a substrate and maintaining cutting ability while using abrasives.
5. Select an abrasive for tasks commonly completed in dentistry.
6. Describe principles of safe, effective abrasive use.

▼ DEFINITION OF ABRASIVES ▼

Abrasives are small, hard particles in a liquid, paste or solid binder.

▼ COMPOSITION ▼

Abrasives are composed of natural minerals or synthetic substitutes.

▼ USES ▼

Abrasives are used to remove stains and to finish and polish natural teeth and all types of tooth restorations and replacements. *Finishing* is cutting and smoothing; *polishing* is smoothing the surface further to create a shine. Allied dental personnel do not cut natural teeth deeply enough to reshape them, but do use abrasives frequently to remove stains from, smooth and polish natural and artificial surfaces. Smooth surfaces promote oral cleanliness, a major factor in prevention of oral disease.

▼ MECHANISM OF ACTION ▼

Rubbing hard abrasive particles over a *substrate,* a softer material, wears the substrate away. The wearing process also creates heat and debris.

▼ CLINICAL CONCERNS ▼

In order to accomplish a wearing task effectively, an abrasive must be selected that has appropriate cutting ability for the job to be completed, is supplied in a convenient form for reaching the area of interest, can retain its cutting ability during use, and stay on the tooth or restoration surface long enough to accomplish its task. At the same time it must not cut too deeply or damage the tooth or material.

Appropriate Cutting Ability

The purpose of using an abrasive may be to finish or polish. Abrasives wear substances by rubbing harder particles over a softer surface to create a myriad of small cuts. Finishing requires relatively larger, deeper cuts; polishing, relatively smaller, shallower ones.

How large and deep the cuts made by an abrasive will be depends in part on the size and regularity of its particles. Manufacturers have developed a *grit* system to inform users of the size and smoothness of abrasive particles. They are rated as coarse, medium, fine, and then X, XX, XXX or XXXX—extra fine to extra, extra, extra, extra fine. Coarse abrasives have rough, large particles that get smaller and smoother as they go toward the fine grits.

Coarser abrasives are used first. Progressively finer grit abrasives are then used to produce the smoothest surface possible. Rough surfaces encourage plaque formation, reflect light poorly and appear dull. Smooth surfaces are less receptive to plaque attachment, reflect light evenly and appear shiny. Patients are particularly interested in the results of abrasive use. They see immediately the benefits that shiny, stain-free teeth provide in improved appearance and they feel improved smoothness with their tongues.

As noted, abrasives wear substrates by rubbing harder particles over a softer surface to create a myriad of small cuts. Abrasive and substrate hardness varies. Enamel is very hard; dentin and cementum are softer. Stain and restorative material range from relatively soft plastic material and yellow stain to hard metal alloys and resistant black stain. Care must be taken to choose an abrasive that will finish or polish as needed without wearing away too much of the tooth or material substrate. Accordingly, abrasives of varying hardness are used to ensure adequate but not excessive cutting ability for the task at hand. The hardness of the abrasive used will depend on the hardness of the substrate. Use too hard an abrasive and you risk damaging the surface; too soft an abrasive will not change the surface.

Pressure and speed of application must be factored into the cutting equation. All other things being equal, strong pressure and faster speed cut faster, lighter pressure and low speed cut more slowly.

All other things are *not* equal, however. Speed can be a problem. When an abrasive paste or slurry is used at high speed on a rotating instrument, an outward force is created that flings the abrasive away. Without abrasive, cutting activity ceases.

Rubbing movement also creates heat, with faster speed creating greater heat. Heat can be conducted to the substrate and tooth, where it may create size and shape changes in the restorative material or injure the pulp. A good rule of thumb is to use low to moderate speed to maintain abrasion efficiency, prevent pulp injury and maintain material integrity.

Additional protection can be obtained by the use of a liquid in the abrasive to absorb heat, thereby cooling the area and avoiding unwanted temperature rise. A liquid also acts as a lubricant, helping the abrasive to move over the material surface and assisting in the removal of the debris that accumulates as the material layers are rubbed away.

Strong pressure is problematic, too. Heavy pressure causes deeper cutting where the pressure is applied. Deep cuts next to uncut areas create a rough surface that encourages plaque attachment and appears dull, the opposite of what is desired as a final result. Strong pressure also slows movement of the abrasive particles over the surface of the substrate. Slower particles cut less efficiently. Light to moderate pressure balances the depth of cutting and movement factors well.

Retention of Cutting Ability

As most abrasive particles are used they become smaller and rounder, thereby becoming less abrasive and less effective until they are finally used up. Some newer abrasives break up into smaller pieces that retain their rough edges, but even these will become less and less effective as they are broken into smaller and smaller units. An abrasive must be frequently renewed to maintain its effectiveness. Abrasives, even if not worn, can be dislodged from the substrate and this will lessen the cutting ability as less abrasive is left on the surface.

▼ HOW ABRASIVES ARE SUPPLIED ▼

Various methods are employed to carry abrasives to, and retain them on, a surface of interest. Abrasives are supplied as powders; in pastes, stones, points, cakes and polishing cups; or bonded to disks, wheels, strips, or stones. *Powders* are mixed with a liquid such as water or glycerin to make a thin paste termed *slurry*. *Stones* and *points* are mixtures of abrasive and binder pressed into various shapes and mounted on a *mandrel,* a metal rod that fits

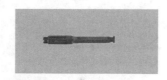

FIGURE 5-1 Mandrel. Mandrels are available with square and round ends. Some have a screw on the end to hold an abrasive wheel.

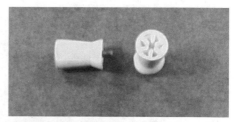

FIGURE 5-2 Abrasive cups. These cups have no abrasive in them. They are meant to hold abrasive for polishing. Some types of cups are impregnated with abrasives.

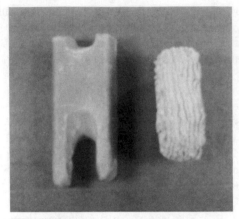

FIGURE 5-3 Cakes. You can see how inexperienced students have worn a groove in the cake on the left with the wheel at right. It is more efficient to move the cake side to side to wear it down evenly.

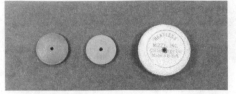

FIGURE 5-4 Disk, stone, and wheel. Each is attached to a mandrel for use in a handpiece or angle as a rotary instrument.

into the dental handpiece or angle (Figure 5-1). Points tend to have long thin shapes; stones, wider, more varied ones. *Cups* (Figure 5-2) are mixtures of abrasive and binder pressed into small round shapes hollowed out on one side and mounted on a screw or mandrel. They may also not be manufactured with any abrasive in them and simply have the hollowed-out area to *hold* abrasive slurry. Mandrel-mounted cups are attached to handpieces and angles. *Cakes* (Figure 5-3) are also pressed shapes, but are larger, hand-held, and for laboratory use. *Disks* and *wheels* (Figure 5-4) are round pieces of paper, plastic, metal or rubber covered or impregnated with abrasive particles. They are placed on mandrels and used in handpieces and angles. *Strips* (Figure 5-5) are relatively long, thin pieces of plastic or metal with abrasive particles attached to one side. They are hand rubbed on proximal surfaces.

▼ MATERIAL SELECTION FOR SPECIFIC NEEDS ▼

It is important to match the abrasive with the surface. The harder the surface is, the harder the abrasive that must be used. Using an abrasive softer than the surface will result in the wear of the abrasive, not the surface. Table 5-1 is a chart with the hardness numbers of common dental abrasives, restorative materials and different tooth layers. Hardness numbers are relative, with diamond, the hardest substance, given a value of 10 and talc, the soft-

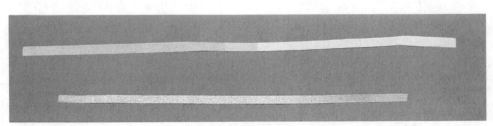

FIGURE 5-5 Abrasive strips. The top strip has a mylar backing. On this strip the center has no abrasive and each end has a different grit. The lower strip is diamond bonded to a metal backing.

TABLE 5-1 Hardness numbers of common dental abrasives. This is an arbitrary scale with diamond at 10.

Material	Mohs Hardness
Diamond	10
Tungsten Carbide	9
Aluminum Oxide	9
Zirconium Silicate	7.5
Quartz	7
Tin Oxide	6.5
Pumice	6
Chalk (Calcium Carbonate)	3
Gypsum	2
Talc	1

est substance, given a value of 1. Other materials are ranked between diamond and talc according to whether they are able to scratch the surface of a substance of known value.

Commonly used abrasives include pumice, tin oxide, quartz, emery, aluminum oxide, diamond chips and rouge.

Pumice (Figure 5-6) is ground volcanic glass that is supplied as a gray powder or a component of various pastes. It is used for finishing and polishing natural and artificial surfaces.

Tin oxide (Figure 5-7) is a very mild abrasive supplied as a white powder. It is mixed with water to form a slurry and used for polishing enamel and metals.

Quartz, also called *sand* or *cuttle*, is a natural mineral supplied as particles on disks or strips and used for finishing gold, plastic and composite. Composite is a plastic esthetic material used extensively for direct restorations.

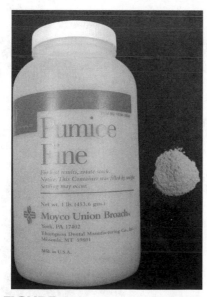

FIGURE 5-6 Pumice. Pumice can be obtained in different grits. This is a pile of fine powder next to the container.

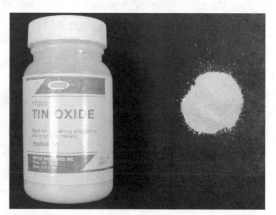

FIGURE 5-7 Tin oxide. Tin oxide has a higher hardness number and finer grit than pumice, making it ideal for putting a high polish on metal restorations.

Emery, also termed *corundum,* is a natural mineral supplied as particles on strips and disks. Most people are familiar with emery as the abrasive used on emery boards for shaping fingernails. In dentistry, emery is used for finishing natural teeth.

Aluminum oxide is a natural mineral supplied as particles bonded to disks, wheels, strips, stones and points, and as a component of pastes. It is used for polishing natural teeth.

Diamond (Figure 5-8) is a natural mineral or synthetic substitute supplied as chips bound to metal wheels and points or as a component of polishing pastes. Diamond is an extremely hard abrasive and is used to cut natural teeth. Diamond wheels and points generate significant heat; the tooth must be cooled with water while they are being used. Diamond paste is used for polishing composite.

Rouge (Figure 5-9) is iron oxide, a natural mineral, supplied as a reddish-brown cake. It is usually used in the laboratory for polishing gold.

▼ PRINCIPLES OF ABRASIVE USE ▼

A series of principles for abrasive use can be derived from the chapter discussion:

- Use coarsest abrasives first and progress to the finest last. This gradually reduces the size of cuts until the smoothest possible surface is obtained. A smooth surface appears shiny and promotes cleanliness.
- Never use large, irregular, coarse abrasives on natural teeth. The danger of removing too much tooth structure, especially cementum, is too great. Only medium or fine materials should be used on natural teeth.
- Position the abrasive carefully to avoid soft tissue damage. Maintain position control whenever the abrasive is moving.
- Apply abrasives with low to moderate speed. This keeps the abrasive on the instrument and decreases the production of unwanted heat.
- Keep the abrasive moist. The liquid will cool the area, help the particles move over the surface and assist in removing accumulated debris.
- Use low to moderate pressure. This will help prevent surface roughening and allow the abrasive particles to keep moving.

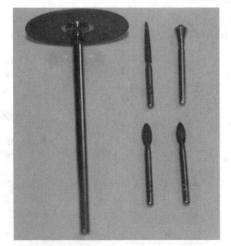

FIGURE 5-8 Diamond. Diamond can be bonded to metal in a variety of shapes to produce some very different-looking abrasives.

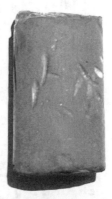

FIGURE 5-9 Rouge. This is used for a final polish of metal restorations.

- Move your hand so the abrasive moves from one area of the tooth to another. Cutting occurs when the abrasive is in contact with the tooth. Prolonged contact in one area causes deeper cutting there, roughening rather than smoothing the surface.
- While working, use a dabbing motion to apply and release the abrasive. Prolonged application in one area localizes and concentrates heat production, creating greater potential for pulp injury and material degradation.
- Renew your abrasive frequently. As the abrasive is used it wears and finally disappears. Renewing the abrasive provides fresh cutting ability.

KEY POINTS

✓ Abrasives are hard particles used to rub away a softer surface, called the substrate.

✓ Abrasives are used to cut, smooth, remove stains from and polish teeth and materials.

✓ As abrasives are used, they are worn away.

✓ Larger, rougher particles cut; as particles become progressively smaller, they become smooth and round, and polish rather than cut.

✓ Using abrasives generates heat and debris.

✓ Heat can damage teeth and materials.

✓ Staying in one area and using higher speed create greater heat.

✓ Higher speed and stronger pressure cause faster, deeper cutting

✓ Abrasives can easily shred soft tissue.

✓ To protect tissue and materials, use abrasives as follows:
- Position abrasive carefully.
- Use coarsest abrasive first, finest last.
- Use only medium or fine abrasive on natural teeth.
- Apply with dabbing motion and slow to moderate speed.
- Use low to moderate pressure.
- Keep the abrasive moist and moving.

✓ Renew abrasive frequently.

SELF TEST

Questions 1–5: Select an abrasive for the task described. Abrasives are listed below. You may use an answer more than once.

    Tin oxide
    Pumice
    Diamond chips
    Quartz (Sand)
    Emery

1. Polish a full denture

2. Polish an amalgam restoration

3. Polish a composite restoration

4. Remove stains from a natural tooth

5. Smooth a natural tooth

Questions 6–10: Describe how you can safely and efficiently accomplish each task listed below.

6. Avoid soft tissue damage when polishing a natural tooth

7. Avoid hard tissue damage when polishing a natural tooth

8. Achieve the smoothest surface possible

9. Provide a final laboratory polish to a full gold alloy crown before it is delivered to the patient

10. Prevent material distortion

DENTAL SEALANTS

OBJECTIVES

After studying this chapter, you should be able to:

1. Indicate why and how sealants are placed.
2. Describe and differentiate available sealant materials.
3. List and suggest means of controlling pertinent clinical factors that affect sealant placement, assessment and retention.

▼ DEFINITION OF SEALANT ▼

A sealant is a thin plastic coating placed on the pits and grooves of a tooth surface, at the interface of a restoration and tooth, or over the margin of a fixed orthodontic appliance where it is attached to a tooth.

▼ MATERIALS USED ▼

Acrylic resin, glass ionomer and composite are used to make dental sealants.

▼ COMPOSITION ▼

All sealants are polymers. By learning the three materials are polymers, what do you already know about them? (To review polymers refer back to Chapter 4.)

▼ USE ▼

Sealants are used to prevent tooth decay. Sealants are applied to sound surfaces to protect them from caries, to surfaces with incipient caries to prevent progression of the lesion, and to the tooth–restoration or tooth–appliance interface to prevent microleakage and secondary decay.

▼ MECHANISM OF ACTION ▼

Sealants isolate vulnerable areas of the tooth from decay-causing bacteria and acids. Some sealants also help prevent decay by leaching fluoride into adjacent tooth structure.

▼ ACRYLIC RESIN ▼

Because acrylic resin is by far the most commonly used sealant material, most of the remaining discussion in this chapter will be devoted to it. Acrylic resin is composed of bis-GMA acrylic acid monomer, copolymers to increase strength and flow, chemicals to begin the polymerization process, and sometimes glass filler particles to increase strength.

Self-cured acrylic sealant materials begin polymerization by mixing a chemical activator, commonly an organic amine, and an initiator, commonly benzoyl peroxide. The activator is packaged in one container and the initiator in another to prevent polymerization prior to use.

Light cured sealant systems also contain a benzoyl peroxide initiator but use a different method of activating it: exposure to visible light. Light cured acrylic resins are packaged as a single material, usually in a container that does not allow light penetration. A single container can be used because the material will not polymerize until exposed to light. Opaque containers are used to protect the material from light until the operator places it on the tooth.

▼ CLINICAL CONSIDERATIONS ▼

Clinical concerns include adequate isolation, ease of placement, visibility, retention, wear, and the caries resistance of surrounding tooth structure.

Adequate Isolation

Most sealant materials are hydrophobic. For adequate bonding to occur, the tooth must be kept dry throughout the placement and curing process. Any molecules of moisture present can be trapped between the sealant material and the tooth or restoration surface, thereby

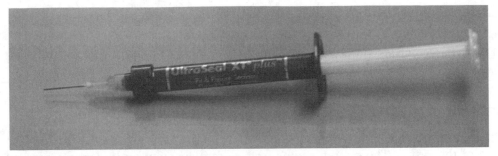

FIGURE 6-1 Multidose syringe. The cylinder needs to be opaque so the material does not set prior to use.

preventing the close contact necessary for bonding. The operator's choice of dental dam, cotton rolls, parotid duct covers, saliva ejectors, and compressed air are available to aid isolation.

Ease of Placement

Both self- and light-cured systems are available. Self-cured systems require the mixing of two materials and take longer to polymerize, but usually cure more completely. Light-cured materials do not require mixing and cure immediately, but not always completely.

Sealant resin is packaged as a viscous liquid to paint on the tooth or restoration, or in a small multidose syringe (Figure 6-1) for ejection of material onto the surface. Brushing the material on takes longer but permits better flow control. Ejection is faster but requires more skill to control the expulsion rate and amount.

Visibility

Clear and tinted sealant materials are available. Clear material is less visible, thus perhaps esthetically more pleasing. White tints (Figure 6-2) have gained favor in recent years because they are more visible to the person evaluating sealant extension and retention.

Retention

Studies indicate the most important factor in sealant retention is prevention of moisture contamination during placement. Adequate isolation is essential.

Wear

Unfilled, lightly filled and filled materials are available. Unfilled materials flow over the tooth surface more readily but are weaker. Lightly filled and filled materials do not flow as well but are stronger. Occlusal high spots on sealants made with unfilled materials will adjust themselves to the patient's bite through normal use; those on lightly filled or filled sealants require adjustment by a dental professional.

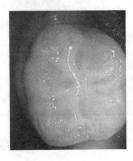

FIGURE 6-2 Sealants. Note how you can see the extension of the sealant material. With clear material this is not evident.

Caries Resistance of Adjacent Tooth Structure

Sealants with and without fluoride are available. Because retained sealants are so effective at preventing decay, fluoride content has not increased sealant effectiveness greatly while the sealant is present, but may be helpful as it is worn away.

▼ SEALANT PROCEDURE ▼

There are three basic application steps: tooth preparation, sealant application, and evaluation of the result. The operator aims for secure placement and adequate but not excessive extension.

Preparing the Surface: Clean, Etch and Inspect

The object of preparation is to create a clean, rough surface that will facilitate bonding. A rough surface has many tiny depressions that aid mechanical interlocking of the sealant and tooth structure. A clean surface permits direct contact between the molecules of the tooth and the material, and aids material flow into the depressions.

The usual cleaning method is polishing with plain pumice slurry to remove pellicle, plaque and stain. Plain pumice is used because it contains no fluoride or flavoring agents that would interfere with bonding. Other methods are also used for cleaning: painting with hydrogen peroxide, an oxygenating agent that breaks up surface molecules; washing with plain water to remove surface debris; removing surface deposits with a sharp instrument tip or toothbrush; or polishing with an air polisher. An air polisher (Figure 6-3) is a small mechanical device that directs a focused stream of sodium bicarbonate particles under pressure to the tooth surface to polish it. Studies indicate all of the cleaning methods discussed are similarly effective.

Once the tooth is clean, it must be etched to create the multitude of tiny depressions into which the sealant material will flow. This is accomplished by painting the surface with an *etchant*. Etchants are weak liquid or gel solutions of acid, usually phosphoric acid, and water that are placed on the exposed tooth surface. The acid will remove some of

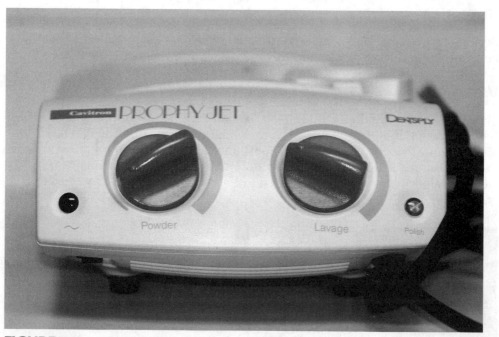

FIGURE 6-3   Air polisher. This unit can also be used to remove stain from the tooth surface.

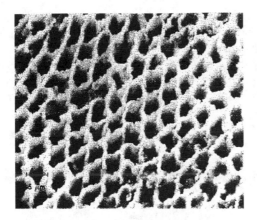

FIGURE 6-4 Etched enamel. This rough surface will mechanically bond to the sealant material. (Photo micrograph reprinted from Daniel S. Harfst: *Mosby's Dental Hygiene: Concepts, Cases, & Competencies,* p. 441, 2002, by permission of the publisher, Mosby Elsevier Science.

the surface crystals. Because of the way enamel is formed some areas are more prone to acid dissolution, so the acid makes a regular pattern of microscopic indentations in the surface.

Etchant action is stopped by flushing the surface with water. Etched enamel is extremely vulnerable. The hydroxyapatite crystals next to the depressions are no longer supported by adjacent tooth structure (Figure 6-4). Since tooth enamel is very brittle the unsupported rods can be easily broken, thus resmoothing the surface that was just roughened. To avoid damaging etched enamel it is not touched with an instrument; inspection is solely visual. The operator is looking for the etched area to be a chalky white color.

Placement and Evaluation

Once etching is adequate, the tooth is isolated and *thoroughly* dried. The sealant material is applied and cured. Finally, the sealant itself is inspected. It should extend slightly beyond the area of interest, be securely attached and not alter either the occlusion or proximal contact areas. Some operators end the procedure by providing a fluoride treatment to protect the edges of the sealed area; others do not. Studies indicate sealants placed without a following fluoride treatment do not experience higher decay rates.

▼ COMPOSITE RESIN ▼

Composite resin is made of the same acrylic polymer material as sealants, but is much more heavily filled. More filling gives it greater strength but also reduces its flow. Composite materials are available in several viscosities. The one used for sealants needs to flow into all the small depressions in the tooth and is the lowest viscosity available. Flowable composites are more viscous than acrylic resin sealant material but less viscous than other types of composite. They flow adequately well for sealant placement but usually must be carefully spread into position with a brush or instrument tip.

Because they are made of the same basic material, etching, inspection, isolation, placement and assessment of a finished sealant are the same for composite sealants as for acrylic resin.

▼ GLASS IONOMER ▼

Glass ionomer is an acrylic polymer as are acrylic resin and composite. It differs because it has fluoroaluminosilicate glass reinforcing particles added to its acrylic polymer base, and tartaric or maleic acid is used as the catalyst (acrylic acid is used in acrylic and composite). The tartaric or maleic acid catalyst attacks the glass reinforcing particles in the glass ionomer, breaking down the outsides of the particles. All of the components in the reaction except fluoride recombine to create a weak polymer matrix with the undissolved portions of the glass particles still serving as reinforcers. The fluoride remains free and is available for leaching into the surrounding tooth structure.

Glass ionomer is also different because when its components recombine it bonds chemically to the calcium in tooth structure. Accordingly, the tooth does not need to be etched prior to material placement. Glass ionomer polymerizes better in the presence of moisture, so thorough drying of the area before material placement is not essential. Glass ionomer has very low viscosity; it flows easily into pits and grooves. It also has poor abrasion resistance and wears away from the tooth or material surface more readily than acrylic or composite.

▼ EFFICACY ▼

Research indicates retained sealants are effective in preventing decay. Reported retention rates range from 45% to 79%, depending on teeth sealed and duration of study, with the single biggest reason for sealant loss being moisture contamination. Choice of liquid or gel etchant does not appear to affect sealant retention, nor does method of surface cleaning. Acrylic and composite sealants are retained at significantly higher rates than those made of glass ionomer, but teeth sealed with glass ionomer experience lower, indeed very low, decay rates. Sealants placed at the tooth-restoration interface clearly reduce secondary decay, and sealants placed over fixed orthodontic appliance margins reduce the incidence of demineralization. Sealants are cost effective. One-surface direct restorations exceed the cost of a sealant. Restorations do not last forever so will need to be replaced a number of times in a person's lifetime. Sealants also require periodic reapplication. Studies show increasing retention times, with current retention expectations for correctly applied sealants ranging up to 17 years.

KEY POINTS

✓ A sealant is a thin polymer coating placed on a tooth surface to prevent dental decay.
✓ Three polymers are used: acrylic resin, composite and glass ionomer.
✓ The vast majority of sealants are acrylic resin.
✓ Bonding mechanism: acrylic and composite—mechanical interlocking; glass ionomer—chemical bond to calcium in tooth structure
✓ Clinical concerns include:
   • Choice of material—filled, lightly filled or unfilled
   • Visibility—clear or tinted
   • Isolation—dryness is essential for acrylic and composite resins, not essential for glass ionomer.
   • Ease of placement—liquid or gel etchant; self- or light-cured material; application with brush or cannula; glass ionomer flows best, composite least
   • Efficacy—sealants prevent decay while in place
   • Wear—periodic replacement required
   • Caries resistance of adjacent tooth surface—glass ionomer leaches fluoride; others do not
✓ Placement procedure: Time steps according to manufacturer's directions
   • Clean, etch, flush, isolate and dry tooth
   • Inspect tooth for adequate etching, signified by chalky whiteness
   • Place and cure sealant
   • Assess sealant for adequate attachment, appropriate height and contour
   • Provide fluoride treatment and postoperative directions

Questions 1–5: Indicate your understanding of the tooth sealing process by answering the questions below.

1. What is the purpose of using a sealant?

2. Why would an operator choose to seal both sound teeth and teeth that have been restored?

3. How can an operator improve the likelihood that an acrylic resin sealant that is to be placed will be retained?

4. Why would an operator choose to place a composite or glass ionomer sealant rather than one made of acrylic?

5. How is sealant material interlocked with the tooth surface?

Questions 6–10: Describe how choice of a particular type of sealant material can contribute to the accomplishment of each task listed below.

6. Maximize sealant visibility to facilitate re-evaluation at subsequent appointments

7. Maximize sealant wear

8. Minimize secondary decay in a restored tooth

9. Minimize decalcification adjacent to orthodontic appliances bonded directly to the tooth surface

10. Maximize sealant cure

TOOTH WHITENERS

HIGHLIGHTS

This chapter discusses the following topics:

1. Definition
2. Use
3. Materials used
   a. Hydrogen peroxide
   b. Carbamide peroxide
4. Mechanism of action
5. Available product types
6. Preparation for bleaching
7. Application schedules
8. Efficacy
9. Troubleshooting

OBJECTIVES

After studying this chapter, you should be able to:

1. Define and describe the tooth whitening process.
2. List materials used as dental bleaching agents.
3. State indications and contraindications for bleaching treatment.
4. Describe common bleaching regimens.
5. Discuss the efficacy of tooth bleaching.
6. Suggest means of preventing or alleviating problems encountered during bleaching.

▼ DEFINITION ▼

Tooth whiteners are bleaching agents. They are extremely popular with patients because everyone wants to have beautiful, white teeth. Dental professionals refer to tooth bleaches as whiteners so as not to give patients the idea of buying household bleach and using it on their teeth. Household bleaches are much stronger and could damage the teeth or soft tissues.

▼ USE ▼

Two types of bleaching are done: internal and external. Internal bleaching is a more powerful process that is done solely by the dentist. It is done with materials of higher concentration. External bleaching employs materials of lesser concentration, can be done at home by the patient, and is often supervised by allied dental personnel.

▼ MATERIALS USED ▼

Teeth are bleached with *peroxides.* Peroxides are combinations of oxygen and some other chemical. The oxygen molecules are not tightly held to the other atoms and therefore easily leave the peroxide. They can then react with another substance. Such materials are termed *oxygenating agents.*

Hydrogen and carbamide peroxides are most often used in dental whitening agents. The carbamide type, also termed urea peroxide, combines oxygen with a nitrogen-based molecule that allows slower release of the oxygen than the hydrogen peroxides. Carbopol and glycerine are added to the material to create a viscous, slow-release gel that can be applied and will stay on the teeth for a relatively long period of time.

▼ MECHANISM OF ACTION ▼

Oxygen molecules from the peroxide enter the tooth and combine with molecules in the tooth structure. The tooth molecules change their chemical structure by the addition of oxygen. This makes formally colored molecules, or pigments, no longer have color, so the tooth becomes lighter.

▼ AVAILABLE PRODUCT TYPES ▼

Three types of tooth whitening products are available for home use: home bleaching agents, whitening dentifrices and mouthwashes (see Table 7-1). Bleaching agents contain higher

TABLE 7-1 Tooth whitening products. You can see how the bleaching agent is basically the same in all systems.

Type	Whitening Ingredient
Whitening dentifrices	Usually abrasives but may have small amounts of hydrogen or carbamide peroxides
Whitening gels	Hydrogen or carbamide peroxides
Polyethyene film	Hydrogen peroxide
Tray systems	Carbamide peroxide
In-office systems	Hydrogen or carbamide peroxides
Light-activated	Hydrogen peroxide

concentrations of hydrogen or carbamide peroxide. Both professionally supervised and over-the-counter home bleaching products are available. Dentifrices and mouthwashes, which contain very small amounts of hydrogen or calcium peroxide, are intended for daily use without professional supervision.

▼ PREPARATION FOR BLEACHING ▼

Home bleaching agents are commonly injected into custom trays (Figure 7-1) and placed over the teeth for varying periods of time, depending on the needs of the patient. For each arch to be bleached, an alginate impression is taken (Figure 7-2) and a gypsum model poured (Figure 7-3). A thin, flexible, polymer sheet is adapted to the model with a vacuum or pressure former (Figure 7-4) and the tray is cut to shape with an electric trimmer (Figure 7-5) or very small trimming shears (Figure 7-6). The edges may be lightly flame polished if sharp edges remain following scissor cutting.

Patients often ask for bleaching. They read about it in magazines, hear about it from a friend or see it advertised on television, and they are sure they are perfect candidates for the process. Are they? Indications for bleaching include:

- Patient interest
- Good oral health and hygiene
- All areas of exposed dentin or open margins of restorations sealed

Contraindications include:

- Smoking or excessive coffee and/or tea consumption. The stains would simply reappear, negating the process.
- Poor oral health or hygiene. As above, the stains would rapidly reappear making it a waste of time and money.
- Inadequate eruption. Bleaching incompletely erupted teeth will cause the tooth color to look uneven. As the tooth continues to erupt through the gingiva there will be a distinct stripe separating the already bleached area from the newly erupted unbleached area.
- Teeth with large pulps. Bleach can travel through small tubes in the dentin and irritate the pulp as it irritates the gingival tissue. Large pulps permit this to occur more easily.

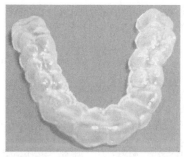

FIGURE 7-1 Bleaching tray. Bleaching trays cover all of the tooth but none of the gingiva to help seal the bleach against the tooth for better bleaching and also to keep the bleach from irritating the soft tissue.

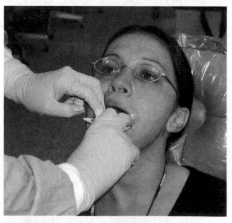

FIGURE 7-2 Impressions. Alginate impressions seem easy but require attention to detail to take well.

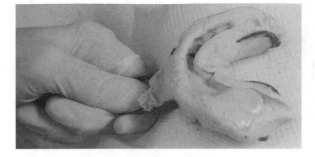

FIGURE 7-3 Pouring a model. Note how the material is started at one end of the impression. This is to avoid voids in the model.

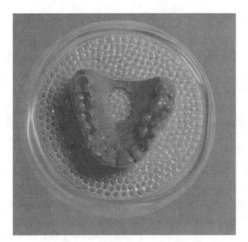

FIGURE 7-4 Pressure forming. The material is well adapted to the model and shows even the ripples in the deck the model rested on.

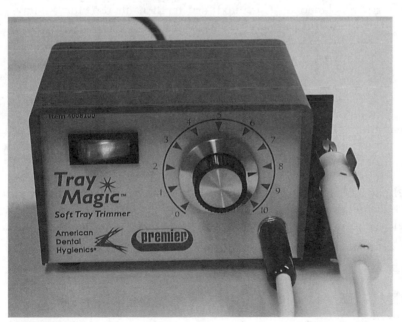

FIGURE 7-5 Electric trimmer. This machine has a small tip that is hot and cuts through the plastic easily without tearing the material.

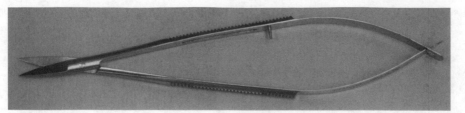

FIGURE 7-6 Trimming scissors. Note how fine the points are and the curvature to trace the gingival margin of the teeth accurately.

- Pregnancy or lactation. No data is available regarding whether bleaching is safe for pregnant women or nursing babies. In the absence of information, avoidance is prudent.
- Allergy to peroxide, carbopol or glycerine
- Concern that patient would aspirate or swallow tray

▼ APPLICATION SCHEDULES ▼

Several application regimens are used to accommodate patients' varying degrees of tooth sensitivity and lifestyles. The teeth are brushed before the tray is inserted. Following insertion, excess gel is removed with a dry brush. Bleach may be applied to the teeth for one or more hours while the patient sleeps, for one or two hours each day or evening, or every so many days for the very sensitive patient. A quick-starting method uses a higher concentration of bleach in-office under professional supervision for the first treatment, then reverts to a more conventional at-home application regimen. The quick-starting method enables the patient to see results from the very first treatment. Conventional regimens may not show results immediately. Most patients see results in a few days, regardless of the method used, and most patients have reached their goal shade in 2–6 weeks.

One over-the-counter method does not require either the use of a tray or brushing of the teeth before the bleaching agent is used. The purchaser buys a box of peroxide gel strips with plastic backing. The backing is peeled away and the gel strip is placed on the teeth for 30 minutes. One strip is placed on the maxillary teeth each day for 14 days, then the process is repeated for the mandibular arch.

Another commercially available method carries the bleaching agent in a gel that is painted on the teeth. This works better than the strips on uneven teeth.

▼ EFFICACY ▼

Overall, tooth bleaching agents are clearly effective and patients like the lighter teeth they create. They are successful most of the time in removing colors present from the time of tooth eruption, or from aging, smoking, diet or poor oral hygiene. Success of varying degrees is reported with bleaching tetracycline stains or the brown areas of fluorosis.

Research indicates bleaches are generally safe and effective at lower peroxide concentrations (10–15%), although some minor side effects have been noted. Dental hypersensitivity and gingival irritation occur in approximately one-third of patients. Temporary white spots on the teeth, clinically insignificant roughening of composite restorations, and color changes in temporary methacrylate restorations have been seen in lesser numbers of cases.

▼ TROUBLESHOOTING ▼

Hypersensitivity may be treated in a number of ways. It may be possible to trim the tray back so that it does not permit the bleach to contact exposed dentin. Exposed areas may be covered with a sealant. The duration or frequency of application may be reduced. A fluoride varnish or potassium nitrate desensitizer may be applied. Fluoride gel may be substituted for bleach in the tray to reduce sensitivity, and bleaching resumed when the teeth have quieted.

Gingival irritation is usually a result of contact with the bleach because the tray was overfilled, does not fit well or extends to the gingival margin. Ensure the tray fits correctly, is correctly filled, and trimmed back to the gingival margin. Bleach reservoirs, if used, should also be ½ to 1 mm short of the gingiva, proximal margins, occlusal surfaces and incisal edges.

Not all teeth respond to bleaching; others seem to respond and then revert to their original shade. Both conditions indicate bleaching failure. Temporary lightening may occur due to tooth dehydration; rehydration causes the color to return. A tooth that has been treated with endodontic procedures also may not whiten. Endodontically treated teeth that do not respond to external techniques may well respond to an internal method.

The cervical third of teeth may appear to be less responsive to the bleach. This is normal and should not be cause for concern. It reflects the normal variation in tooth color throughout its structure.

Esthetic restorations do not whiten. When the new, lighter tooth color stabilizes, and residual peroxide clears from the enamel and dentin, approximately two weeks following bleaching, the patient may choose to replace the restorations.

The contrast between newly lighter teeth and amalgam restorations or cores may cause the amalgam to appear darker following bleaching. Once the new color stabilizes, the patient may elect to have more esthetic restorations placed.

Insufficient data are available to determine whether bleaches of higher concentration (15–40%) are safe over longer periods of time. Some research indicates stronger bleaches may cause irreversible pulp cell changes, and may potentiate the effects of known carcinogens, including alcohol. More research is needed.

KEY POINTS

✓ Tooth whiteners are bleaching agents.
✓ Peroxides, particularly carbamide and hydrogen peroxide, are used.
✓ Peroxides are oxygenating agents.
✓ Oxygenating agents work by breaking down molecules into carbon dioxide and water. Tooth bleaching only partially completes the process, forming intermediate compounds of lighter color then the original pigments.
✓ A custom tray is usually made to hold the bleach on the patient's teeth.
✓ Clinical concerns include
   • Hypersensitivity of exposed dentin.
   • Gingival irritation.
   • Temporary white spots on the teeth.
   • Poor response in the cervical third of the tooth.
   • Temporary response followed by reversion to original color.
   • Lack of whitening by esthetic restorations.
   • Darker appearance of amalgam restorations compared to newly lighter teeth.
   • Differential responses of various types of stains.
   • Time to attainment of desired color.
   • Patient's lifestyle.
   • Need for periodic touch-ups.
✓ The schedule of application varies with patient's lifestyle, the concentration of peroxide selected, and the patient's response to the whitening agent.

Questions 1–5: Select the letter preceding the single best answer.

1. The label of the bleaching product states it has a peroxide concentration of 15%. Is this product for home or professional use?
   a. Home
   b. Professional

2. Your patient's medical history indicates she smokes and drinks red wine. Will this necessitate any changes in her lifestyle if she chooses to undergo home bleaching?
   a. Yes, she will need to stop smoking while bleaching.
   b. Yes, she will need to stop drinking during and after bleaching.
   c. Yes, she will need to stop both smoking and drinking while bleaching.
   d. No, neither of these habits affects the bleaching process.

3. Your patient wants his teeth bleached. He has recession that exposes the root on the facial of the maxillary right central incisor. What potential problem does this create and how can you prevent it?
   a. Gingival irritation; place a plastic strip to dam bleach outflow
   b. Dentin hypersensitivity; trim tray short of cervical margin
   c. White spots on the cementum; continue process as planned
   d. Nonresponse; educate patient about internal bleaching

4. The active ingredient in dental bleach is
   a. Nitrogen.
   b. Hydrogen.
   c. Carbopol.
   d. Oxygen.
   e. Glycerine.

5. Which of the following statements is false?
   a. The cervical third of teeth tends not to whiten as much as other areas.
   b. Fluoride may be applied to decrease dentin sensitivity from bleaching.
   c. Amalgam restorations bleach more rapidly than tooth structure.
   d. Endodontically treated teeth may not respond to bleaching.

Questions 6–10: Describe what should be done in each situation below.

6. The dentist has told the patient she is an excellent candidate for bleaching and that you need to make a custom bleaching tray for her to get the process started. What do you need to do to make the tray?

7. The patient tells you he read in a magazine that the effects of tooth whitening can be seen the very first day the patient starts treatment. What bleaching method is he talking about?

8. The patient is a 12-year-old girl who wants to have her teeth bleached. Her mother has no objection. About what should you talk with them? Why?

9. Your patient has completed the planned bleaching process. He is very happy with the result except that one tooth with an esthetic restoration appears slightly darker. About what should you talk with him? Why?

10. The dentist has asked you to get bleaching material for the patient to take home. There are three products in the bleach storage area, with respective bleach concentrations of 40%, 38% and 15%. Which product should you choose? Why?

ALGINATE

OBJECTIVES

At the conclusion of this chapter, you should be able to:

1. Describe selection, storage and preparation of alginate material.
2. Select and adapt a full-arch tray to fit a patient.
3. Discuss prevention of material preparation voids, patient gagging and impression tearing.
4. Describe proper care of a finished impression.
5. Recognize materials used for wax occlusal registrations.
6. List bite uses.

▼ DEFINITION ▼

Alginate is an elastic impression material.

▼ COMPOSITION ▼

Alginate is an irreversible hydrocolloid. A *hydrocolloid* is a suspension of medium-sized particles in a water-based solution. An irreversible hydrocolloid is one that cannot be softened after setting without damage to the material.

▼ USE ▼

Alginate is used to take impressions that will be used to pour study models, models for patient education, or working casts for making items that do not require highly accurate dimensions.

▼ IMPRESSION PROCEDURE ▼

Alginate powder is mixed with water in a flexible bowl to a soft paste consistency (Figure 8-1), loaded into a tray to carry it to the mouth (Figure 8-2), then placed over the patient's teeth (Figure 8-3) and allowed to set. Once set, it is removed from the mouth; rinsed to remove any adherent saliva, blood or debris (Figure 8-4); disinfected (Figure 8-5); and filled with another soft material that will harden to create a sturdy model of the arch (Figure 8-6). After the model material sets, the impression is separated from the model (Figure 8-7) and thrown away.

▼ WHY ALGINATE IS SELECTED ▼

Alginate is inexpensive, easy to use and fairly accurate at recording the size and shape of mouth structures. Accurate recording enables construction of precise duplicates. Alginate is accurate enough for pouring study models, models for patient education and some types of working casts. It is not accurate enough for pouring casts used to make indirect restorations, which require great precision.

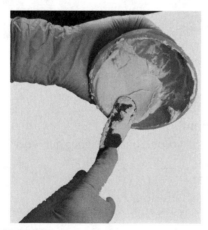

FIGURE 8-1   Mixing alginate. The powder and liquid must be mixed thoroughly by stropping to achieve a creamy consistency without bubbles.

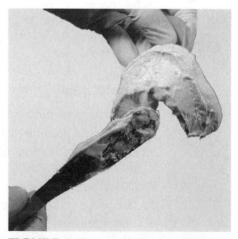

FIGURE 8-2   Loading tray. The material is loaded into the tray in large increments with the spatula. It can be smoothed out prior to inserting in the mouth.

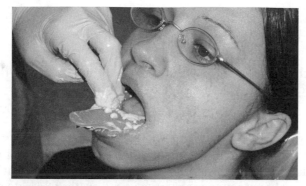

FIGURE 8-3 Impression being taken. Normally the operator would have bilateral pressure on the tray but she moved her right fingers for the sake of seeing the tray better.

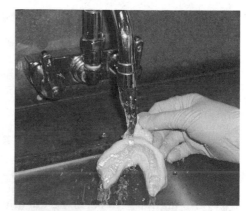

FIGURE 8-4 Rinsing. Rinsing the impression removes any debris and saliva on it.

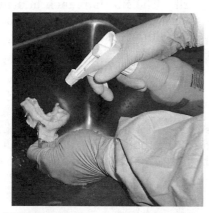

FIGURE 8-5 Disinfection. It is important not to oversoak the material with the disinfectant.

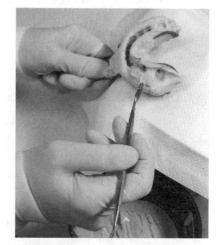

FIGURE 8-6 Pouring the impression. Pouring needs to proceed slowly and carefully to avoid trapped air in the material.

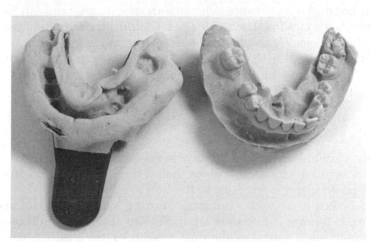

FIGURE 8-7 Model complete. Once the model is separated the impression is discarded. Alginate can only be poured once, so take care to get it right the first time.

▼ MECHANISM OF ACTION ▼

Procedural Level

Alginate hardens around the teeth and associated structures, creating a mold of the structures. This mold can then be filled to construct a duplicate.

Chemical Level

Hydrocolloids have two states: a liquid *sol* and a semisolid *gel*. Think Jello® and you will have the concept. Jello® powder is mixed with water to create a sol. On cooling, it changes from a liquid sol to a semisolid gel. Alginate powder is mixed with water to create a sol. An alginate sol sets by a chemical action rather than cooling, however, so its set is irreversible. Once set, it stays set.

Alginate powder includes particles of potassium alginate, a calcium sulfate reactant, an accelerator, retarder, fillers and other modifiers. When the powder is mixed with water, the potassium alginate dissolves and the calcium sulfate quickly reacts with it to form insoluble particles that clump together and form fibrils. The fibrils branch and intermesh, and water is trapped in the open spaces between them. The accelerator and retarder act to increase and slow the reaction as needed, thereby controlling its speed. The fillers first help distribute the particles in the sol. When it becomes a gel they serve as strengtheners.

▼ CLINICAL CONCERNS ▼

The operator must be concerned about material storage, personal safety, tray selection, proportioning and mixing the material, working and setting time, prevention of voids, patient gagging, impression tearing, and care of the finished impression before it is poured.

Material Storage

Alginate reacts with water and deteriorates when exposed to heat and with aging. The powder is packaged in bulk in tightly sealed plastic containers or in foil pouches to prevent moisture contamination during shipping and storage. Bulk containers should be tightly closed immediately following powder measurement to maintain powder dryness. Some foil pouches contain premeasured amounts of material and are disposable. They provide greater moisture protection and convenience but are more expensive.

Alginate should be stored in a cool area to prevent heat deterioration. A good inventory system should also be in place to ensure adequate alginate is on hand but that it will not be stored longer than 6–12 months. Each container should be completely used before another is opened and the unopened containers should be rotated using a first in, first out system. New containers are placed in the back of the storage area and a container taken from the front for use. This ensures the oldest material is used first and protects material from lingering on the shelves beyond its expiration date.

Operator Safety

A mask and safety glasses should always be worn when working with alginate. The filler material is diatomaceous earth, a natural substance that is the fossilized remains of small animals. It is a very fine powder and is irritating to the lungs and eyes.

Alginate is *fluffed* before it is used. Fluffing is turning a powder container upside down, then right side up, 2–3 times before opening it. Fluffed alginate should be left to sit 2–3 seconds after fluffing to ensure most of the dust created by the fluffing has resettled. Bulk powders are always fluffed before measuring to ensure the particles are separated. Failure to fluff results in too much powder for a good mix, but failure to let fluffed alginate material sit for a few seconds before opening the container results in aerial release of a small cloud of irritating dust. Some alginates are formulated to reduce the dust. These are known as dustless alginates. The manufacturers add a coating of an organic glycol to keep the dust particles together. Manufacturers also have recently been adding antimicrobials to the formula to reduce the chance of infection. The only disadvantage is that these additives tend to make the mixture a little less smooth so they need more careful mixing to become smooth.

Tray Selection

A suitable full arch tray must be chosen before the impression can be taken (Figure 8-8). Maxillary trays extend across both sides of the arch and include the palate. Mandibular trays have an open area for the tongue. Alginate is not adhesive; therefore, trays for alginate impressions have a mechanical lock to hold the material in the tray. Trays are termed *perforated* or *rim lock* depending on the means of retention. The perforations permit some of the alginate to push through the holes when the tray is placed over the teeth. This alginate is locked in position when it is set so the impression does not pull out of the tray when it is removed from the mouth. The rim serves the same purpose as the holes; it helps to keep the material from oozing out, thus locking it in place. Occasionally, these measures alone are not adequate and the tray must be sprayed with an adhesive before the mixed alginate is loaded into it.

Working and Setting Time

Enough time must be available for the mixed material to be inserted in the mouth before it sets. On the other hand, once the tray is inserted, set should not take so long the patient is unable to tolerate the wait.

Working and setting times are partially controlled by the manufacturer. Three basic types of alginate are available, all based on time required for set: *regular set, fast set* and *color indicator.* Exact setting times vary by manufacturer, but it is usual to designate a slow-setting alginate as regular set and a rapid-setting one as fast set. Color indicator materials are one color during mixing, change color when the material is thoroughly mixed and ready to be loaded into the tray and placed in the mouth, and may change color again when the material is set and the impression can be safely removed from the mouth.

The operator may change the standard setting times of any alginate by varying the temperature of the water used for mixing. Alginate is normally mixed with water at room temperature. If the operator judges the patient may be unable to tolerate the wait, warmer water may be used to hasten set. If more time is desired, cooler water slows the process.

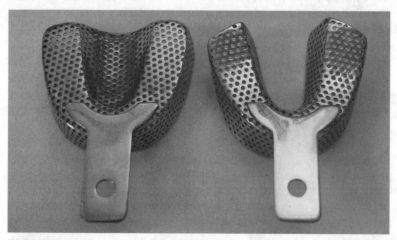

FIGURE 8-8   Impression trays. These trays have numerous, small perforations for the alginate to squeeze through, locking the impression to the tray.

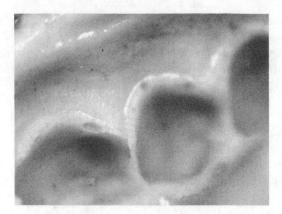

FIGURE 8-9 Voids. You can see numerous voids in the alginate. This both weakens the alginate and spoils the detail necessary for a good model.

Prevention of Voids

Voids are areas of air in the mix. Internal voids weaken the material; surface voids do not record anatomy (Figure 8-9). If important or extensive areas are not recorded, any model or working cast made from the impression will be useless.

Mixing the material correctly will help prevent formation of voids. A flexible bowl and spatula are used (Figure 8-10). Powder is added to water, not vice versa. The particles are first wetted and then stropped against the side of the bowl. The material is periodically gathered against the side of the bowl and mixing resumed. The spatula tip is kept submerged throughout the wetting and stropping process. All of these actions help to prevent incorporation of air in the mix.

Prevention of Patient Gagging

The thick, pasty consistency of mixed alginate can cause some patients to gag. Although gagging has a physical component, it is at least as much psychologically as physically induced. Therefore, how you approach patients has a bearing on whether they gag or not. In most offices the operator whose patient throws up is the one who must clean up the mess, so you want to be sure you become a master at prevention of gagging!

To prevent gagging, avoid anxiety-producing actions or words, be gentle and practice patient distraction. Very occasionally you may need to use a topical local anesthetic, a lozenge, or, in extreme cases, nitrous oxide to prevent the gag reflex.

Educate the patient regarding the upcoming procedure. A simple statement in easily understood language is best. Avoid anxiety-producing words. For example, you might say, "The dentist has asked me to make a duplicate of your teeth. I am going to take an impression of them now so we will have a mold for the duplicate." This tells the patient what will be done and why and does not raise any anxiety-producing thoughts.

You would not say, "I am going to take this bowl full of material and put it in your mouth until it hardens." "Bowl full" indicates that there would be lots of material and

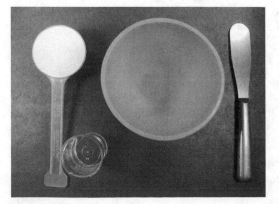

FIGURE 8-10 Alginate armentarium. These items and some practice are all you need to make great alginate impressions.

"hardens" makes the patient think that you will be removing something that is rock solid from around their teeth. This will increase their tendency to gag.

Be gentle as you work. Talk about pleasant subjects. A patient who is treated roughly or hurt will immediately become anxious. Anxiety causes the jaw muscles to tighten, making the impression tray difficult to seat. Pleasant conversation distracts the patient, making your job easier and more enjoyable.

Tipping the patient's head back slightly for a lower impression and forward for an upper impression helps loosen the muscles, thereby permitting easier tray insertion. When inserting a tray, never slide it over the teeth. Position the tray over the arch in question and then press it into place vertically, keeping slight, even pressure on the whole tray.

Some patients will gag despite your best intentions. There are some things that can alleviate the problem. Having the patients lift a leg off the chair helps distract them. Remind them to breathe deeply through their nose and tell them not to swallow their saliva but rather to let it drip onto the bib or a paper towel provided for that purpose.

If all else fails, sometimes a topical anesthetic spray or lozenge will help. Nitrous oxide, a type of inhaled sedative also known as laughing gas, helps relax the patient and can be administered to allow an impression to be taken on even the most sensitive patient.

Prevention of Tearing

Alginate has poor tensile strength, so is easily torn. A torn impression cannot be used. Adequate bulk of material helps to decrease the tendency to tear; place an even thickness of alginate in all areas of an appropriately sized tray and center the tray over the arch to obtain adequate bulk throughout. Never slide a tray into place in the mouth.

Alginate tensile strength can also be improved by leaving the impression in the mouth 1–2 minutes after it sets. Additionally, it helps not to place too much tensile stress on the impression as it is being removed. Hook your finger tip over the top of a set impression and gently pull straight downward to break the seal between the impression and the tissues before attempting to remove the impression. Remove it with one motion; do not rock. Think about a piece of paper. If you want to rip it evenly, you first fold it one direction, then the other. You repeat this several times, then tear. Repeated stress and relaxation at the same place on the paper weaken it, making it easy to tear where it was folded. Jerky, stop-and-start removal of an alginate impression weakens the impression and leaves it vulnerable to tearing just as the repeated back-and-forth folding of the paper weakens and prepares it for tearing.

Care of the Finished Impression

Alginate also has poor compressive strength. The set impression should never be placed impression side down on a flat surface; this may flatten it. Always place it tray side down.

The finished impression is contaminated with saliva and may contain blood and debris. They should all be removed by rinsing it in gently running water. Blood and saliva retard the set of gypsum materials and most alginate impressions are poured with some type of gypsum. Debris also takes up space. It will be recorded in, and lessen the accuracy of, any model poured over it.

Additionally, saliva and blood contain microorganisms. The impression must be disinfected. This is done by spraying it with a disinfectant solution, then placing it in a sealed plastic bag for the time recommended by the disinfectant manufacturer.

Alginate should not be immersed in a disinfecting solution. It is a water-based material and can gain or lose moisture from its environment. If immersed it will absorb water and swell. If left out in the atmosphere it will lose water and shrink. That is why it is placed in a sealed bag. Alginate cannot be autoclaved because high heat converts the water it contains to steam. The steam is then lost to the environment and the impression shrinks.

Gain of fluid from the environment is termed *imbibition;* losing fluid to the environment is *syneresis.* If an alginate impression cannot be poured immediately, appropriate humidity must be maintained to prevent imbibition or syneresis. The impression can be

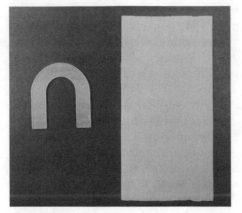

FIGURE 8-11 Wax bites. The flat sheet must be warmed and then bent into the shape of the arch. The other wax is already in the proper shape.

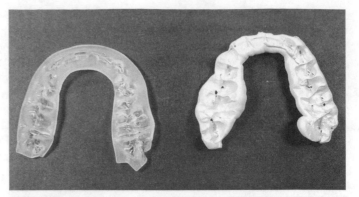

FIGURE 8-12 Bite registrations. Both bites were taken on the same person. The left one was taken using wax; the right one was taken in an elastic impression material. Which will distort more easily?

wrapped in a wet paper towel for a short time to maintain appropriate humidity. The towel should not be too wet or imbibition will occur. It should be wet throughout; dry areas will absorb water from the impression and cause syneresis.

Taking a Bite

Many practitioners also record occlusal relationships between the maxillary and mandibular teeth in wax when they take alginate impressions. Historically, baseplate or bite wax (Figure 8-11) was used for this process but they are being supplanted by vinyl polysiloxane materials (see Chapter 14). Waxes are thermoplastic materials with a broad melting range that can be softened in hot water or over a low flame to just above body temperature and then placed in the mouth. The patient bites on the material and it is allowed to cool and harden. This is termed taking a bite, or fabricating an occlusal registration. The completed bite (Figure 8-12) is used to determine correct positioning of opposing models poured from the impression for trimming or articulation. *Trimming* is cutting models to enhance appearance. *Articulation* is mounting them on an articulator (Figure 8-13), an artificial jaw joint, to stabilize the teeth in proper relationship to their antagonists.

Pouring Alginate Impressions

Alginate may be poured with dental plaster or stone. They are both members of the gypsum family of materials, which will be discussed in the next chapter. Plaster, which is not as strong, less expensive, usually white, and looks quite elegant, is used to pour study models, models for educating patients, or working casts that will undergo minimal processing. Stone, which is usually buff colored, has higher compressive strength and better abrasion resistance, is also used to pour study models and models for educating patients. In addition, it is strong enough to be used for all types of working casts except dies.

KEY POINTS

- ✓ Alginate is an elastic impression material.
- ✓ Impressions made with alginate are used to pour
  - models for study.
  - models for patient education.
  - working casts that do not have to be highly accurate or undergo stressful processing.

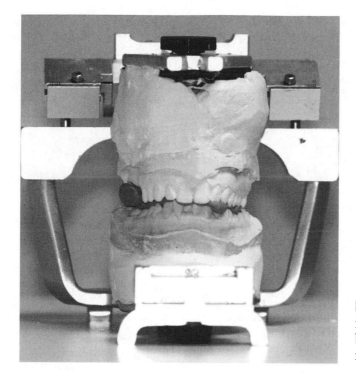

FIGURE 8-13 Mounting models. You can see the bite between the upper and lower models to guide the mounting.

✓ Store alginate in a cool, dry area for no longer than 12 months.
✓ Protect yourself when using alginate by wearing a mask, letting fluffed alginate sit for 2–3 seconds before opening, and replacing the container cover immediately after proportioning powder.
✓ Alginate
  • Reacts irreversibly with water to form a gel.
  • Can fail to record anatomy or be weakened by incorporation of air in mix.
  • Has a thick, pasty consistency that may cause gagging.
  • Has poor compressive and tensile strength.
  • Can react with the environment to gain or lose water.
✓ To use alginate properly
  • Proportion and mix material carefully.
  • Center filled tray over arch before compressing over teeth.
  • Work gently and distract patient during impression procedure.
  • Leave in mouth one minute beyond set.
  • Break suction before attempting impression removal from mouth.
  • Remove set impression with a single continuous pull.
  • Clean and disinfect impression before pouring.
  • Maintain proper humidity until impression is poured.
  • Place impression on flat surface tray side down.

SELF TEST

Questions 1–5: Discuss solutions to each problem described below.

1. The dentist has asked you to take maxillary and mandibular alginate impressions for a patient who is new to you. She greets you with, "I hate impressions. I always gag when they try to take them on me." How can you prevent a possible gagging disaster?

2. How will you select trays for this patient?

3. You are pretty good at what you do. You were able to insert and keep the filled tray in position without incident and the material is now set. How will you remove it from the mouth without ruining it?

4. How will you prepare the completed impression for pouring?

5. How did you protect your own health during the impression-taking procedure?

Questions 6–10: Select the letter preceding the single best response.

6. Regular set alginate sets
   a. rapidly.
   b. slowly.
   c. following a color change.

7. Alginate should be placed in _____ storage for no more than _____.
   a. cool, dry; 12 months
   b. cool, wet; 6 months
   c. warm, dry; 12 months
   d. warm, wet; 6 months

8. Placing a completed alginate impression tray side up on a flat surface may flatten the impression because alginate has poor
   a. tensile strength.
   b. water retention.
   c. void reduction.
   d. compressive strength.
   e. all of the above

9. Select the equipment you will need to proportion and mix alginate.
   a. powder scoop
   b. water measure
   c. flexible bowl
   d. flared spatula
   e. c and d only
   f. all of the above

10. What types of models are poured from alginate impressions?
    a. dies
    b. study models
    c. working casts for indirect restorations
    d. working casts for direct restorations

MODEL AND DIE MATERIALS

This chapter discusses the following topics:

1. Definitions
2. Materials used
3. Composition
4. Use
5. Construction procedure
6. Action
   a. Procedure level
   b. Chemical level
7. Gypsum
   a. Types
   b. Uses
   c. Clinical concerns
      i. Responsibilities of dental team members
      ii. Material storage
      iii. Identification of selected material
      iv. Factors determining ease of pouring
      v. Prevention of voids
      vi. Mixing
      vii. Pouring
      viii. Accuracy of the finished product
      ix. Strength and abrasion resistance
      x. Prevention of fracture

OBJECTIVES

At the conclusion of this chapter, you should be able to:

1. List and differentiate the materials used to construct models, working casts and dies.
2. Describe conversion of mined gypsum to dental plaster, stone and die stone.
3. Describe electroplating of impressions and explain why this is not routinely done in the dental office or clinic.
4. Differentiate the uses and properties of plaster, stone and die stone.
5. List the tasks allied dental personnel perform in model and die fabrication.
6. Describe appropriate conditions for storage of gypsum materials.

7. Indicate how each material can be quickly identified.
8. Discuss factors that affect
   a. Material mixing, pouring and set.
   b. Development and prevention of voids.
   c. Model accuracy, strength, abrasion resistance and fracture.

▼ DEFINITIONS ▼

A model is a replica (duplicate) of oral structures. A die is a replica of one tooth.

▼ MATERIALS USED ▼

Gypsum materials—plaster, stone, and die stone
Metal and metal alloys—plated metal mixtures
Epoxy—a polymer

▼ COMPOSITION ▼

Gypsum—natural mineral
Metal—silver or copper plating
Epoxy—polymer

▼ USES ▼

Gypsum is used to fabricate models, working casts, and dies. It is also used to mount working casts and dies on an articulator. Metal and metal alloys are used to fabricate dies for selected types of final impressions. Epoxy is used to fabricate dies.

▼ CONSTRUCTION PROCEDURE ▼

Gypsum powder is mixed with water (Figure 9-1), poured into an impression (Figure 9-2) and left to harden. In the past dies were sometimes made from other materials besides gypsum. *Epoxy* dies are made by mixing the epoxy material and forcing it into the impression, as it is very viscous. *Metal* can also be electroplated onto an impression. Today epoxy dies are rarely used because they shrink when setting and thus are not as accurate as dentists would like. Likewise, although metal dies are accurate, the types of impression materials used to make them are not as accurate as some of the other materials available today. Also, they require a great deal of time to construct and use some hazardous chemicals, so the vast majority of dies are constructed of gypsum. After a model or die is constructed, the impression used to make it is thrown away.

▼ ACTION ▼

Procedure Level

Models and dies are duplications of the oral tissues recorded by an impression.

Chemical Level

Gypsum powders are processed calcium sulfate rock. It is mined from the earth in dihydrate (di = two, hydrate = water) form, which contains two water molecules for each calcium sulfate molecule. The mined rock is ground and heated. The heat drives off much of

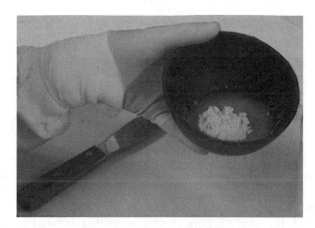

FIGURE 9-1 Mixing stone. Notice that the powder is mixed into the water, never the reverse.

the water as steam, reversing the original proportions. The powder that remains after heating is a *hemihydrate* (hemi = ½, hydrate = water); it has one molecule of water for each two molecules of calcium sulfate. When the powder is mixed with water to pour an impression, the water reacts with the hemihydrate, causing it to revert to a dihydrate. The heat that entered the material when it was heated is liberated as the reaction proceeds.

Gypsum set is a crystal-building exercise, and adding powder accelerates crystal building. The result is a vastly accelerated set in some areas. Setting starts with small areas of reacted (hard) material that serve as scattered hardening centers. The hard centers grow in length and width until they meet each other and water is left in a few spaces between them. Particles and water continue to react to form scattered hard areas. These areas then grow in length and width until they take over almost completely. The few areas of background material that remain contain the excess water that was needed to obtain adequate flow for mixing and pouring, but was not needed for the setting reaction.

Gypsum products for dental use also contain modifiers to control the setting reaction and may contain colored pigments to enable quick identification and selection of material.

Metal alloys are electroplated onto final impressions. The impression is coated with a conducting layer and hooked to one side of an electrical circuit. A rod of metal is immersed in the opposite end and hooked to the opposite pole of the circuit. A conducting liquid is between the two poles. When the electricity is turned on, ions from the metal travel through the solution to the impression and coat it.

When a metal alloy die is desired, the impression is sent to a laboratory because the electroplating process is time consuming and the acid used in the bath can be quite hazardous if used incorrectly. Personnel must be specially trained to do electroplating. Epoxy dies likewise need special equipment to fabricate and are not generally done in the dental

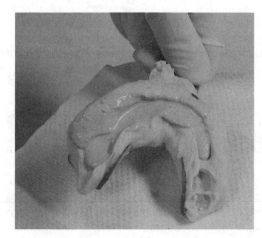

FIGURE 9-2 Pouring a model. The gypsum is always added behind the moving edge so that no air voids are trapped in the model.

office. Since assistants and hygienists do not normally fabricate metal alloy or epoxy dies, the remaining discussion in this chapter will be devoted solely to gypsum materials.

▼ GYPSUM ▼

Types

Three types of gypsum are commonly used in the dental office or clinic: *plaster, stone* and *die stone.* They are created through use of different temperature and pressure combinations when the ground gypsum rock is heated. Temperatures between 110° and 130°C in the absence of pressure form plaster, which has irregularly shaped powder particles and is relatively weak and susceptible to abrasion. A temperature in the 110–130°C range plus pressure forms dental stone, which has more regular particles and is stronger, less porous and less susceptible to abrasion. Temperatures greater than 130°C plus pressure form die stone, which has the most regular particles, and is the strongest, least porous, most abrasion-resistant gypsum. Die stone is also termed *improved stone.*

In addition, the manufacturers add chemicals to achieve certain goals. They can change the setting time of the material by adding retarders or accelerators. Accelerators quicken the set by making the set product less soluble in water and thus the crystals form faster. Another way to accelerate the set is for the operator to add crystals by using water with ground stone in it. This slurry water, as it is known, is obtained from the drain of the model trimmer and provides some already set crystals to act as nuclei for the material setting. Adding slurry water can speed setting considerably.

Retarders will slow down the set. These are usually added inadvertently, as protein-containing solutions are usually the best retarders. Blood and saliva are both protein solutions and as such must be rinsed gently out of the impression prior to pouring. Even some impression materials slow the setting, especially the reversible hydrocolloids.

There are hardening solutions used to increase the hardness of the die stones. These are controlled by the operator and can change the dimensions of the material.

Uses

The type of gypsum selected for a pouring task depends on the use to which the model made from it will be put. Plaster is customarily used to pour study models, models for patient education, working casts on which few processing demands will be made, and articulating models. *Articulation* (Figure 9-3) is fitting models together in correct occlusal relationship on an artificial jaw.

Stone is used for all of the same pouring tasks as plaster, and, because of its greater strength and resistance to abrasion, all manner of working casts except dies. Dies, which undergo the greatest processing stresses, are poured with die stone.

Clinical Concerns

Clinical concerns include the responsibilities of team members; storage and handling of the materials; identification of the type of material selected for use; ease of pouring; void prevention; model accuracy, strength and abrasion resistance; and prevention of fracture.

Responsibilities of Dental Team Members

Assistants and hygienists pour all of the gypsum models in many offices and clinics. Other practices have a commercial dental laboratory pour some or all of them. Those impressions that are sent to the lab must be disinfected and accompanied by a *laboratory prescription* (Figure 9-4), an order from the dentist describing what sort of restoration the laboratory should make and the instructions for what materials to use in the restoration, the colors necessary to match the patient's teeth and any special instructions.

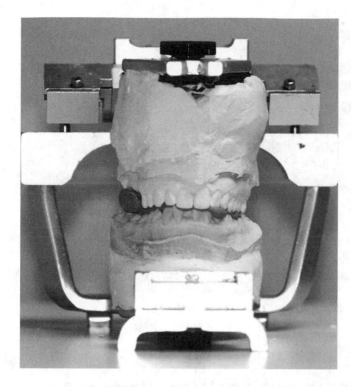

FIGURE 9-3 Articulator mounting. Notice the bite material between the models. This will be removed after the plaster sets.

Material Storage

Gypsum powders react with water to form a hard stone. To protect them from water contamination before use, they are normally packaged in bulk in sealed plastic bags. The bulk powders are heavy, so the plastic may be packaged in paper bags or cardboard boxes to make handling easier. Once a package is opened, the material should be stored in a moisture-proof container. Many practices store gypsum powders in a plaster bin, a compartmentalized metal container that hangs on the wall (Figure 9-5).

Bob's Wonder Lab, Inc
7 Makeatooth Way
Providence, RI
401-111-2032

Doctor Name _Moe Lahr_
Office Address _12 Split Tooth Road, Prov, RI_
Due Date _02/02/02_

Rx

Please make a lower partial denture framework replacing teeth 20,21,24-26, 30 & 31. Rest seats on teeth 19,22,28 & 29. Class I clasps to placed on teeth 19,28 &29. Class II clasp on #22. Please follow survey marks on teeth. Send framework back with bite rims. Thank you.

Signature _Moe Lahr DDS_

FIGURE 9-4 Laboratory prescription. It is important to make very clear to the lab what you expect them to do, as they never see the patient.

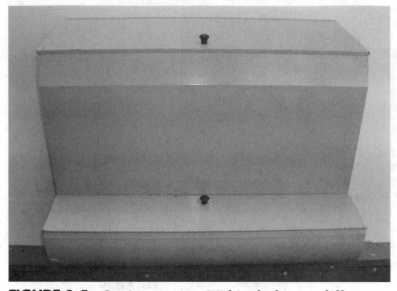

FIGURE 9-5 Storing gypsum. Within the bin are different compartments so that the plaster and stone can be kept separate from one another.

Plaster and stone do not deteriorate as readily from heat and age as alginate; most of them may be kept in moisture-proof storage safely for years without appreciable loss of quality. The one exception is die stone. Stored gypsums deteriorate at a rate of 1–2% a year. Since dies are used in the fabrication of indirect restorations, which must fit precisely, even a 1% discrepancy is too great. Die stone is packaged and purchased in small amounts.

Identification of Selected Material

Color coding is used to differentiate gypsums. Although all forms of gypsum are white powders, plaster is usually left white and color added to stones. Different manufacturers use different colors but it is common for stone to be buff-colored and die stone to be pink, green, blue or yellow. Color coding enables quick identification of the material desired and prevents inadvertent selection of the wrong one.

Factors Determining Ease of Pouring

How easily a model can be poured depends on how well the material flows. Material consistency must be "just right." If it is too thick, flow is impeded; if too thin, the operator cannot control it. Correct consistency is obtained by using the correct water–powder ratio.

How much water a material needs for setting depends on the size and regularity of its particles. When the particles are large and irregular, they have less surface area to react with water. This means they will need more water to wet the surfaces properly as the reactions proceed. Of the three types of gypsum, plaster particles are the largest and most irregular, so they require the most water for setting. Die stone particles are the smallest and most regular, so die stone requires the least water. Stone particle size and shape fall between those of plaster and die stone, so stone requires a "between" amount of water (Figure 9-6).

Regardless of the type of gypsum used, more water is needed for creating a suitable consistency for mixing and pouring than is needed for setting. The amount of water a material needs for easy pouring, then, is the amount required for setting plus the *excess water* required to reach correct consistency for mixing and pouring. Since the amounts required for setting each material differ, the overall amounts required for mixing to correct consistency differ as well. Overall water amounts per 100 grams of powder are 50 milliliters (ml) for plaster, 30 ml for stone, and 18–27 ml for die stone. The exact amount of water required

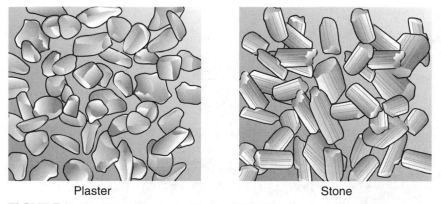

Plaster   Stone

FIGURE 9-6   Particle sizes. Notice how the stone crystals are much better formed.

for die stone differs by manufacturer and will be noted on the package. All water amounts may need to be adjusted to reflect environmental humidity.

Water for model pouring should be measured in a glass graduate (Figure 9-7). Powder should be weighed on a gram scale (Figure 9-8). As a practical matter, weighing takes too much time in daily dental practice. One solution is to purchase premeasured powder packets; another is to weigh a number of proportions during office downtime and package them in sealed plastic bags for later use.

Many dental personnel do not measure either water or powder. They put some water in a bowl and dump what they judge to be the right amount of powder into it. While this may in the right hands result in accurate models, it is totally unacceptable for models that must be accurate consistently. Die stone especially must always be measured carefully. The water–powder ratio affects how much the gypsum expands when set. Too much water leads to larger and weaker models.

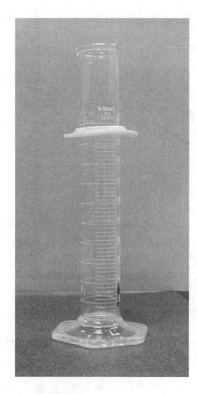

FIGURE 9-7   Measuring water. Water in a graduate cylinder is measured to the bottom of the miniscus, which is the concave shape water takes in a glass.

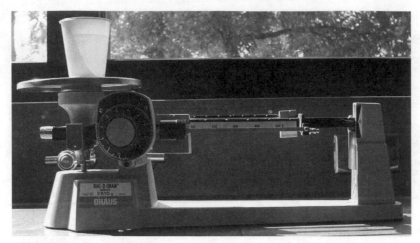

FIGURE 9-8 Weighing powder. Make sure you take the weight of the container into account.

In the "mix-by-the-seat-of-the-pants" office, to obtain the proper flow, more water must be added if the mix is too thick and more powder if it is too thin. When water is added, air accompanies it, creating unwanted voids. When powder is added to partially set gypsum, the new particles increase the number of scattered hard areas in the material. Then they grow. This means greater numbers of growing hard areas quickly cause material thickening. Thickening happens so rapidly that it can be difficult if not impossible to maintain material flow long enough to finish pouring before it sets.

Accelerating material set can be used to good advantage when pouring a model base, however. Once the impression has been filled, extra powder can be added to the remaining material. All of it can then be placed on the slab or in the base former at once, where it will rapidly reach sufficient hardness to support the poured impression without slumping.

Prevention of Voids

Voids are areas of air in the mix. Internal voids (Figure 9-9) weaken the material; surface voids do not record impression anatomy in their areas. If voids are extensive or located in important places, the model will be unusable. Voids are prevented by using correct mixing and pouring technique.

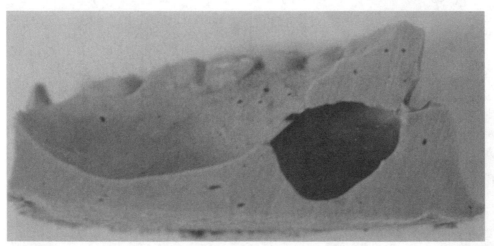

FIGURE 9-9 Voids. Note the large void just under the palate in this model that has been cut in half. There are also numerous small voids.

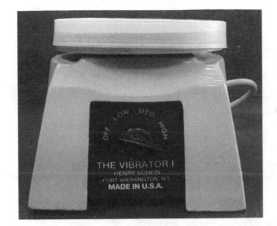

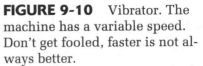

FIGURE 9-10 Vibrator. The machine has a variable speed. Don't get fooled, faster is not always better.

Mixing

A stiff, straight-sided spatula, flexible bowl, and powder and water measures are used. Both water and powder are carefully proportioned and the water is placed in the bowl. The powder is slowly sifted into it. Powder is always added to water, not vice versa. When the opposite occurs, air accompanies the water as it enters the mix. Powder is allowed to settle for a few seconds before mixing begins. This allows air trapped between the particles to escape through the water. The particles are first wetted and then mixed by stirring or stropping. Regardless of motion, the spatula tip is kept submerged throughout. When it is lifted out, air accompanies its reinsertion.

There are also special mixers for gypsum materials that combine an electric motor to drive a blade to mix the material with a vacuum pump to remove all the air from the mixture, thus making a very dense material that will not have voids.

Pouring

Regardless of how carefully mixing is done, some air remains trapped. To remove it, the mixed material is placed on a *vibrator* (Figure 9-10) for up to a minute. A vibrator is a small motor with a flat platform above it. Activating the motor vibrates the platform. The operator holds and periodically taps the bowl on the platform. This brings trapped air bubbles to the surface (Figure 9-11) where they can be popped with the spatula tip. There are

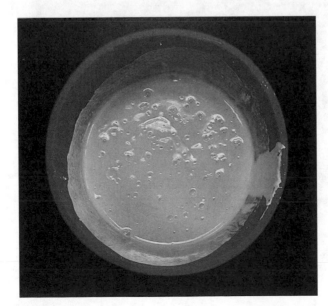

FIGURE 9-11 Vibrating stone. Note the size of some of these bubbles. They are fun to pop.

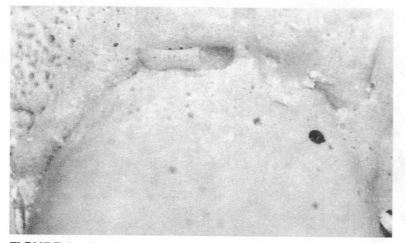

FIGURE 9-12 Overvibration. This is a closeup of a small part of a model where the stone was overvibrated. Notice the great number of small bubbles on the surface of the stone.

also machines that spatulate the material under vacuum to remove all of the bubbles in the material.

Vibration is important for removing air from the mix but it must not continue too long. Overvibration causes the formation of vast numbers of minute air bubbles in the mix. There are so many they cannot possibly all be removed, so they must be poured into the impression. They are so small they rarely affect the detail on the model, but are unsightly. You can tell when voids in a model were caused by overvibration because there will be many, they will be very small, and they will be found throughout the model (Figure 9-12).

Voids may also be caused by hasty pouring. An "empty" impression is actually filled with air. When a model is poured, the incoming gypsum material must push the air out of the way in order to flow into the space the air was occupying. When pouring is too rapid, the incoming material flows over the air rather than pushing it out of the way. The result is a void on the surface of the model (Figure 9-13). Surface voids can be of any size and may

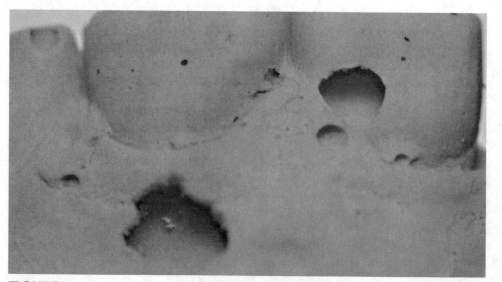

FIGURE 9-13 Surface voids. Here is a closeup of a model with huge voids due to poor pouring technique. Not only does it look bad but it will be unusable.

be quite large. They are always unsightly and if large, extensive or located in critical areas, make the model unusable.

Pouring speed, then, is an art. You must not pour too fast or voids will result; you cannot pour too slowly or the material will thicken and set before you are finished. Pouring experience is the best guide to appropriate speed. Pay attention to your instructor's pouring speed during demonstrations and your own as you practice pouring in the laboratory.

Accuracy of the Finished Product

An accurate model cannot be obtained without a good impression. Select the correct impression material for the job that needs to be done and then care for the completed impression properly before it is poured.

An accurate model cannot be obtained if a good impression is poured poorly. Select the correct type of gypsum material for the job, proportion it as recommended by the manufacturer, mix it correctly and pour it carefully.

An accurate model cannot be obtained if the material poured into it does not reproduce the dimensions of the oral tissues precisely. Gypsum materials expand as they set. Setting expansion slightly enlarges the anatomical details recorded on the model. Any item made on the model will fit the enlarged dimensions. It will not necessarily fit the teeth used to make the impression from which the model was made. Slight working cast enlargement may or may not matter, depending on the use to which the cast will be put. Indirect restorations and implants must fit precisely. Die stone reproduces impression detail most accurately and should be chosen for pouring critical dies.

Strength and Abrasion Resistance

Strong models and dies are needed if stressful processing will occur. Model strength and abrasion resistance are determined by the density of the model material, the water–powder ratio of the mix, and the amount of excess water remaining in the set model.

Denser materials are stronger. Their particles are more regular and fit together more closely, leaving few areas for water. Think fresh and dried fruit. The dried fruit has lost water and is denser and stronger. Die stone is the strongest and most dense gypsum material; plaster the least. As before, stone is "between."

More powder in a mix makes it stronger but also thickens it and lessens flow. Excess water in the set model evaporates as the model reaches complete set, about 24 hours after being poured. Dental personnel talk about the wet and dry strengths of models. *Wet strength* refers to the point when the model reaches initial set, is no longer warm to the touch, and can be safely separated from the impression. At this time much of the excess water has not yet evaporated. Such water weakens the gypsum and so the model does not reach maximum strength until this water evaporates. Evaporation of excess water continues for about 24 hours following pouring. As water evaporates, the model shrinks and increases in density. When evaporation is complete, the model has reached *dry strength*. Dry strength is substantially greater than wet strength. For some materials dry strength may be nearly double that of wet strength.

Prevention of Fracture

All gypsum model and die materials are relatively strong, but can be broken. Fracture may occur from premature separation of the model and impression. To avoid fracture on separation, the material must have reached its initial set and enough excess water must have evaporated for the model to withstand the stresses placed on it when the impression is removed. The setting process is *exothermic.* The heat added to produce the powder during the manufacturing process is released during setting. A surface that is cool to the touch indicates the material has reached initial set and it is safe to attempt separation. Much of the excess water has not yet evaporated, however, and the model remains relatively weak. Lift the impression off the model; do not rock it. Rocking places alternating compressive and tensile stress on the model (remember folding paper in one direction, then the other to tear it?) and the result may well be fracture.

Models also need to be handled carefully. If they drop on the floor, they usually fracture. Store them carefully. Models knocking around in the lab will be pushed from here to there and chipped in the process, but they're too big to fit in the patient's record. Containers of different types or sizes quickly become a jungle. Special model storage boxes are available from dental supply companies to solve the problem. They have enough room to fit maxillary and mandibular full arch models in the same box, are all the same size to facilitate neat stacking, and have a place where the patient's name and the impression date can be written or clipped to permit quick patient and date identification.

KEY POINTS

✓ Most models and dies are poured with some type of gypsum.
✓ Choose plaster for low-strength models, stone for high-strength models, and die stone for dies.
✓ Plaster is usually white, stone is buff, and die stone is a pastel such as blue, pink, green or yellow.
✓ Proportion powder and water accurately.
✓ To prevent voids:
  • Add powder to water
  • Allow powder to settle before mixing
  • Mix without lifting spatula tip out of material
  • Vibrate before pouring
✓ Pour using moderate speed.
✓ Ensure model surface is cool before attempting to separate it from impression.
✓ Wait 24 hours before using finished model.
✓ Handle models carefully.

SELF TEST

Questions 1–2 might well be labeled Food for Thought. What do you think about the situation each describes?

1. Should models be routinely disinfected or sterilized? Why or why not? How would gypsum materials likely react to autoclaving, immersion in a disinfectant or being sprayed with a disinfectant and sealed in a plastic bag?

2. Because models may fracture when dropped, does this mean their compressive or tensile strength is a concern?

Questions 3–8: Select an appropriate word or phrase for the one that is missing.

3. _____ should be selected for pouring a model that will be subjected to high heat.

4. The green powder in a plaster bin is probably _____.

5. Gypsum materials are vibrated before pouring to _____.

6. Gypsum materials _____ when they set. This can result in incorrect fit of an item made on the model.

7. Gypsum materials set by _____.

8. Gypsum materials reach final set about _____ after they are poured.

Questions 9–10. Select the letter preceding the single best answer.

9. Internal voids _____ a model.
    a. weaken
    b. fail to record anatomy on

10. Select the spatula that would be used to mix stone.
    a. A
    b. B
    c. C
    d. D

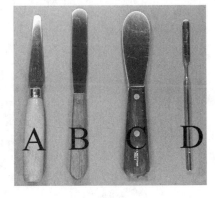

SECTION

III

Materials for Direct Restorations

Teeth lead a hazardous existence. They can be attacked by decay that can destroy parts of the tooth over time. They can be abraded and broken by food, foreign objects and even adjacent or opposing teeth. They can be malformed by fevers, medicines or diseases that affect them before they even erupt into the mouth. Teeth that do not have the correct anatomic formation can be painful, can cause damage to other teeth or the supporting tissue of the teeth, and are often unsightly.

Dentists are called upon to repair tooth damage no matter what the cause. The restorations for these patients ideally need to be strong, easy to place, able to be shaped properly, esthetic, not prone to decay, biocompatible, and preferably inexpensive. The restorations in the next chapters fulfill some of these expectations but not others.

The materials in this section are used in restorations made directly in the patient's mouth. The patient is generally anesthetized, the tooth prepared for a restoration by removing any decay, and shaping the form of the tooth to best accept the material to be used. Any special treatment for the tooth to receive the restoration is accomplished. The material is placed, and after adjustment so that it is the proper shape and size, the patient has, in a relatively short period of time, a functional tooth again.

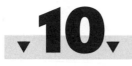

INTERMEDIARY MATERIALS

OBJECTIVES

After studying this chapter, you should be able to:

1. Differentiate a base, varnish and liner.
2. Discuss how the actions of each contribute to pulp protection.
3. Describe controversial aspects of base and varnish placement.
4. List and describe specific materials used as bases, varnishes, liners and bonding agents.
5. Describe dentin bonding.

▼ DEFINITION ▼

Intermediary materials are those placed between the tooth and the main restorative material.

▼ MATERIALS USED ▼

Bases, varnishes and liners are examples of intermediary materials.

▼ TYPE OF MATERIAL ▼

Varies; will be discussed with specific materials.

▼ USE ▼

All intermediary materials protect the pulp but the manner in which they do so varies.

▼ MECHANISMS OF ACTION ▼

Bases

A *base* (Figure 10-1) is a relatively thick layer of material that does one or more of three things: absorb biting forces, insulate the interior of the tooth from temperature changes, or irritate the pulp. Irritating bases stimulate the pulp to make new dentin, thereby thickening the pulp's protective coat under the irritating base.

Some caution relative to base thickness is in order. When a base is too thick, an adequate thickness of restorative material cannot be placed over it without making the restoration too high. Insufficient bulk of restorative material causes restoration fracture. A high restoration also bangs against opposing teeth. Banging forces can be transferred to the pulp and periodontium, causing great discomfort and perhaps serious injury. To protect the pulp, then, a base should be relatively but not unduly thick, and a poor conductor of heat and cold.

The use of bases is now controversial in dentistry, although they are still placed. Bases have traditionally been used to prevent thermal shock and absorb occlusal forces. Many operators now believe pulpal sensitivity is caused by microleakage rather than temperature change, and that the relatively poor support provided to a restoration by a base can lead to cusp fracture. These operators bond materials to teeth rather than placing bases. Bonding effectively seals cut dentin tubules by eliminating the microspace that permits microleak-

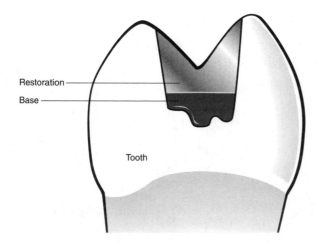

Restoration
Base
Tooth

FIGURE 10-1 Base. In this cross-section of the tooth you can see how the base is used to allow the restoration to sit on a flat surface rather than the uneven surface left when the caries is removed.

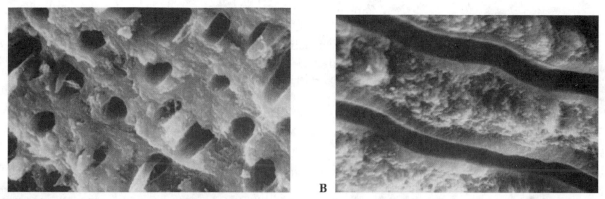

FIGURE 10-2 Dentinal tubules. These photomicrogaphs depict two views of dentin. The tubules are cut across their ends in A and lengthwise in B. (Photos reprinted from Mount, G. J. & W. R. Hume: *Preservation & Restoration of Tooth Structures,* p. 4, 1998, by permission of the publisher, Mosby.

age. It also effectively reduces cusp fracture by creating a single unit of the tooth and restoration. This permits dissipation of occlusal forces through a stronger whole rather than weaker individual sections.

Varnish

Varnish is used to seal cut dentin. Dentin is composed of microscopic tubules that contain fluid (Figure 10-2). When a tubule is cut, this forms an easily traveled expressway to the pulp for anything that reaches the tubule surface. If there is even a microscopic space between the restoration and the tooth, microleakage of acid-producing bacteria, ions from saliva, chemicals and colored pigments from restorative materials readily occurs. Chemical leakage can cause pulp sensitivity, microorganisms can contribute to secondary decay and pigments can result in tooth discoloration. Varnish is meant to seal the cut tubules with a very thin, fluid-impervious layer, preventing microleakage, pulp invasion and discoloration.

Use of varnish is also controversial. It is applied in exceptionally thin layers that can easily be scratched or worn away, leaving the tooth vulnerable. It also dissolves slowly in oral fluids and thus is not permanent. It is used only under amalgam, a metal that corrodes over time in oral fluids. The corrosion products then drift into the microspace between the tooth and restoration, effectively sealing it as the varnish dissolves away. This historically was the use for varnish. The controversy arises because corrosion sealing takes time to occur and newer types of amalgam do not corrode as much as older types do. Thus as the varnish leaves the tooth it is not replaced and an opening develops for microleakage to occur. This is why many dentists now seal cut tubules by bonding amalgam to the tooth surface rather than varnishing.

Liners

A *liner* is a relatively thin layer of material that does one or more of three things: changes the chemistry of the tooth surface, irritates the pulp so that it will form new dentin, or bonds filling material to the tooth.

▼ USES, CHARACTERISTICS AND HANDLING OF SPECIFIC MATERIALS ▼

It is important to note that intermediary materials often have more than one use. As a dental assistant or hygienist, you need to know what an intermediary material is, what types of intermediary materials there are, the names and uses of specific materials, and how each acts on the teeth.

Bases	Zinc oxide and eugenol, zinc polycarboxylate, zinc phosphate, glass ionomer
Varnishes	Copal varnish, universal varnish
Liners	Calcium hydroxide, glass ionomer, zinc oxide and eugenol
Bonding agents	Acrylic resin, glass ionomer

Calcium Hydroxide

Calcium hydroxide (Figure 10-3) is a suspension of calcium hydroxide particles in water and has three characteristics of interest: a basic pH, ready dissolution in oral fluids and an ability to irritate the pulp. As calcium hydroxide dissolves, it raises the pH in the immediate area by releasing its hydroxyl ions. This in turn helps to prevent pulp sensitivity by neutralizing acids that have leaked into the area, and to prevent bacterial growth by providing an environment that is too basic for them to flourish. Less bacterial assault provides time for the pulp to heal itself while it is not being attacked. A high pH also irritates some of the pulp cells themselves, thereby promoting dentin formation. Irritated odontoblasts protect themselves by making new dentin, which then serves as a barrier to the irritation.

Both self- and light-cured forms of calcium hydroxide are available and may be placed under all types of direct restorative materials. When calcium hydroxide is used, it is the first intermediary material placed and is applied only in the deepest part of the cavity preparation. It is not spread over a larger area because it is water soluble and it is not strong enough to provide support to the restoration. If extended to the tooth-restoration interface, it would dissolve and leave the tooth vulnerable to microleakage. If allowed to provide only poor support, it would leave the restoration or tooth vulnerable to fracture. For these reasons it is being replaced in dental practices by the bonding materials which do not have the solubility and tooth weakening effects of calcium hydroxide.

Varnish

Copal Varnish

Copal varnish (Figure 10-4) is a suspension of copal resin or cellulose in a volatile solvent. It is painted on the dentin surface to seal cut tubules. There the solvent quickly evaporates, leaving a very thin, insoluble film. Evaporation occurs so easily that the varnish bottle must be tightly recapped immediately after use or the solvent will be lost. Additional solvent, termed *thinner,* is available if the varnish becomes too thick.

Copal varnish is used under amalgam. It is not used under esthetic polymers as it interferes with bonding and inhibits resin set.

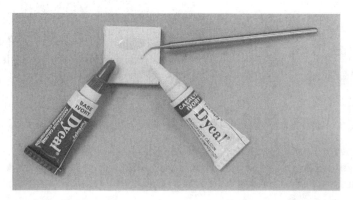

FIGURE 10-3   Calcium hydroxide. Prior to the advent of bonding to dentin, this was the most popular base.

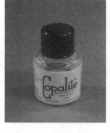

FIGURE 10-4 Copal varnish. This is an antique bottle of a material that was in every dentist's drawer 20 years ago but is rarely seen today.

Universal Varnish

Universal varnish (Figure 10-5) is a suspension of polyurethane, a clear polymer, in a volatile solvent. Rationale for universal varnish use, method of application and mechanism of action are the same as for copal varnish, but universal varnish can be used under any material and is not soluble in water. Its polyurethane component does not inhibit bonding or composite set.

When either type of varnish is used in conjunction with other intermediary materials, it is placed after calcium hydroxide and before all bases. Both types of varnish are, like calcium hydroxide, being supplanted by the bonding materials. It is a very rare office that uses these materials today.

Zinc Oxide and Eugenol

Zinc oxide and eugenol (Z-O-E; Figure 10-6) consists of zinc oxide particles and other additives that are mixed with eugenol (oil of cloves). Eugenol is acidic, so the resulting mixture irritates the pulp, sometimes damaging it but stimulating it to make new dentin in the process. The new layer becomes an insulating barrier for the pulp, lessening microleakage and thermal shock. The net effect is soothing and even though Z-O-E is irritating, it is often described as a sedative. Z-O-E also inhibits resin polymerization; therefore it is not used under composite materials.

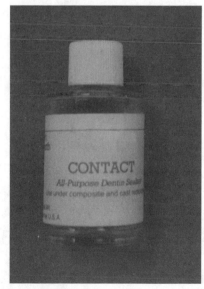

FIGURE 10-5 Universal varnish. This material has no real use since dentin bonding seals the tubules much better than varnish.

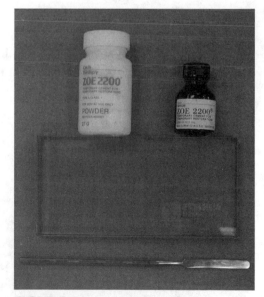

FIGURE 10-6 Zinc oxide and eugenol. This material forms a very weak base.

These materials have been used as liners under amalgam restorations but now are generally used as temporary filling materials. To use such a weak material as a temporary filling it is necessary to reinforce it with acrylic fibers that add some strength, although even then the material is still not near the standards set by the direct restorative materials (covered in the next chapter).

Z-O-E is available in powder and liquid, premeasured capsule or tube form. The powder and liquid are mixed on a fluid-resistant paper pad. It is important that the pad be fluid-impervious because relatively little liquid is mixed with a relatively large amount of powder. Any liquid absorbed by the pad may critically reduce the amount available for reaction. The pad and mixing spatula must be dry, as water accelerates Z-O-E set.

Z-O-E does not have good compressive strength; as much powder as possible is added to the liquid to create the strongest possible mix. Z-O-E mixes are sometimes "worked" to allow incorporation of more powder. Working is repeatedly pressing on the mix while drawing the spatula toward the mixer to ensure the powder particles are well crushed and in contact with the liquid.

A Z-O-E base mix is ready for use when it is thick and putty-like (Figure 10-7). Many operators like to roll prepared Z-O-E into a small ball, place it onto a hand condenser or plastic instrument that has been dipped in a bit of extra powder to keep it from sticking, then tamp and spread the material into a cavity preparation.

Premeasured Z-O-E capsules are small plastic containers (Figure 10-8) that have the correct amount of powder in one end, liquid in the other, and a thin plastic membrane separating the two. They are placed in a *triturator,* a small machine that shakes capsules at high speed. This breaks the thin membrane between the ends and mixes the powder and liquid.

The paste form may be packaged in one or two tubes. Material from a single tube is placed and light cured. Materials from two tubes are proportioned by extruding equal lengths onto a pad, then rapidly mixed with a rotary motion until the material is homogenous in color and consistency.

Set Z-O-E is soluble in oral fluids. This plus its poor compressive strength, porous nature and ultimately sedative effect make it suitable only for temporary applications. If the tooth responds well to Z-O-E, it is more likely to respond well to restoration with permanent materials, and the effect can be seen within the time period that a temporary application is expected to last.

Zinc Phosphate

Zinc phosphate (Figure 10-9) is a zinc oxide powder that is mixed with a phosphoric acid liquid to create a strong but at first quite acidic set material. Zinc phosphate bases are used under amalgam restorations to provide thermal insulation and absorb occlusal forces. They

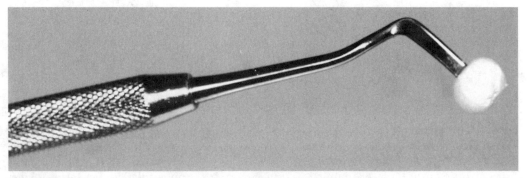

FIGURE 10-7 Mixing bases. Base materials are very firm when mixed properly.

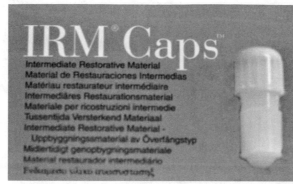

FIGURE 10-8 IRM capsules. IRM is very difficult to mix by hand. It is very convenient to have these capsules around the office.

are not placed in deep cavity preparations until a layer of calcium hydroxide is first placed over the pulp to protect it from the acidity.

Over time, zinc phosphate is soluble in oral fluids. It is also brittle enough to flake away in small amounts. These factors leave the tooth vulnerable to microleakage. To lessen microleakage, varnish is used after calcium hydroxide to seal the cut dentin tubules before a zinc phosphate base is placed.

Mixing technique for zinc phosphate is extremely important. The setting reaction is exothermic; it gives off heat. Heat in turn accelerates the set. A glass slab is used for mixing to help dissipate heat and avoid premature setting. Some operators cool the slab before use by placing it in the freezer or refrigerator until needed, or rinsing it in cool water. A cool slab can absorb more heat as the mixing proceeds. Mixing is also done over a large area of the slab to provide a larger surface for conducting heat away from the mix. It is important to note that any slab used for mixing must be completely dry, as water also accelerates zinc phosphate set.

As for all powder and liquid systems, zinc oxide powder is shaken slightly to remove lumps and air pockets, proportioned with the correct scoop, placed on the slab on the side of the dominant hand, then immediately recapped. The liquid is shaken slightly to ensure all components are distributed throughout the solution, proportioned, placed near the powder on the side of the nondominant hand, and immediately recapped. The powder is then divided into small increments (Figure 10-10). Each increment is separately brought to the liquid and crushed into it.

As much powder as possible is incorporated into the mix to make it as strong as possible. Adding the powder to the liquid is of course what causes the reaction. Adding a large

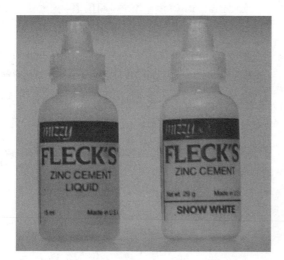
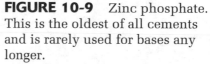

FIGURE 10-9 Zinc phosphate. This is the oldest of all cements and is rarely used for bases any longer.

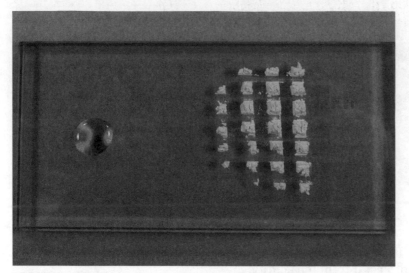

FIGURE 10-10 Mixing zinc phosphate. Not all of these piles will be used but it is better to have extra powder than have to fumble around adding more to the slab during mixing.

amount of powder at once creates more heat at one time, increasing the chance that setting will occur before an adequate amount of powder has been incorporated. Accordingly, the powder must be added to the liquid in small increments. This will avoid creation of a large amount of heat and allow time for dissipation of what is created before another powder increment arrives.

The powder particles must be crushed well to increase the area of surface contact between the powder and liquid molecules that allows the reaction to proceed. Mixing is done with a rotary motion in the early stages; at this point it is easy to crush the particles in the liquid. As mixing proceeds, the mass becomes thicker, and the task of crushing new powder particles into it more difficult. A fold and press motion is then used to ensure thorough crushing.

A zinc phosphate mix is ready for use as a base when it is thick and putty-like (Figure 10-11). As with Z-O-E, many operators like to roll the mixed material into a ball, then tamp and spread it into position with a hand instrument that has been dipped in extra powder.

Zinc Polycarboxylate

Zinc polycarboxylate (Figure 10-12) combines zinc oxide particles with carboxylic acid. The acid can form a polymer component that bonds to the tooth; its metal oxide component provides strength. Although zinc polycarboxylate is acidic, its pH rapidly rises, making it kinder to the pulp than zinc phosphate.

Zinc polycarboxylate can be used under all types of direct restorations but is more likely to be placed under amalgam. It is supplied as two different forms each of powder and liquid. One form has dried acrylic acid bonded to the zinc oxide in the powder and the liquid is plain water. The other, more commonly used form has only zinc oxide in the powder and the liquid is an acrylic monomer solution.

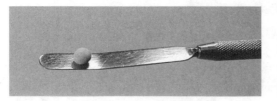

FIGURE 10-11 Finished mix. You can see that the material can be made into a neat ball when it is firm enough.

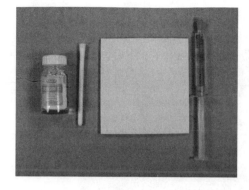

FIGURE 10-12 Zinc polycarboxylate. Like zinc phosphate the main use of this material is as a cement rather than a base.

Mixing is quickly accomplished on a paper pad. The powder is fluffed, proportioned, and recapped. There are two forms of the acrylic acid-containing liquid. One is a typical liquid-in-a-plastic-bottle arrangement. The liquid container is turned upside down several times to ensure thorough distribution of its components, proportioned and recapped. Polycarboxylate liquid is exceptionally viscous, so much so that it is slow and sometimes difficult to proportion. It helps to purchase small containers so the liquid does not evaporate into the unfilled part of the container itself, making the solution even more viscous than usual. The second form avoids the evaporation problem by packaging the solution in a small, calibrated syringe. A plunger pushes the correct amount of liquid out the end and onto the pad. This does not expose the solution to air and provides the careful operator with a more consistent proportion.

The proportioned powder is divided in half, then each half is rapidly and thoroughly incorporated into the liquid until the mix is homogenous in color and consistency. When complete, the mix should still be glossy. Glossy polymers have surface molecules that are still capable of reacting. Loss of gloss indicates the surface molecules have already reacted, working time is over and set is beginning.

Spatulas and instruments used to mix or place polycarboxylate should be wiped clean with a 2 × 2 gauze square and strong pressure *immediately* after use. Once set, polycarboxylate is extremely difficult to remove. An ultrasonic cleaner can be helpful, and soaking followed by scraping with another spatula can be used if absolutely necessary.

Glass Ionomer

As you learned in the chapter on sealants, glass ionomer is an acrylic and maleic or itaconic acid, glass reinforced polymer that bonds chemically and leaches fluoride into the surrounding tooth structure, strengthening it and exerting an anticariogenic effect (Figure 10-13).

Since it is a polymer, glass ionomer also bonds chemically to other polymer materials used in restorations, reducing microleakage at the interface of the bonding agent and restorative material as well as the tooth surface. It can be used under all of the direct esthetic restorative materials and is extremely popular. Self- and light-cured forms are available for use as a base and a dual-cured form for use as a bonding agent.

Acrylic Resin

Acrylic resin intermediary material is an acrylic acid polymer bonding agent. It is the same material used for sealants, but is left unfilled to encourage flow and is not tinted. It is bonded to both enamel and dentin.

Enamel Bonding

As explained in Chapter 6, the tooth is treated with acid to create microscopic depressions. The acrylic resin polymer can then be painted over the roughened surface where it will flow into the depressions. Light-cured resins are placed and exposed to visible light

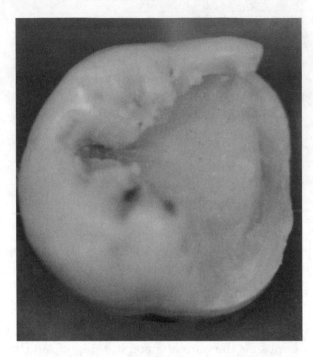

FIGURE 10-13 Glass ionomer base. The base allows the pulpal floor to be flat without removing healthy dentin.

while self-cured resins are mixed, placed and allowed to harden. At the end of the process, hardened resin is mechanically interlocked with enamel (Figure 10-14).

Dentin Bonding

When dentin is to be bonded, an extra step, *priming,* is included in the bonding process after enamel etching. Cutting dentin produces a *smear layer,* a fairly tenacious layer of ground hydroxyapatite crystals and protein debris that coats the surface and partially plugs the cut tubules. Dentin also is approximately 30% fluid. Both factors make it difficult to obtain a strong bond.

The current solution is to increase dentin bond strength by priming the dentin to create a *hybrid layer* that is part dentin, part hardened resin. A *primer,* which is a weak acid solution composed of monomers and wetting agents that can penetrate the dentin surface, is used to lock the material to the dentin (Figure 10-15). This primer is then combined with a polymer to coat and attach the primer to the restorative material. Oxygen in the air over the outer adhesive surface prevents its cure. Placing a polymer restorative material atop this *air-inhibited layer* removes the oxygen supply, allowing the adhesive to bond with the restorative.

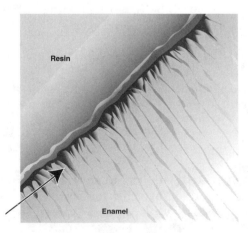

Resin

Enamel

FIGURE 10-14 Resin tags. You can see at the arrow the extension of the resin into the tooth.

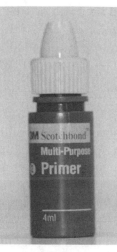

FIGURE 10-15 Dentin bonding agents. There are numerous formulations for sealing dentinal tubules with bonding material. Each has different application instructions. Always read the directions carefully before using a new material.

Dentin Bonding Systems Available

Depending on the brand of material used, there will be different steps involved. Some have separate materials for each step and others combine some or all of the steps. All three components—etch, primer and bond—may now be in one solution. The earliest dentin bonding systems used three materials, one for each step. Intermediate material developments combined more than one step: some have an initial etch, but the priming and bonding are combined into a single step. There are also materials that combine the etching and priming steps then bond as a second step. With the variety of material formats available, it is very important to read the manufacturer's directions to determine the proper technique for the agent being used.

▼ SELECTION OF INTERMEDIARY MATERIALS FOR A SPECIFIC RESTORATION ▼

Not every direct restoration requires the use of intermediary materials. Those that do will need only some of those available. Which ones, if any, are needed for a particular restoration is a professional judgment of the operator.

You may find it helpful to learn some frequent operator choices: Z-O-E when the restoration will be temporary, calcium hydroxide when the cavity preparation is very deep, acrylic resin or glass ionomer as a bonding agent under direct esthetic polymers—composite, glass ionomer, and their hybrids.

It is under amalgam that the choices are not so clear—perhaps varnish or calcium hydroxide, or both; perhaps varnish and one of the bases, with or without calcium hydroxide; perhaps just bonding alone. If amalgam restorations are placed where you are employed, the dentist's philosophy will determine the intermediary materials to be used with it.

In general, however, most dentists will opt for a bonding agent under any restoration that they do, as bonding agents have superior sealing abilities and are not soluble in oral fluids. It is likely the other materials mentioned in this chapter will be replaced completely in a few years at most.

KEY POINTS

✓ Intermediary materials are placed between the tooth and a restoration.
✓ There are several types, all of which protect the pulp in some way:
  • Base—absorbs biting forces and insulates the pulp from temperature changes
  • Varnish—seals cut dentin tubules
  • Liner—reduces acidity, stimulates the pulp and/or is a bonding agent

✓ An intermediary material may have more than one action on the tooth or other materials.
✓ More than one intermediary material may be used in a restoration.
✓ The operator must select which intermediary materials to use for a specified restoration.
✓ What is chosen depends in part on what restorative material will be used.
✓ Common choices:
  • In deep restorations—calcium hydroxide
  • For temporary applications—zinc oxide and eugenol
  • Under esthetic polymer restoratives—acrylic resin or glass ionomer bonding agents
✓ In order to make sound choices for individual patients, the operator must know the purpose of using each material, as well as how it will affect the tooth and other materials.

SELF TEST

Questions 1–5: Suggest suitable intermediary materials for each task listed below.

1. Placing a shallow anterior esthetic polymer restoration

2. Placing a very deep posterior amalgam restoration

3. Bonding an esthetic polymer restoration to enamel and dentin

4. Placing an esthetic polymer restoration for a patient with a high decay rate

5. Placing a strong base under an amalgam restoration

Questions 6–15: Select the letter preceding the material that exhibits each action or property listed below. An answer may be used more than once.

  a. Glass ionomer
  b. Varnish
  c. Zinc phosphate
  d. Acrylic resin
  e. Zinc oxide and eugenol
  f. Zinc polycarboxylate
  g. Primer

6. Cleans and penetrates cut dentin surface

7. Is sufficiently acid that pulp protection must precede its use

8. Seals cut dentin tubules

9. Bonds mechanically to the tooth surface

10. Leaches fluoride into adjacent tooth structure

11. Is acidic but still relatively kind to the tooth

12. Bonds chemically to the calcium in tooth structure

13. Dissolves readily over time in oral fluids

14. Forms a weak base

15. Inhibits resin set

▼11▼

ESTHETIC DIRECT RESTORATION MATERIALS

OBJECTIVES

After studying this chapter, you should be able to:

1. Differentiate composite, glass ionomer and esthetic blends.
2. Discuss how the properties of each contribute to the success of a finished restoration.
3. Differentiate types of curing lights.
4. Describe a core buildup.

▼ DEFINITION ▼

Esthetic direct restorative materials are tooth-colored filling materials.

▼ MATERIALS USED ▼

Composite
Glass ionomer
Blends: Compomer and polyacid modified glass ionomer (PMGI)

▼ PROCEDURAL USES FOR EACH MATERIAL ▼

Composite—Direct restorations, core buildups, veneers, sealants and as a cement
Glass ionomer—Direct restorations, core buildups, sealants, and as a bonding agent and cement
Blends—Direct restorations

▼ TYPE OF MATERIAL ▼

All are polymers with reinforcing particles locked into the polymer framework.

Composite

bis-GMA or urethane dimethacrylate polymer heavily reinforced with glass or silicate filler. The filler is formulated either as discrete particles or as set composite particles that are then ground at the factory and added to the polymer.

Glass Ionomer

Acrylic, tartaric and maleic or itaconic acid polymer reinforced with calcium fluoroaluminosilicate glass.

Blends

Since the basic components of both composites and glass ionomers are polymer chains surrounding inorganic particles, it is possible to combine both into a single substance that will exhibit the properties of both. These blends of composite and glass ionomer exist along a continuum with composite at one end and glass ionomer at the other. As the composition of a material moves closer to the pure type at each end, it is more likely to be known by that name.

Materials that contain about a fairly even split of composite and glass ionomer are known as compomers; those that contain more glass ionomer than composite are polyacid modified glass ionomers, and those with more composite than glass ionomer are composites.

▼ MECHANISMS OF ACTION IN A DIRECT RESTORATION PROCEDURE ▼

Both composite and glass ionomer

Restore form and function in an esthetic manner
Bond chemically with other polymers
Effectively seal cut dentin tubules to eliminate microleakage

Composite

Bonds mechanically and/or chemically to the tooth surface through the use of a polymer bonding agent

Glass ionomer

Bonds chemically with calcium on the tooth surface
Leaches fluoride into adjacent tooth structure

▼ SELECTING COMPOSITE, GLASS IONOMER, OR A BLEND FOR A DIRECT RESTORATION ▼

The type of cavity preparation to be filled (Figure 11-1), as well as material appearance, flow, and ability to set in a moist environment are major criteria for differentiating direct esthetic polymers.

Composite is the workhorse of the direct restoration world because it is strong enough to be used in all types of cavity preparations, closely resembles natural tooth structure, is viscous enough to permit controlled placement, and can be polished to a high shine. On the other hand, it requires a dry environment for set.

Glass ionomer, which can set without adverse effect in a moist environment, is used in gingival areas when moisture control is difficult. Because it leaches fluoride, it may be selected for a patient with a particularly high decay rate. It is also opaque, thus appears less natural. Glass ionomer is weaker than composite and more prone to wear, so is not used where it would be subject to strong biting forces.

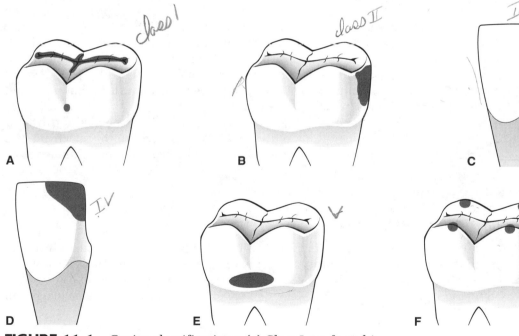

FIGURE 11-1 Cavity classifications. (a) Class I are found in the pits and fissures of a tooth; (b) Class II are smooth surface interproximal cavities on posterior teeth; (c) Class III are interproximal cavities on anterior teeth; (d) Class IV include the incisal edge of anterior teeth; (e) Class V are smooth surface cavities along the gumline; (f) Class VI are abraded areas on occlusal and incisial surfaces.

▼ MECHANISM OF ACTION—CHEMICAL LEVEL ▼

Composite

Composition

Composite is a dimethacrylate or urethane dimethacrylate resin that is heavily filled with glass, silicates or ground, prehardened composite. Additional substances are included as modifiers. The resin and filler form a physical mixture rather than a chemical compound, so silane is added to link the different types of molecules together and prevent the loss of surface filler as the finished restoration wears. An initiator substance is included to respond to a light or chemical activator and initiate polymerization. Benzoyl peroxide is used to respond to chemical activation, and a photoinitiator molecule such as camphoroquinone is used to respond to light activation. These in turn react with an accelerator to cause polymerization of the material. Coloring agents are added to create esthetic shades and opacifiers are added to make the material more opaque to mimic various portions of the tooth structure.

Reaction

Chemically activated systems consist of two pastes, one of which contains a benzoyl peroxide initiator and the other, a tertiary amine such as toluidine. When the two pastes are mixed, the benzoyl peroxide and amine react to form free radicals, which are charged chemicals that are capable of breaking chemical bonds. The free radicals then react with atoms in the resin to begin polymerization. Composite resin hardens through an addition reaction that chains the resin molecules.

Light-activated systems consist of one paste that includes both an amine activator and a photoinitiator molecule such as camphoroquinone. When the material is exposed to visible light, the energy from the light excites the photoinitiator molecules, causing some of their bonds to open and react with the amine. The remainder of the process occurs as in chemically activated resins; it is only the activation, by light or chemical substance, that is different. The important difference between the chemically cured material and the light cured material, then, is the initiation of the reaction. It is important to note that the benzoyl peroxide used as the chemical initiator yellows over time, discoloring the restoration.

Composite is the same material as acrylic resin sealant. It is, however, more heavily reinforced, tinted to resemble tooth structure, and available in a wider variety of viscosity, filler, opacity and packaging options to provide the qualities needed for different types of direct restorations. You can think of the sealants at one end of the spectrum of composites and the packable resins that are very heavily filled as the other end of the continuum.

Glass Ionomer

Composition

Two types of materials are available. In one type, the powder contains ground calcium aluminofluorosilicate glass plus zinc oxide opaquers, and the liquid is a solution of polycarboxylic acid in water. In the other type, the ground glass particles and freeze-dried acid are both placed in the powder, and water or a water-tartaric acid solution is used as the liquid.

Reaction

When the powder and liquid are combined, the acid attacks the glass surface, liberating calcium, aluminum, sodium and fluorine. Calcium and aluminum cross-link the polyacrylic acid chains to form a hard resin matrix with the remaining glass particles scattered throughout as reinforcers. Calcium reactions occur within minutes, but aluminum binding occurs more slowly and is not complete for nearly 24 hours. The sodium and fluorine ions combine to form sodium fluoride, which is also scattered throughout the matrix but not bound to it.

Because it is not bound, this fluoride is available for diffusion into the surrounding area. While the matrix is being formed, carboxyl groups from the acids combine with calcium on the tooth surface, creating a chemical bond between the tooth and material.

▼ SPECIFIC MATERIALS ▼

Composite

Multiple composite products are available. The clinician chooses among them on the basis of material strength, flow, polishability, translucency, ease of use, and wear. Composites are also notoriously technique sensitive. Handling procedures affect voids, depth of cure, and bond strength. Various material options are available to address all of these concerns.

Viscosity Options

The proportion of resin to filler determines material flow. As the number of filler particles increases, viscosity decreases. This can be an advantage when flow needs to be controlled, as, for example, when a Class IV restoration is being constructed and there are no walls available to contain the material at the incisal angle. It can be a disadvantage when flow is needed, such as when a material must flow into small retention areas in the cavity preparation floor or walls.

Three types of materials are available to meet different flow requirements: flowable, packable and conventional. *Flowable composites* contain fewer filler particles and more resin. Accordingly, they flow well and form a strong bond with underlying polymer bonding agents, but are not very strong. *Packable composites* contain more filler and less resin. They do not flow well, but are stronger and sufficiently viscous to be pushed into a preparation. Because of these characteristics, dental personnel also refer to packable materials as *condensable composites* or *high-viscosity resins*. *Conventional composites* follow a middle ground; the material flows, is of sufficient viscosity that an operator can mold it with a hand instrument, but is not viscous enough to be packed.

Operators tend to use conventional composites alone for an entire restoration, and to use flowable and packable composites in combination. The flowable resin is placed in a layer on the cavity floor, where it will flow into small retention areas and bond well with the underlying polymer bonding agent. Packable material is then placed over it. Pushing the packable material into place helps prevent voids that may occur between the bonding agent and restorative material, in the body of the restoration or at the restoration margin.

Filler Options

Filler particles provide body and strength to composite. To understand how the filler changes the composite properties we need to look at three properties of the filler: type, particle size and amount.

Type

Fillers are composed of silicates such as quartz or very fine colloidal silica particles, or they are one of a number of glasses. The glasses often contain radiopaque elements such as barium, strontium or zinc to make the restoration visible on radiographs.

Size

The size of the particles affects strength and polishability. Generally, the larger the particles the greater the strength, although the amount of the filler has a greater effect. The size of the particles greatly affects the polishability of the surface. The resin is softer and when abraded disappears faster than the filler. Thus the larger the filler particle the rougher

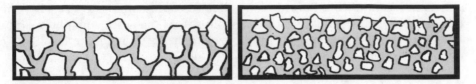

FIGURE 11-2   Particle sizes. As you can see, the larger particles protrude further through the resin (gray), thus giving a rougher surface.

the final result (Figure 11-2). So there is a tradeoff between beauty and strength. Often this means that the larger particle materials will be used in the posterior where high shine is not as important and the smaller particle materials will be used on the anterior teeth where the surface needs to be smooth.

Amount

The filler amount changes the strength and polymerization shrinkage properties of a composite. More filler increases strength. It also leaves less polymer between the particles. The ideal restoration would be 100% filler, similar to an indirect porcelain restoration, but that is not possible in a direct restoration that must flow into the cavity preparation. The greater the amount of filler that can be incorporated, then, the better the strength and the less the polymerization shrinkage. The filler particles do not change in the setting reaction; only the resin shrinks significantly as it polymerizes.

The number of particles that can be placed in a specified amount of resin is limited by the increase in viscosity of the material as particles are added. It is like adding flour to cake batter; as the flour is added the mixture thickens and becomes more difficult to stir. This is due to the frictional effect of the particles within the resin. The more surface area of filler involved the greater the viscosity. Although it is not intuitive, it is true that the smaller the particles the greater the surface area they will have in a given weight or volume. So the smallest particles, colloidal silica, can only be added in small amounts. To overcome this problem the manufacturers sometimes incorporate large particle loads and cure the material in the factory, then grind it into particles that can be incorporated into resin, thereby enabling larger filler loading.

The final properties of the composite will also depend on the particle sizes. They are found along a continuum, as was the case with the filler amount. Originally composites had been divided into two categories, conventional and microfilled. The conventional had larger particles and more filler, while the microfill had small particles. Because of the large surface area of their small filler particles, microfilled composites could not contain as much filler. Thus the conventional composites had greater strength but were not as smooth when polished. Manufacturers then learned to mix the two particle sizes to form hybrid composites that had grater strength than the microfills and greater polishability then conventional, macrofilled composites. Today most manufacturers use ranges of particle sizes in their materials, blurring the lines completely.

Opacity Options

Different tissues and areas of natural teeth vary in their opacity. Enamel is translucent and dentin is opaque. Thick areas of either tissue are more opaque, thin areas, more translucent. Accordingly, various tooth structure translucencies occur even on a single tooth. Composite materials are available in various formulations to simulate the translucency differences of natural teeth. Materials classified as opaque are available in dentin shades and those classified as translucent, enamel shades. Operators often skillfully employ composites of varying translucency and opacity to simulate tooth structure so well it is difficult to differentiate the restored portion of a tooth from the remaining natural area.

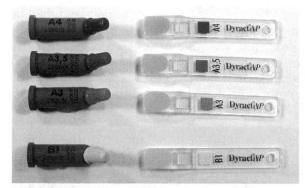

FIGURE 11-3 Composite material. Notice how the manufacturer has keyed the color of the caps to the shade guide.

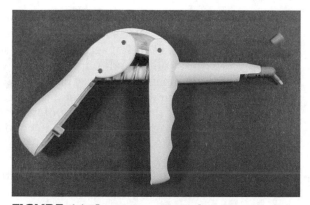

FIGURE 11-4 Using compules. Here is the compule loaded in the gun and ready for use.

Packaging Options

Packaging indicates type of material and affects cost and ease of placement. Self-cured, light cured and dual cured paste systems are available.

One paste is available in compules or syringes and will be light cured. A *compule* (Figure 11-3) is a disposable unit dose container. It is snapped into a hand-held, gun-type syringe applicator and the material is ejected into the cavity preparation (Figure 11-4). The great advantages of a compule are convenience, color standardization, and infection control. It is easy to slip a prepared compule into the syringe and shades are mixed by the manufacturer under precisely controlled conditions. After use, the compule is thrown away, although the applicator will be reused and must be disinfected. The disadvantage of compules is cost. They are relatively expensive to purchase, any unused material is thrown away and a variety of shades must be kept on hand to match tooth shades for different patients.

A syringe (Figure 11-5) is a disposable multidose container of a single shade of material. Some syringes have a screw-type mechanism that must be turned to eject a high-viscosity paste. Others have a plunger that is pushed to dispense a flowable material through a cannula.

High-viscosity paste is dispensed onto a small paper pad, then carried to the mouth, pushed into position and sculpted to correct form with a hand instrument. The advantages of multidose syringe use are placement control, the ability to make custom color blends and cost. The material does not flow beyond where it is wanted and there is very little waste. Disadvantages are time required for dispensation, a tendency for the material to harden in the syringe unless it is kept tightly capped, and the difficulty of disinfecting the syringe after use.

Flowable material is ejected directly into the cavity preparation. The advantage of plunger ejection is ease of placement in small areas. Disadvantages are difficulty in controlling the flow and again the difficulty in disinfecting the syringes used.

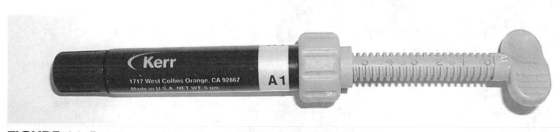

FIGURE 11-5 Composite syringes. Syringes are another popular way of dispensing composite materials.

Two pastes (Figure 11-6) are packaged in small, round plastic containers and may be self-cured or dual set. One paste is a base, the other a catalyst. A small, double-ended disposable spatula is used to place approximately equal amounts of the two pastes in close proximity on a small paper pad. They are then mixed rapidly with a fold and press motion to a homogenous color. The double-ended spatula calls attention to the need to keep the pastes separate; an end that has been in base paste should not be placed in catalyst paste, or vice versa. If paste in one container is contaminated with the other type, a setting reaction will begin in the contaminated container.

Self-cure pastes require only mixing; dual cure pastes require both mixing and exposure to light. It is important to read the label of any two-paste material you are using to determine whether it is self- or dual cured.

The advantage of a dual cure system is quick and thorough curing. Self-cured materials cure more completely but require a longer time to harden. Light cured materials cure immediately but may not harden completely. Dual cure systems seek the advantage of an immediate cure followed by a complete cure over time. They are usually used in deeper areas of the restorations or areas that are difficult to access. As you know from earlier in the chapter, the benzoyl peroxide initiator in self-cured composites may cause discoloration of this material, limiting its use in esthetically demanding areas.

Placement of a Composite Restoration

A direct restoration procedure follows a similar course regardless of the restorative material used. Variations for specific materials occur only in the filling and finishing steps. The tasks of the allied dental health student when considering direct esthetic materials, then, are to learn the filling and finishing steps of each material, and why it is handled as it is. This will enable the assistant to anticipate the operator's needs, saving valuable time in the restorative process; the operator to receive properly prepared material; and patients to receive correct information about direct esthetic materials.

Composite placement seems simple and quick but is in reality technique-sensitive. The basic process is etch, prime, bond, fill, finish. Newer materials may combine some or all of the etch, prime and bond steps. The tooth is isolated to facilitate etching, priming and bonding and when indicated, a thin plastic or metal matrix strip is placed to retain the composite in position while it is soft and to create a smooth restoration surface. Light cure composites are inserted and sculpted until the operator is satisfied they are correct, then

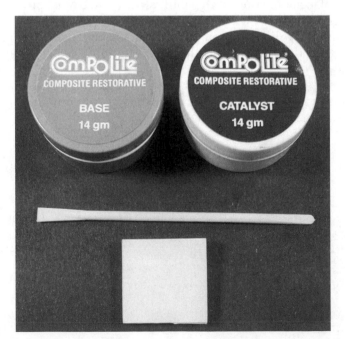

FIGURE 11-6 Self-curing composite. These systems are useful in areas that complete curing with the light might not be feasible.

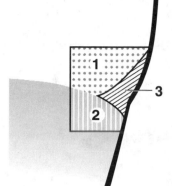

FIGURE 11-7 Placement of composite. Diagram of the placement order for a Class V composite to lessen strain on the tooth.

the material is light cured. Because of the limitations of light passing through the material, composites cannot be put into a deep restoration in one increment. They must slowly be built to the surface, curing each layer in turn. Another problem encountered is that because of the normal shrinkage of composite material, if it is inserted in large amounts, the bulk shrinkage will be higher. This can lead to tooth sensitivity, due either to bending of the cusps, the restoration's pulling away from the tooth or fracture of the tooth enamel under stress. To lessen the amount of internal stress in the restoration caused by this shrinkage the composite is not only layered but ramped against one wall at a time (Figure 11-7) during the buildup.

Once the restoration is completely built up and the material is set, the restoration is finished and polished. The process described above is the same for self- or dual cure composites, except insertion and sculpting time is limited and layering for setting reasons is no longer important. In the self-cure materials there is also naturally less internal stress because the entire mass of the material is setting at the same time, unlike the light cured materials in which curing starts closest to the light source and progresses deeper.

▼ CURING LIGHTS ▼

As noted above, cure in light-activated materials is controlled by the ability of the light to start the chemical reaction leading to polymerization. Light can cure only as far as it penetrates. Conventional high-intensity visible lights and newer types of halogen, LED and laser lights are all used for curing; each has different abilities to penetrate material. The opacity of the material also matters as opaquing agents within it block light. Each type of light source also emits characteristic wavelengths that penetrate at different speeds to different depths. The initiators in the material also are tuned to certain light frequencies, which need to match the frequency of the curing beam. This is normally at the blue end of the light spectrum. Conventional lights have filters to limit the light to those frequencies. Some light sources may not contain the correct frequencies for certain materials. The compatibility of the material and the light source, then, is an important issue when using any type of curing light. For maximum polymerization of the material, curing lights should be held as close as possible to, but not touching, material to be cured for the time determined to be optimal for the material and type of light in use.

Curing lights may lose efficiency through use and each should be frequently checked. Inexpensive, reliable assessment devices are available (Figure 11-8). Training for their use requires only a few minutes and the actual assessment procedure requires less than a minute. Allied dental personnel should monitor the efficiency of all curing lights in the office or clinic at least weekly.

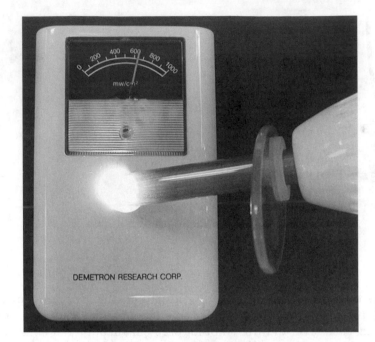

FIGURE 11-8 Light tester. This light is ready to go.

▼ FINISHING ▼

Finishing methods differ from operator to operator but the order always goes from finishing to polishing. Sharp instruments, diamond burs, carbide burs, abrasive disks and stones can be used to remove any excess material, then to shape and smooth any overcontoured areas. Once the shape of the tooth and the occlusion with the opposing tooth is correct, the restoration is polished. Polishing is done with silicon dioxide abrasive disks, fine-fluted carbide burs or a diamond dust polishing paste. In keeping with principles of abrasive use, progressively finer disks are used as the finishing progresses. A lubricant may be used to ensure that unsightly debris formed by the polishing process does not stain the newly placed composite.

▼ CLINICAL CONCERNS ▼

A composite restoration is strong, with better tensile than compressive strength. It is attractively translucent and can be polished. It is bonded to the tooth surface, thereby creating a single strong unit and eliminating microleakage. Composite restorations are, however, subject to wear, discoloration and loss of marginal integrity.

All composites wear, but at different rates depending on the strength of the material itself, the adequacy of the silane bond between the resin matrix and filler particles, and the nature of opposing teeth. Material strength and silane bonding are under the manufacturer's control. Porcelain, metal and natural antagonists wear composite; acrylic antagonists do not.

The resin portion of a composite restoration can sorb fluids and dissolved coloring agents. The edge of the restoration, with its thin film of bonding agent that is pure resin, is the most likely place to see staining. The large quantity of fillers in the filling material keeps this to a minimum, but material discoloration can occur over time. As mentioned earlier, all self-cure composites will yellow over time naturally. Excellent oral hygiene prevents surface staining.

Marginal integrity can be lost through bond breakage, material wear or as secondary decay undermines adjacent areas. The edges of composite restorations may be sealed to assist in maintaining marginal integrity.

On balance, composite restorations are esthetically pleasing, adequately strong, relatively quick and inexpensive to place, and provide excellent service.

▼ A NOTE CONCERNING COMPOSITE SAFETY ▼

Unreacted monomer in composite is hazardous. Exposure can result in soft tissue irritation, contact dermatitis, allergy, respiratory difficulty, nausea, liver or kidney damage, and central nervous system depression. It is flammable. Dental procedures require use of very little monomer, but common sense must be employed and appropriate precautions taken.

- Work in a well-ventilated area.
- Keep containers tightly closed when not in use.
- Avoid using near an open flame.
- Store containers in a flammables cabinet that is not near a heat source.
- Although dental masks do not protect against monomer fumes, a mask, gloves and safety glasses will protect against contact. If resin is spilled on soft tissue, wash the area thoroughly; if on a glove, follow new glove procedure: discard gloves, wash hands, and replace gloves. If the material is spilled on a cabinet, floor or other inanimate surface, clean the area with an organic solvent cleanup kit. It is also important to use tinted safety glasses whenever light curing a material. Long-term use of curing lights without tinted-glass protection presents the potential for damage to the retina of the eye.

▼ GLASS IONOMER ▼

Packaging Options (Figure 11-9)

Class I material is used as an adhesive and Class II material for direct restorations. The adhesive material is supplied as a powder and liquid in two separate containers and is dual cured. The restorative material may be supplied as separate containers of powder and liquid or as a single capsule or applicator tip containing a unit dose of premeasured materials. A capsule is placed in a triturator and shaken at high speed. A thin membrane separates the powder from the liquid so the shaking breaks the membrane and mixes the two materials. Material in an applicator tip is placed and light cured.

Safety

Glass ionomer is not a hazardous material.

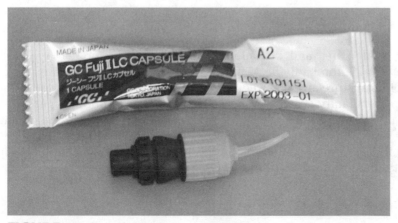

FIGURE 11-9 Glass ionomer capsule. This is placed in an amalgam triturator and inserted into a special gun to extrude the material through the tip and into the tooth.

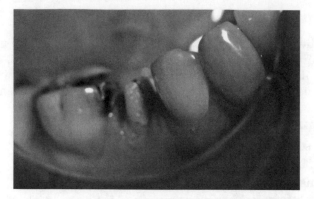

FIGURE 11-10 Core. Most of the crown of this tooth was missing. The remaining tooth is darker than the composite used for the build-up.

Preparation of Powder and Liquid Systems

Use a paper pad and flexible spatula. Fluff powder, measure level scoops, place powder on pad on side of dominant hand and replace cover. Ensure all powder lumps have been removed and powder is neat. Proportion liquid and recover. Bring powder to liquid and mix rapidly to homogenous color and consistency. The mix should be completed while the material is still glossy.

Clinical Considerations

Because glass ionomer can set without adverse effect in a moist environment, total moisture control is not necessary. Puddles of water are unacceptable, however, as they will cause voids in the material.

Because glass ionomer bonds directly to the tooth, separate etching and bonding agents are not required, although many systems come with a primer to enhance the bonding.

Because glass ionomer flows readily, flow control can be difficult.

Because aluminum binding in the matrix occurs slowly, glass ionomer set is not complete for nearly 24 hours. During this time, it remains vulnerable to drying. Dry material is subject to cracking and crazing. Glass ionomer restorations should be protected from contact with the oral environment for several days following set. Protective glass ionomer coatings, termed *varnishes,* are available for this purpose. Rather than use the varnish, many operators place a protective layer of bonding agent over the material.

The set glass ionomer restoration is nearly insoluble in oral fluids and, particularly in its early months, leaches fluoride into the surrounding tooth structure. It wears readily, but if placed in a nonstress bearing area may provide years of faithful service.

▼ CORE BUILDUP ▼

Both very strong composites and a reinforced form of glass ionomer are used for core buildup. When a tooth is too badly broken down to retain a crown, the dentist may shape the remaining tooth structure and place composite, glass ionomer or amalgam over it to create adequate support capacity. The procedure is called a *core buildup* (Figure 11-10). Cores created this way are subject to chewing forces and must be strong; reinforcing metal or filler is added to glass ionomer to make it strong enough. Added metal tints the material dark gray and the heavily filled material is generally tinted blue, so this form of glass ionomer is never used for esthetic direct restorations.

KEY POINTS

✓ Composite, glass ionomer and blends of the two are used as esthetic direct restoration materials.

✓ All are polymers that bond to the tooth and decrease microleakage.

✓ Composites are strong, translucent, polishable and can be used to restore all classes of cavity preparations, but are subject to wear, discoloration and loss of marginal integrity.

✓ Glass ionomer is useful where moisture control is difficult, chewing forces are minimal and fluoride diffusion is desired.

✓ Composite products with a variety of options are available.
  • Flowable, conventional or packable viscosity
  • Fillers of different sizes and opacities
  • One-paste light cured systems in disposable multidose syringes or unit dose compules
  • Two-paste self- or dual cured systems

✓ Restoration placement procedure—etch, prime, bond, fill, finish. Newer materials may combine some or all of the etch–prime–bond steps.

✓ Curing lights should be assessed for efficiency at least weekly.

✓ Hold curing light as close to material as possible, but not touching, during curing procedures.
  • Protect eyes by wearing tinted safety glasses when curing.

✓ Glass ionomer set is not complete for approximately 24 hours.
  • Glass ionomer material should be protected with a glass ionomer varnish or a thin coat of bonding agent until set is complete.

✓ Once set, glass ionomer is nearly insoluble in oral fluids and leaches fluoride, but is opaque and readily wears.

SELF TEST

Questions 1–12: *Select the letter preceding the best answer.*

1. This is the material of choice for Class V restorations where biting forces are absent and moisture control is difficult.
   a. Composite
   b. Compomer
   c. Glass ionomer

2. Which type of composite has the lowest viscosity?
   a. Condensable
   b. Flowable
   c. Packable
   d. Conventional

3. A limit on the amount of filler that can be included in a composite is set by the
   a. Agent used to link filler and matrix
   b. Type of matrix cure employed
   c. Filler particle size and amount
   d. Both *a* and *c*
   e. All of the above

4. Given filler size, polishability would logically be expected to be greatest for a _____ composite.
   a. Conventional
   b. Microfilled

5. Free fluoride is available to leach into adjacent tooth structure from set glass ionomer material because of the type of _____ the powder contains.
   a. Filler
   b. Repeating polymer molecule
   c. Bonding agent

6. Composite materials are used for _____ in addition to direct restorations.
   a. Core buildups
   b. Veneers
   c. Sealants
   d. Both *a* and *c*
   e. All of the above

7. All of the esthetic direct restorative materials can adhere mechanically to the tooth and chemically to other polymers. Only esthetic direct materials containing glass ionomer bond chemically to tooth structure.
   a. Both statements above are true.
   b. The first statement above is true; the second is false.
   c. The first statement above is false; the second is true.
   d. Both statements above are false.

8. This class of restoration requires the _____ of _____ material.
   a. Polishability; composite
   b. Strength; composite
   c. Flow; glass ionomer
   d. Fluoride release; glass ionomer

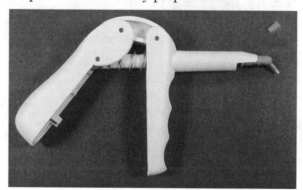

9. How will the material in this container be placed in the cavity preparation?
   a. Ejected from this syringe tip
   b. Injected through a cannula
   c. With a hand instrument

10. Composite material packaged in a single container will be
    a. Chemically cured.
    b. Light cured.
    c. Dual cured.
    d. Either *a* or *b*.
    e. Either *b* or *c*.

11. Why does it matter that there is a limit on the amount and type of filler that can be incorporated into a composite material?
    a. Less polymer creates a better bond to calcium.
    b. Less polymer enables better color matching.
    c. More filler enables better material flow.
    d. More filler creates a stronger material.

12. The catalog from which you will be ordering esthetic direct restorative materials lists five types of composite: packable, flowable, microfil, hybrid, and small particle. What should you order for anterior restorations if your dentist employer prefers to use only one material?
    a. Packable
    b. Flowable
    c. Microfill
    d. Hybrid

Questions 13–17: *Discuss each concept listed below.*

13. The relative usefulness of composite and glass ionomer for Class II, IV and V restorations

14. The relationship of amount and type of filler to the ability to create a high shine on a composite restoration

15. The role of itaconic acid in formation of a glass ionomer polymer

16. How curing shrinkage can be controlled

17. How the translucency or opacity of an esthetic direct restorative material relates to the naturalness of its appearance

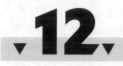

NON-ESTHETIC DIRECT RESTORATION MATERIALS

This chapter discusses the following topics:

1. Materials used
2. Amalgam
   a. Definition
   b. Type of material
   c. Uses
   d. Mechanism of action
   e. Placement procedure
   f. Clinical concerns
      i. Safety
      ii. Material selection and preparation
      iii. Prevention of microleakage
      iv. Fracture
3. Reinforced zinc oxide and eugenol
   a. Definition
   b. Type of material
   c. Use
   d. Preparation
   e. Mechanism of action
   f. Clinical concerns
      i. Replication of tooth anatomy
      ii. Assessment of tooth response

OBJECTIVES

After studying this chapter, you should be able to:

1. Discuss amalgam alloy, including available types, composition and selection.
2. Describe amalgam uses, preparation, placement and setting reaction.
3. Describe safe amalgam use and disposal.
4. Discuss prevention of restoration and tooth fracture when amalgam is used.
5. Describe the uses, preparation, mechanisms of action and clinical concerns related to zinc oxide and eugenol temporary restorative material.

Only one nonesthetic material is commonly used for permanent direct restorations: amalgam. Two materials are used for temporary direct restorations: acrylic resin and reinforced zinc oxide and eugenol (Z-O-E). Z-O-E, which is not esthetic, is used for temporary direct restorations and is discussed in this chapter. Acrylic is an esthetic material used for temporary coverage of teeth that have been prepared for an indirect restoration. It will be discussed with indirect restorations in Section IV.

▼ AMALGAM ▼

Definition

Amalgam is a mixture of silver, copper, tin and sometimes zinc or a small amount of other metals with mercury.

Type of Material

Amalgam is a metal alloy.

Uses

Nonesthetic direct restorations
Core buildups
Retrograde restorations (Figure 12-1): A *retrograde restoration* is an amalgam restoration placed from the root end of a tooth following an apicoectomy. An *apicoectomy* is surgical removal of the apical portion of a tooth root.

Mechanism of Action

Mercury is a metal that is liquid at room temperature. When mixed with alloy particles, it dissolves their outer layers. The metal ions in solution then recombine to form a mercury–silver background matrix with particle cores scattered throughout. The cores serve as reinforcers.

Procedure for Placing an Amalgam Restoration

The tooth is prepared and isolated. Amalgam is mixed in an amalgamator (Figure 12-2), placed in an amalgam well or disposable cloth (Figure 12-3), loaded into an amalgam car-

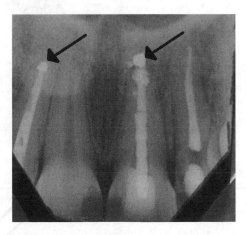

FIGURE 12-1 Retrograde fillings. Radiograph of two retrograde amalgams (shown by the arrows). Notice the amalgam is more dense than the other items in the radiograph.

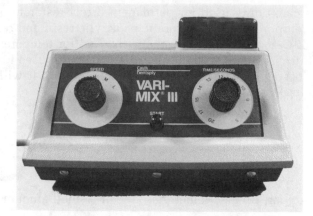

FIGURE 12-2 Amalgamator. The machines can be used to mix other materials that come in capsules also.

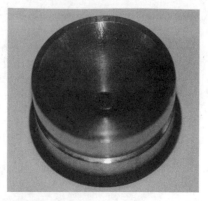

FIGURE 12-3 Amalgam well. The sloped sides cause the amalgam to fall to the base where it can be picked up more easily.

rier (Figure 12-4), inserted into the cavity preparation, then condensed, carved and burnished with hand instruments. *Condensing* (Figure 12-5) is pushing into position with heavy pressure, actually causing the material to be denser. *Carving* is sculpting to correct shape and *burnishing* is hand polishing. Before the patient is dismissed, occlusion and contacts of the new restoration are checked and any remaining stray bits of amalgam removed.

Clinical Concerns

Clinical concerns include safety, material selection and preparation, prevention of microleakage and fracture.

Safety

Mercury is a hazardous material. It is liquid at room temperature and vaporizes at slightly above that level. It can be inhaled, ingested or cross the skin or mucous membrane. In the body, it can cause a wide variety of gastrointestinal, neurological, oral and other disturbances.

There are two basic types of mercury: organic and inorganic. The inorganic type used in dentistry is by far the less toxic. Although dental personnel do not use large amounts of mercury at one time, we frequently use small amounts. This leaves us vulnerable to chronic mercury poisoning. Some of the symptoms of mercury poisoning are gingival soreness, in-

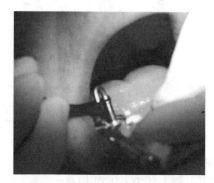

FIGURE 12-4 Amalgam carrier. The carrier is used to place the amalgam in the preparation.

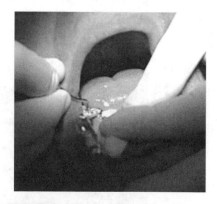

FIGURE 12-5 Condensing amalgam. The condensation is done with a plugger and plenty of pressure.

creased salivation, fetid breath, tooth loosening, abdominal cramping, and diarrhea. Chronic exposure can cause irreversible neurological damage. Risk is greatly reduced by using mercury correctly.

Safety Precautions

- Use disposable, preloaded capsules of mercury and alloy
- Wear mask, gloves, safety glasses and lab coat
- Use a no-touch technique
- Close the cover on an amalgam triturator before activating it
- Use high-volume suction to evacuate
  - excess mercury that rises to the surface when amalgam is being condensed
  - bits of excess amalgam left from carving procedures
  - mercury fumes that arise when old amalgam restorations are being ground away
- Seal contaminated disposable items and scrap amalgam in plastic bags and use regulated waste carrier to collect it periodically
- Retrieve amalgam from dental unit water line traps on a regular basis and discard as described above
- Using a mercury spill kit, clean spills immediately
  - hand vacuum into a plastic bag or absorb with commercial mercury-absorb products
  - do *not* sweep or use regular vacuum
  - seal disposable cleanup items in a plastic bag, then store and discard as regulated waste
- Dispose of mercury-contaminated items through a reputable hazardous waste contractor

Material Selection

Composition of Alloy. Amalgam alloys are mixtures of varying amounts of silver, tin, copper, and sometimes zinc or small amounts of other metals. The user selects from among zinc, nonzinc, conventional and high-copper types.

Zinc alloys contain approximately 1% zinc; *nonzinc alloys,* none. Zinc adds plasticity to an amalgam mix, thereby making it easier to push into all areas of the cavity preparation. If zinc-containing alloys are contaminated with moisture during placement, the zinc may cause the amalgam to enlarge excessively as the amalgam sets. Complete setting requires several days. Thus overenlargement may not be immediately apparent and is referred to as *delayed expansion.*

Expansion beyond the cavity preparation walls leaves unsupported amalgam that is prone to edge fracture. Thus moisture contamination leaves the restoration weaker and the restoration prone to fractures. These fractures create a visible space at the restoration margin, a process termed *ditching.* This leaves the tooth vulnerable to increased microleakage and secondary caries.

Enlargement in the body of the restoration, where the material is confined within hard tooth walls, places uncomfortable pressure on the walls and moves the fluid in adjacent dentin tubules. Fluid movement results in pain. Accordingly, zinc-containing amalgams must be placed in a dry environment. This is not to say that zinc-free amalgam should be placed in a wet area either, as all moisture incorporated into amalgam weakens it.

High copper alloys contain a minimum of 13% copper and have better compressive strength than *conventional alloys,* which contain 4–5% copper. When the silver and tin particles in conventional alloys are dissolved in mercury, tin combines with silver to create silver–tin particles, and silver combines with mercury to create a silver–mercury background matrix. When the same chemicals plus the extra copper in high copper alloys are dissolved, the silver–mercury matrix is again formed and the copper combines partly with tin and partly with silver and tin. The resulting copper–tin and silver–copper–tin compounds are much stronger than the silver–tin formed in conventional amalgams.

Copper is also less vulnerable to electrochemical assault. High copper amalgams are not only stronger, they are also less likely to tarnish and corrode. Corrosion weakens material. High copper amalgams, then, are stronger to begin with and less likely to weaken during use.

Mercury–Alloy Ratio. More mercury is needed for preparation and handling of amalgam than is needed for setting. This means *excess mercury* is present in the mixed, unset amalgam. As the operator condenses amalgam into the cavity preparation, this excess mercury rises to the surface and needs to be removed with a high volume evacuator.

Free mercury is hazardous. Set amalgam is not, for nearly all the mercury in a set restoration is bound to other metals. Operators aim to keep the amount of excess mercury as low as possible and still have a workable mix. This can be accomplished by using only slightly more mercury than is needed for setting, that is, a less than 1:1 ratio of mercury to alloy.

Shape of Alloy Particles. Two basic particle shapes, lathe cut and spherical, are used to make three types of alloys: lathe cut, spherical and admixed. *Lathe cut alloys* are made by grinding a solid metal alloy bar on a rotating lathe. This creates rough, irregular particles, termed *filings,* of various sizes. *Spherical alloys* are made by spraying molten alloy into a vacuum and letting the drops fall. Gravity rounds the drops into balls as they descend. *Admixed alloys* contain mixtures of lathe cut and spherical particles.

The shape of alloy particles is important because it determines what size condenser the operator will need for pushing soft amalgam into a cavity preparation and affects the strength of the finished restoration.

Remember that particle cores and newly formed particles are in the mixed amalgam mass. The operator needs to condense the material into the cavity preparation by hand. If he or she pushes hard on spherical particles with a small condenser, the instrument will slide between the spheres rather than pushing them down. Think of a jar full of peanut M&M® candies and your finger. If you push your finger hard into the jar of fairly spherical M&Ms, it will go right through to the bottom; the candies will not be pushed down at all. On the other hand, if you used the palm of your hand the larger size of your palm would push them down rather than sliding through. The operator who is using spherical particles has the same sort of problem and needs a large-size condenser.

Irregular lathe cut filings, either alone or in admixed alloys, can be pushed down with a smaller condenser. Think about a box filled with twigs of all sizes and shapes. If you tried to push your finger through them, it wouldn't work very well. Your finger would keep getting caught on the irregular shapes unless you moved it around in several directions. Your finger, then, pushes the twigs down. When an operator pushes down on the irregular shapes of lathe-cut particles, they react similarly. Even a small condenser gets caught on the particles and pushes them down.

Most alloys sold today are spherical or admixed, not solely lathe cut. Why? The spherical particles serve as reinforcers. The spherical particles are regular in shape, thus can be more closely packed. Closely packed particles provide more reinforcement in the same amount of space. Since amalgam is chosen where strength is needed, the increased strength is desirable.

Material Preparation

The operator needs to condense the amalgam into all areas of the cavity preparation, including any undercuts that may be present. A sufficiently plastic mix is needed to accomplish this. Amalgam mixing, termed *trituration,* is carefully controlled to ensure appropriate plasticity.

Amalgam is packaged in premeasured capsules. Capsules containing different amounts of material are the same size, but color coded to indicate which is which. Dental personnel refer to the sizes as a *single-, double-,* or *triple-spill mix.* This terminology is a remnant of the days when mercury and powder were measured by pushing a plunger on a mercury–powder container that allowed a roughly standard amount of each material to spill into a reusable capsule held underneath it. This type of measurement is no longer used, but the one-spill, two-spill terminology remains. In fact, the premeasured double-spill capsule only contains 1½ times as much material as the single spill. The three-spill capsule contains twice as much as the single.

The manufacturer suggests the number of seconds that each type of mix should be triturated in a particular model machine. The amalgamator is set on the appropriate speed and number of seconds, and the capsule shaken for the full time. A single capsule of material may not fill the larger cavity preparations, but larger mixes set before they can be completely placed. If more amalgam is needed, additional mixes are made rather than using larger batches.

Mixed amalgam should be one mass, shiny, and should squeak when pushed into the carrier. If it is dull and wet, it was overmixed; if dry and crumbly, it was undermixed (Figure 12-6). A poor mix is unusable and should be thrown out. Make a new mix; never try to correct a poor one.

Assistants and hygienists should be aware that some premeasured capsules are just duds. Not every poor mix is due to poor trituration; some are from incorrect capsule loading. When a poor mix occurs, observe what happens when you throw it out and make a new one. If the second mix is good, the first capsule was probably a dud. If several mixes are poor, the problem is likely to be due to a problem at the office, usually incorrect amalgamator timing or speed.

Prevention of Microleakage

Amalgam does not bond directly to tooth structure. This means microleakage will exist at the restoration margin unless steps are taken to control it. One step is taken by nature. Amalgam, as a metal, is subject to tarnish and corrosion. As a restoration corrodes, fragments drift into the adjacent microspace and ultimately fill it. This self-sealing process may take months to years, especially with high copper alloys that corrode very little, if at all.

Some operators bond the amalgam to the tooth surface. This effectively seals the area and prevents microleakage. Generally a dual-cure bonding agent is placed in the cavity preparation, then the amalgam is condensed into position over it while the bonding material is still wet. However, the bonding agent does not bind to amalgam as strongly as it will bind to composite. The other problem with this technique is that when the amalgam is condensed the bonding agent is pushed up into the amalgam, weakening it.

Other operators prefer not to bond to the amalgam but rather use the bonding agent as a sealer. The bonding material is placed in the cavity preparation and cured, sealing the dentin tubules. There might still be microleakage between the amalgam and the bonding material, but the tooth itself is sealed. This should eliminate postoperative sensitivity.

In the past most operators sealed the dentin tubules with varnish to prevent diffusion of unwanted ions and microorgansims toward the pulp during the time required for self-sealing to occur. Varnishes were covered in Chapter 10 and their limitations were discussed there.

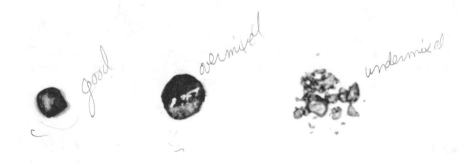

FIGURE 12-6 Amalgam. The amalgam on the left was triturated properly, the middle one is too wet, and the right side too dry.

When varnish is applied, an insulating base may be placed as well. Amalgam, a metal, is a good thermal conductor. Sharp temperature changes relayed to the interior of the tooth expand and contract fluid in the dentin tubules, stimulating the pulpal nerve endings that register pain. To prevent this, a material that conducts heat and cold poorly is placed between the restoration and the tooth as an insulating base. The base provides a physical barrier to rapid thermal transfer, thereby reducing the fluid movement and resulting pain. These materials were also covered in Chapter 10.

Prevention of Fracture

Amalgam creeps; it flows after set. If it creeps over an unsupported area, such as a microspace at the margin, the restoration edges may fracture. Amalgam is also subject to corrosion. As restoration edges corrode, they weaken, disintegrate and fracture. Clinicians are familiar with amalgam *ditching* (Figure 12-7), the presence of a visible open area around an amalgam restoration. Ditching is the end result of a complex process that assaults amalgam with fluids, ions, electrochemical attack and chewing forces. Creep and corrosion contribute to the process.

Amalgam restorations may fracture for other reasons. Insulating bases placed underneath it are weaker than the amalgam itself; poorly supported restorations are prone to fracture. Large amalgam restorations that are not bonded to the tooth do not transfer occlusal forces to the surrounding tooth well; these restorations may also weaken and fracture. Insufficient bulk of material in any area may cause fracture. Bonding an amalgam restoration to the tooth creates a single, stronger unit from its three parts—restoration, bonding agent, and tooth—but amalgam bonds are not strong.

The restoration is not always what fractures; teeth break too. When a large amalgam restoration is placed, there may be insufficient tooth structure to support it and the tooth may fracture. Amalgam also has a much higher coefficient of thermal expansion than tooth structure, and repeated pulling and pushing on the tooth as the amalgam expands and contracts may weaken and break the tooth.

Overall, the dental profession considers amalgam to be a safe, inexpensive, effective restorative material for areas that require strength but not esthetics. Patients, however, are not necessarily convinced that it is safe. Television and print media have presented material that casts doubt on amalgam safety, suggesting that it may be linked to development of systemic disease. Patients are concerned that it may cause or worsen multiple sclerosis, cancer, arthritis and a host of other problems. It is important to note that responsible health organizations have found *no* link between mercury and any of these diseases. Although some mercury does escape from the restorations over time, it is not in quantities that the body cannot effectively eliminate.

What is known is that dental amalgam contributes to the mercury load in the environment. Amalgam from dental unit waste lines enters public sewage systems and eventually ends up in our lakes, streams and soil. Dental assistants and hygienists should clean unit waste line traps of amalgam scrap on a regular basis, store it properly, then dispose of it through a reputable regulated waste contractor. Units are available to remove amalgam from suction lines. Of course, this amalgam needs to be disposed of properly. The American Dental Association and other responsible health, manufacturing and governmental bodies are cooperating on continued research in the field.

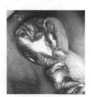

FIGURE 12-7 Ditching. Notice the large gap between the amalgam and the tooth.

▼ REINFORCED ZINC OXIDE AND EUGENOL TEMPORARY RESTORATIVE MATERIAL ▼

Definition

Metal oxide powder and oil of cloves liquid. This is a different form of the same material that is used in an intermediary capacity for bases and liners.

Type of Material

Reinforced cement

Use

Temporary restorations

Procedure

Powder and liquid are available in pure form in separate containers, as a component of base and catalyst pastes and in preloaded capsules.

Powder and Liquid

Fluff powder, proportion onto a paper pad, and divide it into one half and two quarters. Proportion liquid drops. Quickly and thoroughly incorporate the powder half, then each quarter, into the liquid.

Oil of cloves is sticky. Many operators prefer that a small amount of extra powder be available for coating the placement instrument so the mixed material will not stick to it.

Base and Catalyst Paste in Tubes

Place equal lengths in close proximity on a paper pad. Mix quickly with rotary motion until the material is homogenous in color and consistency.

Premeasured Capsule

Activate at speed and for number of seconds recommended by the manufacturer.

Mechanisms of Action

Irritation of the Pulp

Irritated cells in the pulp accelerate their production of dentin to protect themselves. Newly formed dentin increases the thickness of the insulating layer between the pulp and the material. The net effect is soothing to the tooth.

Form and Function Maintenance

A temporary restoration protects cut tissue and maintains the anatomy of a prepared tooth until a busy dentist is able to see the patient or while an inlay is being made.

Clinical Concerns

Clinical concerns include accurate replication of the normal tooth anatomy and assessment of tooth response to the restoration.

Anatomy

Allied dental personnel place many temporary restorations. Care must be taken to ensure the cavity is completely filled and there are no overhangs or occlusal high spots. Incomplete coverage results in open margins and microleakage. Material overhangs create plaque traps. Occlusal high spots can result in inflammation of the periodontal ligament.

Assessment of Tooth Response

If pulp irritation is the motivation for placement, then pulp quieting will be the principal assessment concern. Quieting may take some weeks and the patient may be seen more than once for assessment.

If form and function maintenance is the placement motivation, then time available in the dentist's schedule or arrival of the indirect restoration will signal successful termination of the procedure.

The student should understand that pulp quieting, and form and function maintenance, are not mutually exclusive concerns. Form and function maintenance are necessary while a pulp quiets.

Regardless of placement motivation, patients need to understand that the Z-O-E temporary will not be as strong as a final restoration. If large pieces, or the entire restoration, are lost the patient should contact the practice to arrange for professional examination of the area.

KEY POINTS

✓ Amalgam is inexpensive, easy to use, and strong, but not esthetic.
✓ It is used for direct restorations, retrograde restorations and core buildups.
✓ High copper alloys are stronger and less likely to weaken during use.
✓ Mercury is toxic and must be handled and disposed of properly.
✓ Amalgam restorations
  • creep, ditch, corrode, fracture, and may contribute to tooth fracture.
  • prevent microleakage by self-sealing over time.
  • whether amalgam should be bonded or the tooth varnished and a base placed to protect it while waiting for self-sealing to occur is controversial.
✓ The safety of amalgam restorations is
  • of concern to patients who are aware of media presentations implying it causes or contributes to an array of chronic diseases.
  • well researched, and supported by responsible dentists and dental organizations.
✓ Reinforced zinc oxide and eugenol is used for temporary restorations.
✓ It maintains tooth form and function while the patient is waiting for an appointment with the dentist, an inlay to be made or a pulp to quiet down.

SELF TEST

Questions 1–5: *Provide the short answers requested.*

1. Why would an operator choose amalgam for a direct restoration?

2. Suggest a reason for choosing each of the available types of amalgam alloy.

3. When amalgam alloy and mercury are mixed, what happens?

4. What mechanisms are available for the operator to prevent microleakage around an amalgam restoration?

5. What can the operator do to lessen the chance of fracture when a tooth is restored with amalgam?

Questions 6–10: *Select the letter preceding the best answer.*

6. Define *trituration*.
   a. Proportioning
   b. Pushing into position
   c. Sculpting to shape
   d. Mixing by shaking

7. A zinc oxide and eugenol restoration may be placed to provide
   a. Strength.
   b. Esthetics.
   c. Healing time.
   d. All of the above.

8. Amalgam is placed over a bonding agent when the agent is
   a. Wet.
   b. Firm.
   c. Clear.
   d. Wrinkled.

9. Overmixed amalgam is
   a. Dry and crumbly.
   b. Wet and dull.
   c. Shiny and squeaky.

10. How can mercury enter the body?
    a. Inhalation
    b. Ingestion
    c. Through the conjunctiva
    d. Across the skin
    e. All of the above

SECTION IV

Materials for Indirect Restorations

When a material requires processing that cannot be completed in the mouth, any restoration constructed using it must be made outside the mouth and cemented or bonded in place. Such items are indirect restorations, and a number of different materials are used in their construction. An understanding of the basic fabrication process helps to put these materials in perspective.

The tooth is prepared, and a precise impression and occlusal registration are made. The impression and bite are sent to a dental laboratory, accompanied by a laboratory prescription specifying what is desired in the finished product. Because the patient will not receive the restoration immediately, the tooth must be temporarily covered to maintain its form and function until the permanent restoration is available. At the laboratory, a technician pours a highly accurate model and constructs a restoration to meet the dentist's specifications, finishes and polishes it, and returns it to the office or clinic. The dentist then tries it on the tooth preparation, makes any indicated adjustments, provides a final polish and cements or bonds it in position.

There is variation in how dentists complete the precise impression step. Some dentists take a preliminary impression with alginate, then an office staff member or a dental laboratory technician constructs a custom tray. This tray is then used to take a precise final impression. Other dentists omit the preliminary alginate impression, model pouring and custom tray fabrication. They use a stock impression tray with a firm material in the tray and a thinner material on the preparation or a dual impression tray technique that allows one to take a simultaneous final impression and occlusal registration.

This section discusses the materials used in the indirect restoration process: custom tray materials, final impression materials, materials for temporary coverage, materials for the restorations themselves, and cements used for attaching these restorations to teeth.

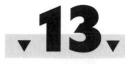

IMPRESSION TRAYS

OBJECTIVES

At studying this chapter, you should be able to:

1. Differentiate stock and custom trays.
2. Select a tray for use in a specified procedure.
3. Identify materials used to make custom trays.
4. Describe custom tray fabrication techniques.

▼ DEFINITION ▼

Stock tray — one purchased ready-made from the manufacturer
Custom tray — one made specifically to fit an individual patient

▼ USES ▼

Stock trays — all types of impressions
Custom trays — very accurate final impressions

▼ TYPES ▼

For a single arch:

Full arch tray (Figure 13-1) — covers entire arch
Quadrant tray (Figure 13-2) — also termed a *posterior tray;* covers half an arch (one quadrant of the mouth)
Sextant (Figure 13-3) — also termed an *anterior tray;* covers canine to canine (one-third of an arch; one-sixth of the mouth)

For both arches:

Dual impression tray (Figure 13-4) — also termed a *triple tray*
Bite tray (Figure 13-5) — records occlusion

▼ MATERIALS USED ▼

Polymer sheets (Figure 13-6)
Polystyrene beads (Figure 13-7)
Light cured polymer (Figure 13-8)
Self-cured resin

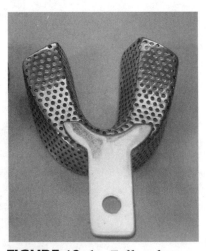

FIGURE 13-1 Full arch tray. This is a lower tray. The upper tray covers the palate.

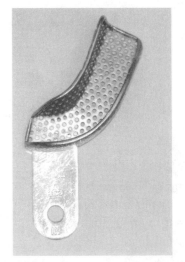

FIGURE 13-2 Quadrant tray. This tray obviously will only cover one half of the arch.

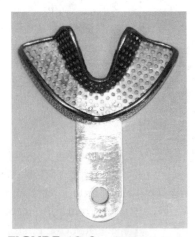

FIGURE 13-3 Sextant tray. This tray will only take an impression of the anterior sextant.

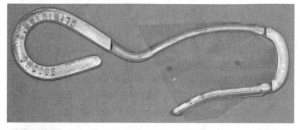

FIGURE 13-4 Triple tray. Note how much this looks like the bite tray in Figure 13-5, but it is made of metal and therefore much stiffer.

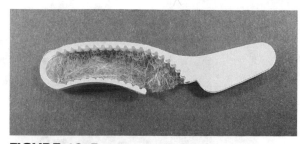

FIGURE 13-5 Bite tray. The thin gauze holds the material while allowing the teeth to come together.

▼ ITEMS MADE ▼

Sheets — used for custom trays, bleaching trays, athletic mouthguards
Beads, light cured polymer, and self-cured resin — used for custom trays

▼ SELECTION OF MATERIAL ▼

Which material is chosen depends partly on the task to be accomplished and partly on the operator's preference. *Custom trays* can be fabricated using any of the materials, and different operators find they have more success with one material than another. *Custom trays* need to be stiff, and are fabricated from light cured materials; polystyrene beads; thick, stiff polymer sheets; or rolled resin dough with sufficient thickness not to flex when impression material is inserted.

Some other dental appliances are also formed using some of the same materials. These include custom *athletic mouthguards* that are made with a thick sheet of relatively soft and flexible material, often vinyl acrylic, which absorbs and distributes forces well. Custom *bleaching trays* are fabricated with thinner but still flexible polymer sheets, again often vinyl acrylic, for case of insertion and removal.

▼ CUSTOM TRAY PROCEDURE ▼

In order to make a custom tray, an alginate impression must be taken and a gypsum model poured. If needed, a spacer and stops are made (discussed in the next section of this chap-

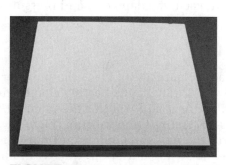

FIGURE 13-6 Polymer sheet. These sheets are very stiff plastic.

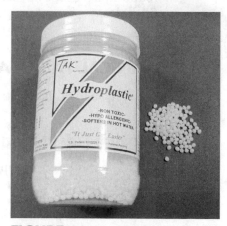

FIGURE 13-7 Polystyrene beads. These are very easy to use but the resulting tray can be difficult to trim.

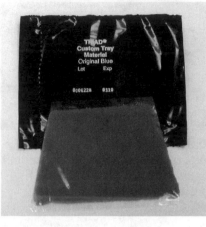

FIGURE 13-8 Light cured material. This material must be kept in the black pouch or the room light will cause it to set.

ter). The custom tray is then fabricated. During the fabrication process, the dentist may want small holes placed in the body of the tray with a lab bur to relieve pressure as the impression is taken. This allows the material to flow through to the outside, lessening the chance that the tray will flex as the impression is taken. Should the tray flex outward and then return to its original shape when the impression is removed from the mouth, the resulting model will be distorted. Perforations also help mechanically interlock the set material and tray. Following fabrication, a completed custom tray is always cleaned, disinfected, and replaced on the model. All types of custom trays may be scrubbed with soap and water and immersed in disinfectant solution.

Custom trays that will be used with rubber impression materials (discussed in the next chapter) must be painted with rubber base adhesive before use. This coating must dry completely prior to taking the impression.

Spacers and Stops. Custom trays that are used for some types of final impressions need a spacer and stops. This allows for a sufficient bulk of impression material to capture all the detail without ripping.

A *spacer* is a layer of wax between the model and the tray. It saves space for impression material. If the tray were tightly adapted to the teeth on the model, there would be no room left for impression material.

Stops are small projections of material into the space on the tissue, or inner, side of the tray. Their purpose is to stop it from being seated too deeply during the impression procedure. If the stops were not present, the operator could push the tray too far in and end up with no impression material between the tray and the tissue. Stops are made by cutting round holes in the spacer with a warm spatula or lab knife, then pushing tray material into the holes.

▼ MECHANICAL FABRICATION TECHNIQUES ▼

Two mechanical fabrication techniques are used: vacuum adaptation and pressure forming.

Vacuum Adaptation

Place the model in the middle of the flat surface (Figure 13-9). Place the polymer sheet in the open frame and lock it in position (Figure 13-10). Swing the heating element into position directly over the polymer sheet. Activate the heat and wait for the material to soften evenly and sag just below the frame (Figure 13-11) Activate the vacuum (Figure 13-12), deactivate heat, and quickly lower the frame over the model, being careful not to touch the heating element. The heating element can then be swung out of the way. Wait 30 seconds and deactivate the vacuum. Let model and tray cool prior to removing the tray from model. Trim to shape with scissors or heat (Figure 13-13).

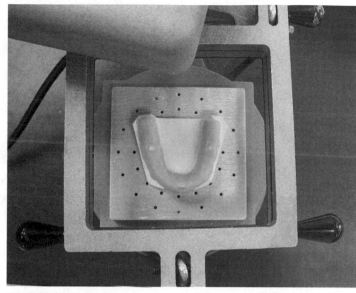

FIGURE 13-9 Vacuum former. The more holes uncovered the better the vacuum can work on the polymer. Note also the holes made for stops.

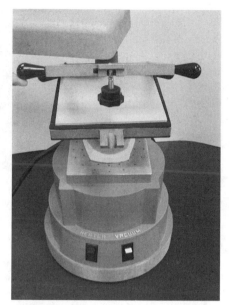

FIGURE 13-10 Placing sheet in frame. Care must be taken to square the sheet in the frame so it doesn't pull out and ruin the vacuum.

Pressure Forming

Pressure forming is not very different from vacuum forming. The only difference is that rather than the material being pulled down over the model it is pushed down on top of it. The machine will have a timer for heating the material and use the office air pressure to push a piston down onto the model. The advantage of this approach is that with large bulky models a vacuum is not always effective in pulling the material completely down onto the model because there is no path for the vacuum to exert force on it. The pressure former will exert even force everywhere.

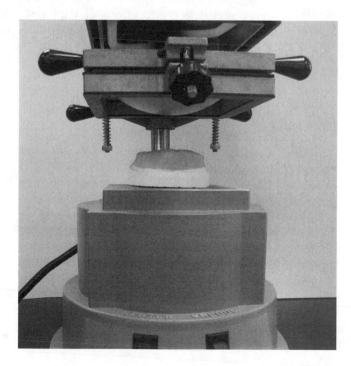

FIGURE 13-11 Softening sheet. See how the once-stiff sheet sags when warmed.

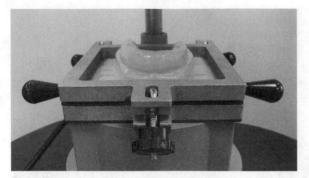

FIGURE 13-12 Adapting sheet. The vacuum has pulled the sheet tightly over the model.

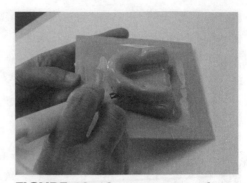

FIGURE 13-13 Trimming. The heat trimmer can be used after the tray cools. Scissors require use prior to the materials becoming cool and hardening.

Hand Molding

Three types of hand molded trays are made: polystyrene bead, light-cured polymer, and rolled acrylic dough. The first step for each process is construction of a spacer and stops if necessary. Many operators choose to make three stops in a full tray, two in a quadrant tray. To avoid interference with tissue detail recording, stops are always placed away from the tooth of interest.

▼ POLYSTYRENE BEAD TECHNIQUE ▼

Polystyrene beads are thermoplastic. One-half scoop of beads is recommended for a quadrant tray and a full scoop for a full arch tray. The operator may choose to adjust these amounts based on whether the arch is maxillary or mandibular and its overall size.

Place a thin coat of lubricant on the spacer. Soften the beads in warm water (Figure 13-14), gather material into one mass, and knead it to homogenous consistency. Form the mass into a flattened shape that approximates but is slightly longer front-to-back than the area of interest on the model. Adapt the material to the model and push it into the holes in the spacer to form stops. Adapt the excess material anteriorly to form a flat, smooth handle (Figure 13-15). Smooth the tray edges. When the material has cured sufficiently to be handled lightly without deformation, remove and discard the spacer. Readapt the tray to the model, using light pressure so as to maintain the space for impression material. Allow the material to cool completely. If the tray is not quite right, the material can be reheated and readapted.

▼ LIGHT-CURED POLYMER TECHNIQUE ▼

This material is supplied in strips and preformed arch shapes. Paint the spacer with a thin layer of lubricant to facilitate later spacer removal. Adapt the material to the model and spacer holes, then trim as indicated (Figure 13-16). Cure lightly, remove from the light box and remove the spacer. Paint the tray with the supplied air barrier coating (Figure 13-17). Place the model back in the light box and complete the cure according to the manufacturer's directions (Figure 13-18). Although the material is light cured it will be quite hot on removal so it needs to be allowed to cool prior to trimming, smoothing and polishing. Scrub away any remaining air barrier coating as necessary.

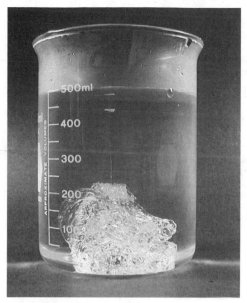

FIGURE 13-14 Melting beads. You know the beads are ready when they become translucent and cling together.

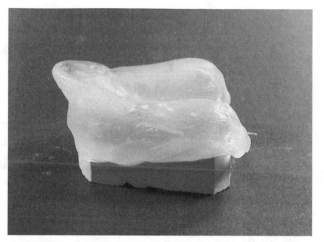

FIGURE 13-15 Polystyrene tray. Notice how you can see the spacer wax underneath the still-warm tray. This is the time to neaten the edges.

▼ ROLLED ACRYLIC DOUGH TECHNIQUE ▼

The acrylic tray material is self-cured acrylic and therefore consists of a monomer liquid and a polymer powder. It sometimes contains fillers for stiffness. To make an acrylic custom tray, the model is prepared as for the other materials. The material is then measured and mixed according to the manufacturer's directions. Make sure to recover the monomer immediately after pouring as the fumes are hazardous. Another caution is that the acrylic monomer will seep into paper so it is important to use a waxed paper or glass cup for this material. Most offices use wooden tongue depressors to mix the material. This makes cleanup easier as the material shrinks onto metal spatulas, making it difficult to remove from them.

As the material starts to polymerize, it will go through four stages prior to setting: runny, sticky, doughy and stiff. Once the material has passed through the first two stages it is placed on a lubricated board and flattened with a rolling pin. The board has an indentation of fixed depth between two ridges, which keeps the thickness of the material consistent from tray to tray.

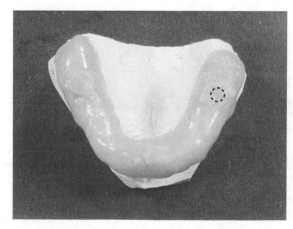

FIGURE 13-16 Stops. A dotted line has been added to this picture to demonstrate stop size, shape and placement. If you look carefully, you can see a completed stop, into which the tray material has been pushed.

Rolled Acrylic Dough Technique **159**

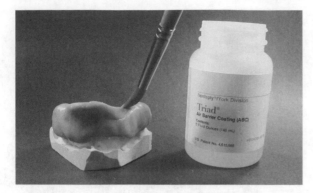

FIGURE 13-17 Air barrier coating. This coating gets rid of the air-inhibited layer.

At this point the material is lifted off the rolling board and draped lightly over the model. Adapt it very lightly to the model, trim off the extra material, use it to make a handle and attach it to the tray.

While setting the material will get very hot. Once it has cooled and is hard it can be removed from the model and trimmed as necessary. These trays will continue to polymerize for many hours and as they do they still continue to shrink slightly. Since highly accurate models are the goal, rolled acrylic dough trays should not be used for impression taking for at least 24 hours after they are made.

KEY POINTS

- ✓ Both stock and custom trays are used for final impressions
- ✓ Full arch, quadrant, sextant, dual impression and bite trays are available
- ✓ Which tray type is selected depends on the use to which it will be put and the size of the area to be duplicated
- ✓ An alginate impression must be taken and a gypsum model poured before a custom tray can be fabricated
- ✓ All custom tray materials are polymers
- ✓ Which material is used depends on the thickness and flexibility needed in the completed tray, and the operator's preferences

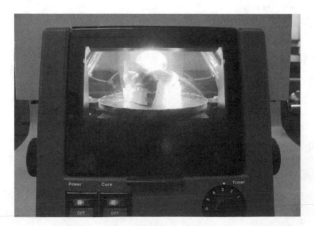

FIGURE 13-18 Light box. The platform rotates similar to a microwave oven.

✓ The following custom tray fabrication techniques are used:
  • Vacuum adaptation
  • Pressure forming
  • Hand molding of
    • polystyrene beads
    • light cured polymers
    • rolled acrylic dough
✓ Polymer sheets are vacuum adapted or pressure formed; other materials are hand molded, then self- or light cured
✓ Athletic mouthguards and bleaching trays are also made using polymer sheets and vacuum adaptation or pressure forming technique

SELF TEST

Provide the short answers requested.

1. Differentiate stock and custom trays.

2. Describe the process you would follow to make a custom tray.

3. Discuss tray selection for a final impression for a posterior three-unit bridge.

4. The dentist will be using a stock tray for a dual impression for a full crown. Indicate the type of tray you will need.

5. You are to make a bleaching tray. The patient will be treating the four maxillary incisors. What type of material will you need and what type of tray will you make?

6. You must set up for an occlusal registration procedure. How many of what type of tray will you need?

7. You will be making a quadrant custom tray with polystyrene beads. Describe what you will need to get started.

8. How will you make the bead tray?

9. Discuss why some custom trays are pierced with small holes when they are made.

10. Indicate why and how stops are sometimes made in a custom tray.

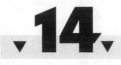

FINAL IMPRESSION MATERIALS

OBJECTIVES

After studying this chapter, you should be able to:

1. Define and state the use of final impressions.
2. Compare rubber base and hydrocolloid materials.
3. Describe how each works in the mouth.
4. Discuss the relationship of viscosity to selection of material for use.
5. Assess packaging and describe how the material in each type is prepared.
6. Describe procedures for using rubber base and hydrocolloid materials.
7. Differentiate polysulfide, polyether, silicone and vinyl polysiloxane on the basis of characteristics and handling.
8. Discuss impression disinfection.

▼ DEFINITION ▼

Materials used to take an impression for pouring an accurate working cast. Final impressions are also termed *secondary impressions* and *mucostatic impressions*.

▼ DESIRABLE CHARACTERISTICS ▼

Final impression materials must flow well, record tissues accurately, be dimensionally stable and be flexible. Flow enables the material to travel to all areas of interest to record tissue detail. Accuracy and dimensional stability enable the final restoration to fit the patient precisely. Excellent fit is possible only when a working cast is carefully made from an accurate impression. Flexibility enables the set impression to be removed from the mouth and from the set cast without damage. Tooth ridges and proximal contacts are larger than cervical areas and prepared undercuts. The set impression must stretch to slide over them, then return to its original dimensions for pouring. Once the cast is poured the material must be able to be removed without breaking the cast.

▼ MATERIALS USED ▼

Rubber bases—polysulfide, polyether, condensation silicone, addition silicone
Reversible hydrocolloid (also termed *agar*)

▼ TYPE OF MATERIAL ▼

Rubber bases—all are synthetic rubber polymers
Reversible hydrocolloid—suspension of polymer particles in water

▼ MECHANISM OF ACTION—PROCEDURE LEVEL ▼

Material hardens in and around prepared tooth to form a mold for pouring an accurate working cast.

▼ MECHANISM OF ACTION—CHEMICAL LEVEL ▼

Reversible Hydrocolloid. Just from the name, what do you already know about reversible hydrocolloid? Think back to what you learned about alginate. A hydrocolloid is a suspension of particles in a water-based solution and this type will have a reversible, therefore thermoplastic, set. It will have gel and sol phases. Suspended particles in the sol will aggregate into fibrils with water in the spaces between as the material sets to form a gel. The set material will be weak, soften when exposed to heat and harden when cooled.

Rubber Bases. Rubber bases are a group of nonaqueous, elastomeric synthetic rubber polymers. Once you know this, what else do you know about them? Think back to what you learned about polymers in the sealant chapter.

Polymers are chained monomers. They contain an initiator to start the chaining process, as well as accelerators and retarders to control its speed. Their set is chemical and irreversible. Since rubber base polymers are nonaqueous, they do not contain water. This is an advantage since they will not imbibe or release water while being stored. It is a disadvantage in that most nonaqueous materials are hydrophobic. As elastomeric polymers, they will be flexible, although the flexibility varies among materials.

Rubber base materials as a group are strong, flexible, accurate and dimensionally stable. They are far more commonly used than reversible hydrocolloid.

▼ RUBBER BASE MATERIALS ▼

Types

There are four basic types of rubber bases: *polysulfide, polyether, condensation silicones* and *addition silicones.* The condensation silicones were on the market before the addition ones and are generally known as silicones, while the addition ones are known as polyvinyl siloxanes. Although any rubber base material can be used for any type of final impression, each has advantages and disadvantages for use in specific procedures.

Clinical Concerns

Viscosity

Several different viscosities—light body, regular body, heavy body, putty and single phase—are available for use in different techniques. *Light body* has low viscosity, and *regular body,* medium viscosity. *Heavy body* and *putty* (also termed *extra heavy body*) are highly viscous. *Single phase* materials are thixotropic, so do not flow until pushed. When compressed over the teeth, single phase material flows well in the area of greatest pressure, that is, in and around the teeth, but does not flow in other areas.

The lower its viscosity, the better a material flows. The better it flows, the better its detail reproduction. Light body materials, then, are used when excellent flow is required for excellent detail reproduction. They do not provide bulk for impression handling and must be used in conjunction with high viscosity material that does.

Regular body materials provide adequate but not excellent detail and enough bulk for handling. They are used alone when detail reproduction is less critical.

Heavy body and putty materials provide bulk for easier handling. They do not record detail well and are used in conjunction with light body materials, which do.

Single phase materials combine flow around the teeth with stasis in other areas, thus provide both detail and handling ease. They are used alone.

Flexibility

All rubber base materials are relatively flexible, but there are differences among them. Polysulfide is the most flexible, polyether the least.

Packaging and Preparation

Two Tubes of Paste. Light, regular and heavy body materials may be packaged as two pastes in tubes, one containing the base material and the other the catalyst (Figure 14-1). Equal lengths of the two materials are placed close to each other on a large paper pad and a flexible, tapered spatula used for mixing. All of the catalyst is picked up at once and placed on

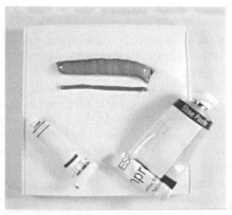

FIGURE 14-1 Tubes. Advances in packaging have made this once-common sight quite rare in the dental office.

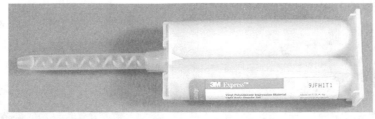

FIGURE 14-2 Cartridge. Cartridges are much easier and cleaner to use than the tubes.

top of the base. The spatula tip is moved in circles to incorporate the catalyst into the base, then the flat side of the blade used with a figure-eight motion to mix the combined materials to homogenous color and consistency. Periodically, the material is picked up and repositioned near the center of the pad to ensure that all of it is included in the mix and the mixing activity is not too close to the edge. Some brands of rubber base material include a third tube, termed *thinner,* which can be included in the mix to prolong its working time and/or thin the material.

Cartridge. Base and catalyst pastes may be packaged in separate compartments of a single cartridge (Figure 14-2). The cartridge is placed in an impression syringe and an automix tip affixed. Squeezing the syringe handle moves two plungers, forcing the materials through a spiral device in the tip that mixes them. The finished material is extruded through a hole in the tip (Figure 14-3). Because of the convenience of this method mixing pads and spatulas are rarely used at present.

Multi-use Disposable Pouches. Base and catalyst pastes may be packaged in large, polyethylene pouches (Figure 14-4). The pouches are placed in a mixing machine (Figure 14-5). A button is pushed to activate material mixing and extrusion into a tray held underneath the exit point (Figure 14-6).

Paste or Putty and Liquid. Base and catalyst materials may be packaged as one tube of paste or tub of putty and a bottle of liquid catalyst. Base paste is placed on a pad and the correct amount of catalyst dropped on the surface. Base putty is proportioned in level scoops, flattened on the pad, scored and catalyst dropped on the scored surface. The edges of the base material are folded and pressed toward the center to enclose and incorporate the liquid. The mass is then picked up and kneaded to homogenous color and consistency. This formulation is rarely seen today.

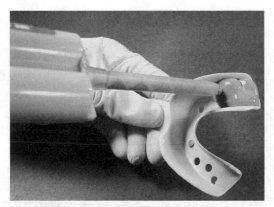

FIGURE 14-3 Filling tray. The material should be flowed into the tray in one batch to reduce voids.

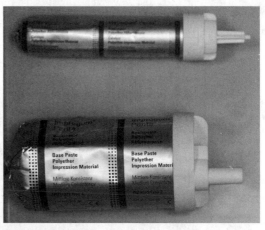

FIGURE 14-4 Pouches. This is the same material as in Figure 14-1. Notice the pouches are different sizes, just like the tubes.

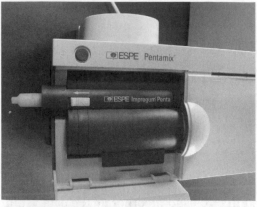

FIGURE 14-5 Loading the machine. The silver pouches are now under the covers and ready to go.

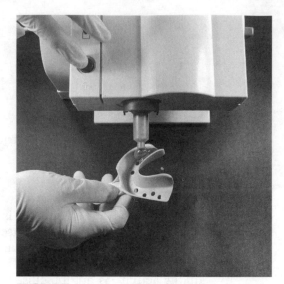

FIGURE 14-6 Filling tray. You can see how simple it is to get mixed material this way.

Two Putties. Rubber base putty is similar in consistency to Silly Putty®. Base and catalyst pastes are packaged in small round plastic tubs (Figure 14-7), and a spatula and scoop used to proportion level scoops of material. They are kneaded together until homogenous in color and consistency (Figure 14-8). The mixed material is adapted to the tray by hand (Figure 14-9).

Impression Techniques

Four basic techniques are used for rubber base impression-taking procedures: syringe, tray, putty-wash and direct placement.

Syringe Technique. In this technique light body material will be placed around the tooth using a syringe tip to get the maximum amount of detail. The light body material can be mixed by hand and placed into an impression syringe, or mixed with the automix tip and extruded directly into the syringe or by using a small extension at the end of the automix tip. The dentist then places the material around the tooth preparation(s) and a tray filled with heavier body material (heavy body or putty) is placed over it.

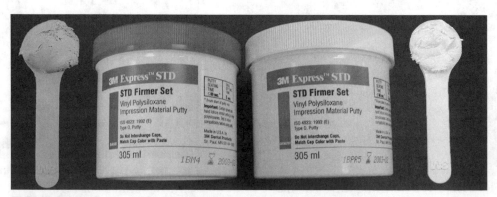

FIGURE 14-7 Putty. The contrasting colors make it easy to tell when a good mix is achieved.

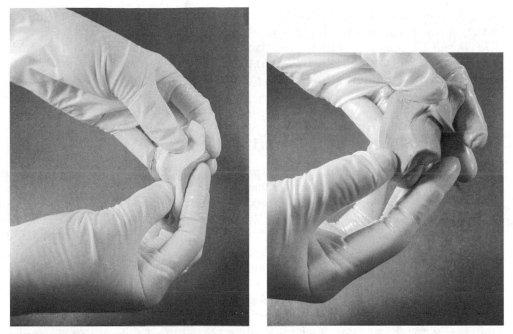

FIGURE 14-8 Mixing putty. You can see how the colors blend into a homogeneous color.

Tray Technique. Regular body material is placed in the selected tray and passed to the dentist to take the impression. This is used when great detail is not needed.

Putty-Wash Technique. The putty is mixed, placed in the selected tray and an indentation made where the tooth of interest is located. The indentation can be made either by taking an impression with the putty material or poking it with an instrument or gloved finger.

When a putty impression is taken, the material does not flow well. The teeth make a deep indentation but detail is not recorded. A second impression made with light body material is necessary to record tissue detail. The dentist may also elect to enlarge the indentation with a knife or lab bur to provide more room for the light body material in the second impression. Enlarging the indentation is termed *relieving* the impression.

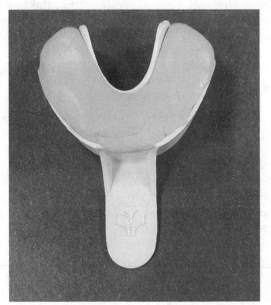

FIGURE 14-9 Filled tray.

However made, the indentation is filled with light body material, in this instance termed a *wash*. The second impression is then taken.

Direct Placement Technique. A cartridge and tip are affixed to the automix syringe and the material is ejected directly onto the area of interest without the use of any impression tray. This technique is commonly employed for making occlusal registrations.

Selecting a Rubber Base Material

Polysulfide. Polysulfide, also termed *mercaptan,* is the oldest of the rubber base materials. However, both base and catalyst pastes contain sulfur, which has an objectionable odor, and the catalyst is lead dioxide, a hazardous material. Excessive lead exposure causes mental deficiency in children and mental deterioration in adults.

Polysulfide was a great advance for its time but has now been superseded for many applications by newer materials. Today, polysulfide is used primarily with regular body material and tray technique to take full denture impressions. Light and heavy body material are available, though, and some operators still use them with the syringe technique because they are inexpensive and have a long history of good service.

Operators who do not use polysulfide object to its smell, the time it takes to prepare and set, its messiness and the fact that there is no known solvent to remove it from clothing. It has a tendency to shrink after removal from the mouth so models must be poured quickly or the material will lose its dimensional stability. Additionally, many patients object to its taste and long setting time, and dentists do not want to alienate their patients.

Polyether. Polyether was the next rubber base material developed. It quickly became popular and remains so today. Polyether enjoys several advantages over polysulfide. It is not hazardous, has no taste or odor, is quick and easy to prepare and does not stain clothing.

Polyether is available in light, regular and heavy body forms and is used in syringe and tray techniques. Its principal disadvantages are stiffness, which makes it difficult to remove from the mouth once set; poor tear strength; a tendency to sorb fluids, which suggests it should not be immersed in disinfectant solution for a long time; and a set that is so rapid, experience is needed to prepare, load and transfer it in time when the syringe technique is being used.

Silicone. There are two types of silicone: condensation silicone and addition silicone. *Condensation silicone* is also termed *polysiloxane,* or simply *silicone.* It is less popular because it gives off water and condenses, or shrinks, excessively as it sets. This means it does not maintain impression dimensions as well.

Addition silicone is also termed *polyvinyl siloxane,* or simply *vinyl.* The addition of vinyl to polysiloxane formulations changes the setting reaction such that the molecules are added together to be chained, rather than combining with each other and giving off a byproduct as happens in the condensation silicone reaction. This means vinyl material experiences almost no shrinkage as it sets. Accordingly, it is more accurate and dimensionally stable. Vinyl is also tasteless, odorless, colorless, can be tinted a variety of colors, is not messy, does not stain clothing and is quick and easy to use.

Vinyl polysiloxanes have become the most popular final impression material because of their great accuracy and ease of use. They are also more costly but dentists apparently believe their characteristics justify the expense. Vinyl material is available in cartridge, putty, two-tube and single-phase forms, and is used with syringe, putty-wash, tray and direct application techniques for all manner of final impressions.

Some cautions are in order. Latex gloves can inhibit vinyl set, so nonlatex gloves should be worn if mixing putty. The set material is hydrophobic, and most impressions are poured with gypsum, a water-based material. Gypsum may flow poorly over a vinyl impression surface, trapping air bubbles and reproducing them on the working cast. Lately, manufacturers have been formulating more hydrophilic materials that do not have this disadvantage. Another solution is to paint the impression surface with a wetting agent to increase pouring success.

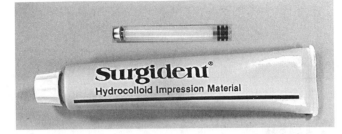

FIGURE 14-10 Hydrocolloid. Here are the tube and carpule forms of hydrocolloid.

▼ REVERSIBLE HYDROCOLLOID MATERIAL ▼

Reversible hydrocolloid, also termed *agar,* and commonly called *hydrocolloid* by dental personnel, is a suspension of polysaccharide polymer particles in a water-based solution. The particles were originally derived from natural seaweeds. Hydrocolloid set is reversible.

Hydrocolloid is supplied in semisolid gel form in carpules, tubes and small, round tubs containing cylinders of material the size and shape of short cigarettes (Figure 14-10). It must be heated before use to assume its liquid sol form. In the sol, particles are individually suspended in the solution. In the gel, the particles have aggregated into fibrils and water fills the spaces between them. In either case, the material has a high water content. Water is inexpensive and flows well but deforms readily under load. Polysaccharide fiber chains are also not strong. As a result, hydrocolloid is an accurate, inexpensive but weak material. Light and heavy body materials are available and used with the syringe technique.

Material Preparation and Use

The material is prepared in a *hydrocolloid conditioner* (Figure 14-11). Notice it has separate water compartments, termed *baths.* The one on the left is the *liquefying bath;* water in it is kept at 100°C. The gel-filled tube and syringe or carpule are boiled in this bath for 8–12 minutes to soften the hydrocolloid. The center one is the *storage bath;* its water temperature is 65°C. Softened material may be stored here for up to several hours. Before use, the tube material must be placed in a tray and the filled tray placed in the *tempering bath.* Water here is kept at 46°C, slightly above mouth temperature. Notice the tray. It has two tubular extensions that insert into rubber tubes to be attached to a water source in the conditioning machine or dental unit (Figure 14-12). Tray and syringe remain in the tempering bath for approximately five minutes to cool the material to a level that will not burn the patient. Hydrocolloid should not remain in the tempering bath too long because the sol will slowly set at this temperature. Once tempered, the syringe material is ejected in and around the prepared tooth. While this occurs, the assistant scrapes the waterlogged surface off the tray ma-

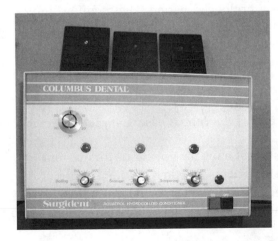

FIGURE 14-11 Hydrocolloid conditioning unit. You can see the hatches for the three different baths and of course the seperate temperature controls.

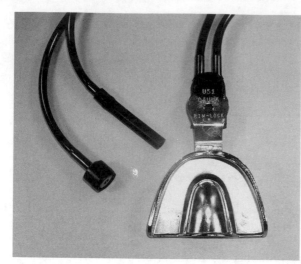

FIGURE 14-12 Hydrocolloid tray. The thin end hooks to the water line. The other end is weighted so it stays in the sink to drain the tray of the cooling water.

terial with a knife or sharp instrument, then the dentist compresses the tray over the syringe material. After the tray is positioned, cool water is circulated through the tubes and tray to set the hydrocolloid.

Care of a Hydrocolloid Impression

High water and polysaccharide content make the hydrocolloid impression weak; it may deform if pressed, or rip if not enough material bulk is present or the impression is removed from the mouth too rapidly. Hydrocolloid impressions should always be handled carefully and placed on a flat surface tray side down.

High water content also renders hydrocolloid susceptible to imbibition and syneresis, with resultant swelling and shrinkage. To avoid unwanted dimensional change, hydrocolloid impressions should always be disinfected and poured immediately.

▼ DISINFECTION OF IMPRESSIONS ▼

All impressions must be disinfected before they are poured. Just as with any item, blood, saliva and debris must first be cleaned away to allow the disinfectant to contact the impression surface. Completed impressions are rinsed in gently running water, then shaken slightly to remove the excess. Rubber bases may be immersed in glutaraldehyde or iodophor solution for the manufacturer's recommended time. Polyether, however, sorbs fluid and should not be immersed for a prolonged period. Hydrocolloid impressions will swell if immersed. They should be sprayed with iodophor or bleach solution and sealed in a plastic bag for the manufacturer's recommended time.

KEY POINTS

✓ Final impressions are taken with one of the rubber base materials or reversible hydrocolloid
✓ They are used to pour working casts that must have accurate dimensions
✓ Rubber bases are nonaqueous, elastomeric, synthetic rubber polymers
✓ Reversible hydrocolloid is a suspension of polymer particles in water
✓ Low viscosity final impression materials are used for accurate detail and high-viscosity materials, to provide handling bulk

- ✓ The vast majority of final impressions are made with rubber base materials
- ✓ From lowest to highest viscosity, rubber base materials are available as light body, regular body, heavy body and putty
- ✓ Single phase rubber base material combines two flow rates—higher near the teeth and lower near the tray
- ✓ Rubber base materials are used with syringe, tray, putty-wash, automix and direct application techniques
- ✓ Basic rubber base types are polysulfide, polyether, silicone and vinyl
- ✓ All except vinyl require that two materials be mixed
  - Proportion equal *lengths* of each material
- ✓ Polysulfide has many disadvantages and is now used mostly with regular body material and tray technique for full denture impressions
- ✓ Polyether is available in light, medium and heavy body, and is used with syringe and tray techniques for all types of final impressions
- ✓ Silicone can be used for all types of final impressions but is prepared with a time-consuming type of putty-wash technique and shrinks excessively during curing
- ✓ Vinyl is available in materials of any viscosity, can be used with all of the techniques, for all types of final impressions, and is the most accurate and most popular
- ✓ Special water-cooled trays are used for reversible hydrocolloid material
- ✓ It is prepared by boiling and tempering in a hydrocolloid conditioner
- ✓ All final impressions should be disinfected
  - Rubber base impressions may be sprayed or immersed
  - Hydrocolloid impressions are highly subject to imbibition and should be sprayed
- ✓ Hydrocolloid impressions are also highly subject to syneresis and should be poured immediately following disinfection

SELF TEST

Select the letter preceding the best answer option.

1. The name *reversible hydrocolloid* tells you this material
   a. Is a suspension of particles in water.
   b. Forms extremely accurate working casts.
   c. Has a thermoplastic set.
   d. Both *a* and *c*
   e. All of the above

2. Describe single phase final impression material.
   a. Has a medium flow rate
   b. Can be mixed easily
   c. Tastes foul
   d. Is thixotropic

3. A _____ body rubber base material is used in a syringe.
   a. Regular
   b. Medium
   c. Light
   d. Heavy
   e. Extra heavy

4. What is the purpose of using a wash?
   a. To provide ease of impression handling
   b. To record anatomic detail well
   c. To prevent surface contamination
   d. To wet impression to improve gypsum flow

5. Impressions made with _____ should not be immersed in disinfectant solution.
   a. Polysulfide
   b. Polyether
   c. Silicone
   d. Vinyl
   e. Hydrocolloid

6. The dentist has asked you to set up the items needed for a final impression for an implant. A high degree of accuracy will be required. What will you get ready?
   a. Alginate
   b. Polysulfide
   c. Vinyl
   d. Hydrocolloid

7. The dentist will be using regular body polysulfide for an impression for a full denture. How will you proportion the materials?
   a. Squeeze out equal lengths
   b. Measure level scoops
   c. Pour to the bottom of the meniscus
   d. Count drops

8. Water-cooled trays are used with reversible hydrocolloid because
   a. Its strength is poor.
   b. Syneresis is a danger.
   c. Immersion disinfection cannot be used.
   d. Its set is thermoplastic.

9. Select the material that is less accurate because it shrinks excessively as it cures.
   a. Silicone
   b. Polyether
   c. Vinyl
   d. Polysulfide

10. Automix cartridges are used only for _____ materials.
   a. Polysulfide
   b. Polyether
   c. Vinyl
   d. Silicone

▾15▾

MATERIALS FOR TEMPORARY COVERAGE

OBJECTIVES

After studying this chapter, you should be able to:

1. Define temporary coverage and discuss why it is used.
2. List and describe the materials used for temporary restorations.
3. Select a material for a specific use.
4. Discuss temporary restoration fabrication and placement techniques.

▼ DEFINITION ▼

Restoration designed to be placed on a prepared tooth for a limited time

▼ USES ▼

Maintain tooth form and function
Protect tooth from the oral environment

▼ RATIONALE FOR USE ▼

Final impressions are usually sent to a commercial laboratory, where the necessary models and restorations are fabricated. This process may require days to weeks. In the meantime, prepared teeth must continue to function and be protected from the oral environment. Temporary restorations are placed to meet this need.

▼ MATERIALS USED ▼

Acrylic resin — for temporary inlays, onlays, crowns and bridges
Composite — for temporary inlays, onlays, veneers, crowns and bridges
Preformed crowns — for temporary full crowns

▼ CLINICAL CONCERNS ▼

Temporary restorations should reproduce tooth esthetics, form and function. They should be quickly and easily made and removed. They should be durable enough to last several weeks if necessary, but not so durable the patient will not return for placement of the permanent restoration. As a temporary measure, they should be inexpensive.

Criteria for selecting a material for a particular restoration, then, are placement location, material strength, ease of use and cost.

Anterior restorations must be made of esthetic materials. Esthetics are less critical but still important posteriorly. Ability to withstand biting forces is necessary for use in Black's Class I, II and IV restorations, but not necessary for those of Class III and V. All of the current materials are relatively inexpensive and used in simple, quick techniques. Where more than one material could be used, operator preference may be the deciding factor.

▼ CHARACTERISTICS OF SPECIFIC MATERIALS ▼

Table 15-1 summarizes the characteristics and uses of temporary restorative materials.

▼ TECHNIQUES FOR USE ▼

Acrylic Resin

There are many different ways to make an acrylic temporary, depending on circumstances. All methods, though, have the same end result. It must be kept in mind that acrylic setting is exothermic and the material shrinks significantly during this time. It is important when using the material in the mouth not to leave it on a tooth for too long; there is a danger of irritating the pulp of the tooth or the cells of the periodontal ligament with the heat. The material contracts as it sets, and this contraction plus undercuts on adjacent teeth can cause

TABLE 15-1 Characteristics of temporary restorative materials.

Material	Properties	Clinical Significance
Acrylic	Esthetic	Suitable for all areas of the mouth
	Inexpensive	May be material of choice when cost is important
	Fabrication techniques are relatively simple	Can be completed quickly by allied dental personnel
	Discolors and wears readily	Most suitable for temporary restorations
Polymer	Sold as preformed shell crowns	Keeping a variety of sizes on hand requires storage space and money to be idle in inventory
	Crown is transparent and is lined with an esthetic polymer	Suitable for all areas of the mouth
	Fitting crown cervix to prepared tooth requires time and expertise	Time and training are expensive
	May be bulky as compared to natural teeth	Appears less natural and is less comfortable
	Available only in shell crown form	Not suitable for temporary bridge fabrication
Stainless steel	Sold as preformed shell crowns	Keeping a variety of sizes on hand requires storage space and money to be idle in inventory
	Non-esthetic silver color	Suitable only for posterior, lingual or palatal areas
	Fitting crown cervix to prepared tooth requires time and expertise	Time and training are expensive
	May be bulky as compared to natural teeth	Appears less natural and is less comfortable
	Subject to tarnish and corrosion	Should be polished routinely
	Available only in shell crown form	Not suitable for temporary bridge fabrication
	Has no polymer components	Suitable for patients who are allergic to plastics
All	Are cemented or bonded into position	Margins must be examined regularly and frequently for continued integrity

the material to get locked to the teeth in such a way that only a bur can remove it. So remember, only place material on the teeth in the early doughy stage and slip the temporary on and off the tooth until it is completely set. Water can be used to cool the material when it is removed for those brief periods to protect the teeth and lessen the shrinkage.

Replacing a Missing or a Badly Broken-Down Tooth

If the restoration is being planned to replace a missing tooth or one that is badly broken down, two methods can be employed. In the first (Figure 15-1), an alginate impression must be made at an appointment prior to the preparation appointment. Using denture teeth, wax, or composite to fill in the edentulous area, or restore the missing tooth contours, one can modify the study model to look like the desired result. A thin sheet of vacuum or pressure forming material can be adapted to the modified model. This *stent* can then be used over the prepared teeth at appointment time to make the temporary by filling it with acrylic. Alternatively, a rough preparation of the teeth can be made on the model and the stent filled with acrylic or composite, then a temporary made in the laboratory. This temporary can be filled with acrylic and placed over the restoration. Filling a cavity in the temporary and readapting it to the tooth is termed *relining*.

The second method is called making a block temporary. In this case (Figure 15-2), the acrylic is mixed and when doughy is formed into a block that is the same length and width as the temporary. This block is then placed over the preparations and the patient is in-

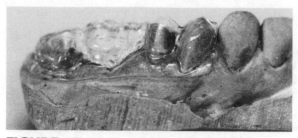

FIGURE 15-1 Stent. This clear acrylic pattern will be filled with resin. Note the teeth in the bridge have been prepared on the working model so the temp can be made before the patient comes in for the appointment.

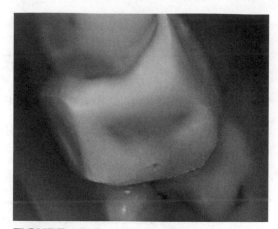

FIGURE 15-2 Block temporary. You can see why it is called a block temp. It will take some time to carve this crude form into a tooth.

structed to bite down on the soft material. The temporary is trimmed roughly to size with scissors and then slipped on and off the tooth as described for all acrylic materials until completely set.

While both of these techniques can handle any sort of tooth temporary situation, the first one takes up less of the patient's time in the chair. It also allows the introduction of reinforcing wires or fibers to strengthen temporary bridges plus better control of the temporary shape and size. However, when the patient shows up as an emergency with a broken tooth the block technique will get them a replacement in a short period of time.

Replacing a Mostly Intact Tooth

Prior to tooth preparation, take an impression of the arch of interest or make a small custom tray. This technique only works if the tooth in question is intact or close enough for the missing area to be corrected quickly with wax or composite. An impression is made of the tooth prior to preparation. This can be done with alginate, bite registration material, softened polystyrene beads or even a rubber impression material (Figure 15-3). After the tooth is prepared, fill the impression where the tooth or teeth are being restored with resin. Rein-

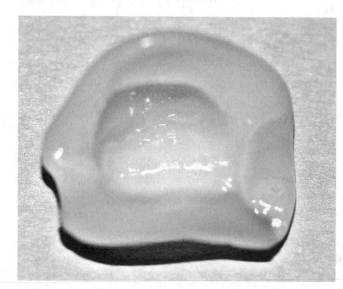

FIGURE 15-3 Tooth form. This one happens to be polystyrene but impression or bite materials also work.

sert the impression. When the resin is sufficiently cured to permit light handling, remove the restoration from the impression. Handle the restoration lightly as it is still incompletely cured and can be easily deformed. Quickly trim the excess material, termed *flash,* away. Cool the temporary in water, reposition the restoration in the mouth and have the patient bite. The restoration is then removed, cooled and replaced until set, then finished as described in the previous section.

Composite

Because composite materials are really reinforced acrylics there are composite-based temporary materials that can be used to make temporary crowns. They can be lightcured, self-cured, or, most commonly, dual cured. They are packaged either in syringes like composite direct filling material, or in a dual cartridge system with mixing tips to place them. The basic principles are the same for making a composite temporary crown as an acrylic one.

Composite materials (see Chapter 11) are also used for both temporary and permanent veneers. Dental personnel often term composite veneers *bonded veneers,* even though veneers made of other materials may also be bonded in position.

Permanent veneers may be made of composite or a type of glass termed *porcelain.* Porcelain must be processed at very high temperatures, restricting its use to indirect restorations. Temporary composite veneers are placed for patients waiting for porcelain veneers. Unlike permanent veneers, composite veneers need to be placed so that they can be removed without disturbing the preparation. Dentists generally use mechanical locking interproximally to keep them in place.

Preformed Crowns

Preformed polymer and stainless steel crowns are available in a variety of shapes and sizes (Figure 15-4). Polymer crowns may be either polycarbonate or polyacrylate. Both materials are esthetic, used in the anterior, and prepared for attachment similarly. Stainless steel crowns (Figure 15-5) are nonesthetic, able to withstand biting forces, placed in the posterior usually for pediatric patients, and prepared for attachment using a slightly different technique.

Polymer Crown Technique

Select a crown of appropriate size and shape. Try it in the mouth to ensure fit. Fill selected crown with acrylic resin or composite and position it on the tooth. When the flash material is doughy, remove the crown from the mouth and cut the flash away with scissors. Just as in the other techniques described earlier, the crown should be placed in water for a short time to cool it and reduce curing shrinkage. Replace the crown on the tooth to ensure continued fit and continue to remove it periodically and cool it until the material is completely cured. Smooth and polish the completed crown. Isolate and dry the tooth, then cement the crown in position using temporary cement.

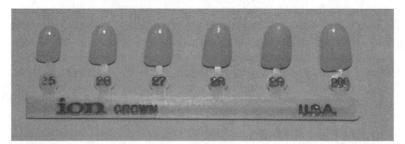

FIGURE 15-4 Polycarbonate crowns. Here is a selection of upper left lateral incisors. Of course, there are selections for the other anterior teeth and the premolars.

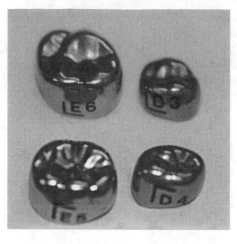

FIGURE 15-5 Stainless steel crowns. Notice the marking on the side denoting the tooth and the size.

Stainless Steel or Aluminum Alloy Crown Technique

Select a crown of appropriate size and shape. Fit it to the tooth cervix by bending and crimping it with pliers. Roughen the inside of the crown using microabrasion (directing a stream of aluminum oxide particles at the material) or a bur. Fill the crown with cement. A permanent cement (see Chapter 17) will probably be used because the "permanent restoration" a child is waiting for is eruption of the permanent tooth. A stainless steel crown will be used until the new tooth erupts. However, a reinforced zinc oxide and eugenol cement can be used to cement the crown temporarily. Position the crown on the tooth and stabilize it with a cotton roll or bite stick until the cement is set. Remove any excess cement, check the proximal contacts and occlusion, and adjust if necessary.

KEY POINTS

✓ Temporary restorations protect and maintain the function of prepared teeth
✓ Resin is used for crowns and bridges, composite for veneers, and preformed crowns for full crowns
✓ Polymer crowns are esthetic and used in both the anterior and posterior
✓ Stainless steel crowns are nonesthetic and used in the posterior for children
✓ Resin crowns are made by taking an impression, then using it as a mold for the restoration
✓ Composite is placed as learned for direct restorations: etch, bond, cure
✓ Preformed crowns are selected for size and shape, fitted to the tooth and cemented in position
  • Polymer crowns are fitted by lining the crown with resin
  • Stainless steel crowns are fitted by bending and crimping with pliers

SELF TEST

Select the single best answer option.

1. The patient's tooth has been prepared for a full crown for a second molar. Why will a temporary crown be placed until the permanent crown is available?
   a. To assure the patient's appearance remains unchanged
   b. To prevent migration of the anterior tooth
   c. To maintain the patient's comfort and chewing ability
   d. To prevent caries development in the adjacent teeth

2. The patient is having permanent porcelain veneers made. What material will need to be set up to place temporary veneers while awaiting the permanent ones?
   a. Acrylic
   b. Composite
   c. Porcelain
   d. Preformed alloy

3. Why is it **not** a good idea to place a durable temporary restoration?
   a. Tooth preparations will not be protected by adequate bonding.
   b. Tooth preparation margins may discolor too readily.
   c. Patient will believe he has been overcharged for the restoration.
   d. Patient may not return for delivery of the permanent restoration.

4. Why is a temporary acrylic restoration periodically dipped in water and slipped on and off the tooth when it is constructed?
   a. Curing heat may damage the pulp and periodontal ligament.
   b. Curing speed may be retarded by prolonged contact with calcium.
   c. Curing shrinkage may lock the restoration to the tooth surface.
   d. Both a and c
   e. All of the above

5. What is a stent?
   a. An individualized mold that can be relined to construct a temporary restoration
   b. A cooling device that is applied to temporary restoration material periodically to prevent heat formation
   c. A type of cannula that can be used to extrude temporary restorative material onto a prepared tooth surface
   d. A specialized bur used to design cavity preparations for indirect restorations

6. Describe the texture of the flash material when an acrylic temporary crown is ready to be removed from a tooth and trimmed.
   a. Flowable
   b. Doughy
   c. Stiff
   d. Drippy

7. What types of checks should be made after a temporary crown has been placed initially to assure it will function correctly?
   a. Proximal contacts should meet adjacent proximal contacts
   b. Cervical margin should be completely filled with cement or bonding agent
   c. Usual occlusion should be maintained
   d. Both a and c
   e. All of the above

8. Which type of preformed crown is used primarily for pediatric patients and why?
   a. Stainless steel; strength
   b. Polycarbonate; appearance
   c. Aluminum; ease of construction
   d. Acrylic; esthetics

9. You are setting up for construction of a temporary bridge. Which type of material will you select?
   a. Aluminum
   b. Stainless steel
   c. Acrylic
   d. Polycarbonate

10. What instrument will be necessary if a preformed metal alloy crown is to be fitted to a prepared tooth?
    a. Periodontal probe
    b. Explorer
    c. Lab engine and bur
    d. Vitalometer
    e. Crimping pliers

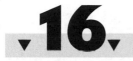

MATERIALS FOR PERMANENT INDIRECT RESTORATIONS

OBJECTIVES

After studying this chapter, you should be able to:

1. List and describe the materials and techniques used to construct permanent indirect restorations.
2. Discuss the following in relation to indirect restorations:
   a. Appointment scheduling
   b. Reasons for clinical failure
   c. Clinical examination
   d. Selection of polishing agents and fluoride treatment materials

▼ DEFINITION ▼

Materials for restorations that are made outside that mouth, cemented or bonded in place, and expected to last for a substantial time

▼ MATERIALS EMPLOYED ▼

Metal alloys—combinations of metals
Ceramic—a type of glass
Resin—acrylic polymer

▼ USES ▼

Ceramic—veneers, crowns, onlays and inlays
Metal alloys—crowns, bridges, inlays, onlays, substructures that will be veneered
Resin—inlays, ceramic repairs

▼ MATERIAL SELECTION ▼

Allied dental personnel do not select or design permanent indirect restorations, nor do the vast majority of assistants and hygienists fabricate them. The dentist selects and designs based on an assessment of material characteristics and known record of service in relation to observed patient conditions. Highly skilled commercial laboratory technicians construct each restoration to meet the dentist's specifications.

Assistants and hygienists do need to be aware of the fabrication process and characteristics of each type of finished indirect restoration. This enables effective restoration examination, patient education and appointment scheduling. Additionally, the knowledgeable operator is better prepared to avoid damaging indirect restorations while scaling, polishing or providing a fluoride treatment.

▼ SPECIFIC MATERIALS ▼

Ceramic

Composition

Ceramic is a glass material composed primarily of feldspar, silica (quartz) and kaolin. *Kaolin* is clay, the fine-grained soil found along riverbanks and at the bottom of streams that becomes cohesive when wet. *Feldspar* and *quartz* are natural minerals mined from the earth that can be ground into powders. Most people are familiar with such particles as ingredients of common sand.

When subjected to high temperatures, feldspar particles fuse to form glass of the same shape, but silica particles do not change. This means adding water to dental ceramic powder will form a cohesive mixture that can be molded to shape, will not lose its shape when processed, and contains silica reinforcing particles. Coloring agents, which are various types of metal oxides, are added to modify the natural gray to pink tint of feldspar and yellow to orange tint of silica. Opaquers and a fluorescing agent may be added to further simulate different types of natural tooth structure. The result is an esthetic material that has both the advantages and disadvantages of glass.

Types

Different proportions of feldspar, kaolin and silica are used to create two basic glass materials: porcelain, which is fired, and ceramic, which is cast or machine milled. *Firing* is baking at a high temperature. *Casting* is liquefying and pouring or injecting into a mold. *Machine milling* is grinding a pre-cast block of ceramic to the proper shape for the restoration.

Characteristics

Porcelain. Porcelain is more familiar in the form of fine dinnerware. Porcelain restorations are similar in properties: esthetic, translucent, hard, insoluble, great compressive strength, dimensionally stable, and able to expand and contract in response to thermal change at a rate very close to that of natural teeth. Unfortunately, they are also brittle, have poor tensile strength and a different surface texture than natural teeth. Tensile strain from biting forces may cause small brittle fractures that crack or craze a porcelain restoration, similar to the way compressing the two sides of a soda cracker results in a tensile fracture in the middle.

The different surface texture reflects light slightly differently, rendering an exact color match to natural teeth difficult. Very close matches can be achieved, however, and the ability to do so is more art than science. Laboratory technicians who fabricate excellent color matches are much in demand and much valued.

Ceramic. Ceramic is familiar as the pottery used in less expensive dinnerware. It has more opaque clay and fewer translucent feldspar and silica particles. As a result, ceramic restorations possess the basic characteristics of glass, but are opaque. Since tooth enamel is translucent, ceramic restorations appear less natural.

Fabrication of Restorations

Technique for Fired Porcelain Restorations. A final impression is taken and poured in die stone. A matrix, which is a thin layer of platinum foil similar to aluminum foil, is carefully fitted over the die (Figure 16-1). The correct shade of porcelain powder is mixed with distilled water and applied to the matrix. The applied mixture is condensed by vibrating or pressing it, then blotting away the water that rises to the surface with a towel or dry powder. Application and condensation of powder layers to simulate various tooth body and surface shades and opacities continue until the correct shape and esthetics are obtained. The crown is then fired two to three times, depending on the firing technique selected. Before the final firing, the restoration, including the matrix, may be returned to the office or clinic to be checked for fit. The final firing uses porcelain that melts at a lower temperature than the body ceramic. This glaze layer melts completely and creates a thin, smooth surface glaze. The matrix, which served to hold everything in position throughout, will be removed when the restoration is complete.

This painstaking, time-consuming, technique requires much knowledge and skill, as well as special equipment. It requires an initial appointment for preparing the tooth, taking

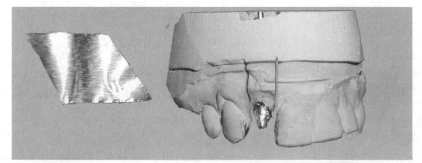

FIGURE 16-1 Platinum foil. The thin sheet of foil is adapted to the die.

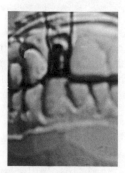

FIGURE 16-2 Wax coping. The die is covered with a thin sheet of wax that will be replaced by metal in the casting process.

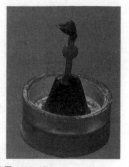

FIGURE 16-3 Spruing. The wax is placed on the sprue, which has a reservoir so that as the casting shrinks it can pull enough metal in to avoid porosity.

the impression and bite, and placing a temporary restoration; appointments for one or more try-ins for fit; and an appointment for final delivery. Fired porcelain restorations therefore tend to be costly, but the expense is rewarded with esthetics and comfort.

Technique for Fired Porcelain-Fused-to-Metal Restorations. A final impression is taken and poured in die stone. A coping (cover) of castable metal alloy is made by the lost wax technique. The lost wax technique utilizes a special casting wax that is shaped into the form that the metal will take (Figure 16-2). The wax is then attached to a sprue, which acts as a funnel for the melted alloy (Figure 16-3). Once the sprue is made the wax mold is placed in a strong metal ring and casting investment material is poured around it. Once the investment is set the casting ring is warmed in an oven. This melts the wax out of the investment, leaving a space where the wax was. When it reaches the proper temperature it is loaded at one end of a spring-loaded arm (Figure 16-4). Next to it is a ceramic crucible that contains the metal. The metal is melted and then the arm is released. As the arm spins the melted metal is thrown into the open area in the investment where the wax was. When it all cools down the metal can be removed from the investment (Figure 16-5), the sprue cut off and the metal finished.

Once the metal is finished a layer of very opaque porcelain is placed to cover the metal coping (Figure 16-6). At that point the body porcelain is applied as for a pure ceramic crown (Figure 16-7). The key to making the technique work is having the coefficients of expansion and contraction in the metal and the ceramic match. Otherwise, when fired in the oven at high temperature stresses will be created that will result in fracturing the porcelain.

Technique for Cast Ceramic Restorations. A final impression is taken, a die is poured, and the restoration is cast using the *lost wax technique.* In this technique (which is also used for casting metal), a wax pattern is made on the die, surrounded with a hard material, removed to make a mold, and replaced with a liquefied permanent material (Figure 16-8). After the permanent material hardens, the mold is broken away and the casting cleaned.

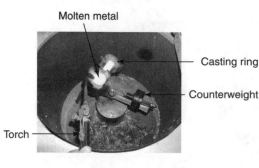

Molten metal

Casting ring

Counterweight

Torch

FIGURE 16-4 Casting machine. The machine has a strong spring in the base. It is wound and held in place by a pin. When the metal is completely melted, the pin is released and the rapid rotation of the arm shoots the molten metal into the pattern.

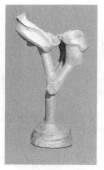

FIGURE 16-5 Casting. This is how the casting looks when it is taken out of the investment. To save time and effort, three castings are attached to this one sprue.

Clean cast ceramic restorations must be heated to crystallize and harden them, a process termed *ceramming.* Before casting, coloring agents cannot be dispersed in a material so as to simulate the varying shades of a natural tooth. This means cast, cerammed glass is clear. The final step in fabricating a cast ceramic restoration is to veneer it with the correct shades of glass and fire it.

Technique for Machine Milling Ceramic Restorations. Computers are used to design and cut ceramic restorations. This is usually termed *CAD-CAM,* an acronym for *computer aided (or assisted) design and manufacturing.*

Special equipment is used for this technique (Figure 16-9). A digital image of the tooth preparation is made and stored in the computer. The operator uses graphics software to create a three-dimensional image of a total restoration that will fit the preparation and contact both adjacent and opposing teeth properly. The image is then used to control rotating diamond burs to cut a ceramic block to the correct size and shape. Final adjustments are made by hand. The restoration is then stained to match adjacent teeth, polished and cemented in place.

CAD-CAM technique can be used for blocks of resin or metal as well as ceramic. Allied dental personnel can be trained to define existing parameters and mill the material once the dentist has constructed the proper image. Only one appointment is required to fabricate and deliver the restoration.

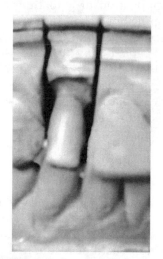

FIGURE 16-6 Opaque layer. The metal is covered with opaque porcelain to mask the metallic color. Notice that it is a very thin layer.

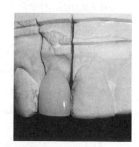

FIGURE 16-7 Crown. The body and incisal porcelain are applied and glazed to produce the final crown.

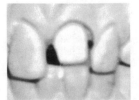

FIGURE 16-8 Porcelain cores. This is a Ceristore® coping. Special porcelain will be added to produce the proper shape.

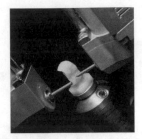

FIGURE 16-9 CAD-CAM. The machine is cutting the restoration out of a block of porcelain.

Selection of Porcelain or Ceramic

The excellent esthetics and brittle nature of porcelain mean it appears natural but is not suited for posterior areas subject to high biting forces. It is used for anterior jacket crowns, where biting forces are lower; Class III or V inlays, where they are minimal or absent; and veneers for natural teeth or unsightly metal substructures. Ceramic, which is opaque, is more suited for the posterior but is also placed in the anterior. It can be used alone for crowns, but more commonly is chosen for veneering metal substructures of crowns and bridges.

Clinical Concerns

Surface care, secondary decay and *fracture repair* are the everyday concerns when ceramic restorations are present. The surface glaze produced by final porcelain firing enables the restoration to reflect light in a manner similar to natural tooth structure. The glaze is also very smooth, but the material below the glaze is coarse and porous. Surface integrity must be maintained if the restoration is to appear natural and not provide ready anchorage for plaque attachment.

Surface glass can be scratched or chipped with a scaler, roughened by polishing with abrasives that are too coarse, or etched by acid fluorides. Allied dental personnel should position and activate scalers carefully so as not to scratch the glaze or chip the cervical margin; use fine abrasives for polishing; and avoid application of acid fluorides to ceramic restoration surfaces. Neutral fluorides are available and should be used.

The cervical area is of additional concern because all indirect restorations are cemented or bonded in position. Bonds may break and cement may slowly dissolve, exposing the tooth preparation and the inside of the restoration. This provides protected anchorage for plaque and a pathway for bacteria to reach the tooth surface to initiate secondary decay. Careful examination of all indirect restoration surfaces, particularly the cervical margin, to detect scratches, chips, fractures and open margins should be an integral part of every dental examination.

Fracture Repair

Small chips and fractures should be promptly repaired with an acrylic resin composite material. Dental dam is placed to isolate the area. First, the tooth and restoration are prepared for bonding: the restoration surface is roughened with a bur or intraoral aluminum oxide sandblaster, then etched with either a hydrofluoric acid or acidulated phosphate fluoride solution. Any exposed metal is covered with opaque composite, and any exposed enamel is etched with phosphoric acid solution. Silane linking agent (Figure 16-10) (remember in composite silane linked the matrix and glass-reinforcing beads) is applied to the restoration surface. Second, bonding is done. Adhesive primer is applied to the whole—the silanated area on the restoration and any exposed metal or enamel then an unfilled resin

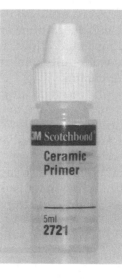

FIGURE 16-10 Silane. This has to be left on the surface for minutes to work properly.

bonding agent is applied and cured. Finally, composite restorative material is applied, cured and finished. Despite all the steps these repairs are not strong and usually the restoration will need replacement.

Metal Alloys

Composition and Properties

Metals are chemical elements that conduct heat and electricity, and are lustrous, malleable, and ductile. *Noble metals,* including gold, silver, platinum, palladium, and others, are what we ordinarily think of as precious metals. They are relatively inert; the lower the reactivity of a metal, the higher its nobility. With the exception of silver they resist tarnish and corrosion well. They also tend to be scarce, valued and expensive. *Base metals,* including copper, chromium, iron, lead, nickel, zinc, titanium and others, are more reactive. Titanium and copper excepted, they are less resistant to tarnish and corrosion. They also tend to be more widely distributed and are often less expensive.

Metal alloys are mixtures of metals that are heated at high temperatures to chemically combine the different elements. Each ingredient brings both desirable and undesirable characteristics to the whole. Metals to include in an alloy are determined by the clinical use to which it will be put, the relative importance of each characteristic to success in that use, and the ability of one metal to counteract the undesirable characteristics of another.

Types

To date, two basic types of mixtures have been developed to bring two basic sets of characteristics to dental restorations. *Noble alloys* combine larger amounts of precious metals with smaller amounts of base metals to create strong, hard, biologically compatible mixtures that are highly resistant to tarnish and corrosion but expensive. *Base metal alloys* combine lesser amounts of precious metals with various proportions of base metals to create mixtures that are biocompatible, silver in color, able to bond acceptably to porcelain and ceramic and very hard, but less expensive, and more susceptible to fracture, tarnish and corrosion.

Fabrication and Use

In dentistry, metal alloys are cast using the lost wax technique to form crowns, bridges, inlays and onlays, as well as crown and bridge substructures, implants and denture frameworks.

Gold is alloyed with silver, copper, platinum and palladium to form gold-based high noble alloys. *Silver and palladium* are alloyed with copper, cobalt, gallium and smaller proportions of gold, or no gold at all, to form silver–palladium noble alloys. Gold-based high noble alloys and silver–palladium noble alloys are both used for all-metal restorations and metal substructures that will be veneered with porcelain or ceramic.

Base metal alloys can be made of pure titanium; titanium alloyed with aluminum and vanadium; or combinations of nickel or cobalt with chromium, molybdenum, and tungsten. Titanium alloys are used for implants as well as crown and bridge substructures, and will be discussed in Chapter 18. Cobalt–chromium alloys are used far more extensively for partial denture parts than crown and bridge substructures, and will be discussed in Chapter 19. Nickel–chromium is a common base metal casting alloy that typically also includes iron or beryllium and small amounts of other metals. It is used for casting metal substructures for porcelain fused to metal crowns and bridges. It is very hard, light and strong, with excellent bonding to porcelain.

Contributions of Specific Materials

Gold is soft, malleable, corrosion resistant, has a distinctive color and for some populations, intrinsic social value based on its historical use in jewelry, decoration and coinage. It is very dense and therefore produces heavy castings.

Copper strengthens but reddens the alloy, lowers its melting temperature and provides corrosion resistance in the finished restoration.

Silver strengthens, hardens and lightens the color of the alloy, but increases restoration susceptibility to tarnish and corrosion. Color lightening is termed *whitening*. All metals except gold and copper whiten alloy.

Palladium and platinum whiten the alloy and raise the melting point, an important consideration when the casting must be heated to very high temperatures for fusing a veneer to it.

Gallium brings a bluish-white color and strength, but is brittle and increases the possibility of fracture.

Zinc may be included in alloys; it will combine with oxygen to remove impurities.

Nickel improves ductility but the incidence of nickel allergy in the general population is approximately 10%. Females are four times as likely as males to be affected and nickel has been associated with development of cancer. The link is not definitive and nickel use in dental alloys is allowed in the United States.

Beryllium improves castability as well as bonding to porcelain and resin cements.

Iron brings strength, ductility and malleability and helps the bond to porcelain but is highly susceptible to tarnish and corrosion.

Clinical Considerations

Appointment Scheduling.   Metal alloy restorations require two appointments, one to prepare the tooth, take the impression and bite, and place a temporary restoration; and one to deliver the finished restoration and educate the recipient regarding its proper care. Try-in appointments for fitting are not required.

Polishing.   It is very important to polish metal restorations to remove tarnish and corrosion, and to ensure the restoration surface is smooth. The selective polishing that is practiced on natural teeth is not appropriate for metal restorations, because surface defects predispose metals to corrosion. Corrosion weakens metal, predisposing it to fatigue and fracture.

It is also important that polishing with fine or extra fine abrasive be the final step. Coarse and medium abrasives roughen metal, leaving in their wake the very defects the polishing was meant to remove. Fine or very fine pumice and tin oxide are mild abrasives that are suitable for final intraoral metal polishing.

Examination. Metal crowns and bridges are not prone to chipping and fracture, but can be scratched. Scratches should be smoothed away using appropriate abrasive technique. In common with all porcelain and ceramic restorations, metal crowns and bridges are cemented or bonded in position. If the bond breaks or cement dissolves, the margin is left open. Open metal alloy margins, unlike amalgam margins, are not self-sealing. As with porcelain and ceramic, open metal alloy restoration margins provide protected anchorage for plaque and easy access to the tooth for initiation of secondary decay. At the dentist's discretion, an open margin may be sealed with a bonding agent or the restoration may be removed and recemented.

Fluoride Treatments. Metal restorations may be treated with either acidulated or neutral fluorides.

Resin

Acrylic composite resin is used with indirect techniques to fabricate inlays, primarily in the posterior. Inlay resin is another form of the acrylic polymer used for sealants and direct composite restorations. As such, it is composed of ingredients and possesses characteristics described in previous chapters (see Chapters 6 and 11).

Resin inlays are an alternative to direct composite restorations. As discussed in Chapter 11, posterior composite material is rough and shrinks excessively as it cures. Layered material placement and curing helps to minimize, but does not completely eliminate, curing shrinkage, and rapid or excessive shrinkage may fracture the bonding material or tooth. Resin inlay material attempts to solve these problems through the use of composite material processed using indirect techniques.

Two techniques are used. One is completely indirect, the other combines direct and indirect methods.

Indirect Resin Inlay Technique. The tooth is prepared. An impression is taken and poured, and a resin inlay formed on the die. The inlay is usually cured initially using light and once initial set is achieved, then heat. Heat curing produces more complete polymerization than light or chemical curing but of course cannot be used in the mouth. Finally, the cured inlay is cleaned and polished. It shrinks using indirect curing methods, but this occurs outside the mouth where it does not adversely affect attachment.

The completed inlay is cemented in position using a thin layer of dual cured translucent resin cement. Its translucency maintains restoration esthetics, its resin nature enables mechanical bonding to the preparation, and its dual cure provides for both immediacy and completeness of cure.

As a polymer, the cement itself will shrink slightly as it cures. Shrinkage will be minimal because the layer is thin. The remaining cement will compensate for the curing shrinkage of the inlay and fill the area between it and the preparation.

The result is an esthetic posterior inlay that is relatively inexpensive but more completely cured, smoother, and at least initially, denser and stronger than a direct posterior composite restoration. Margins are well adapted. Esthetics are excellent because the translucency supplied by composite is present.

Combination Resin Inlay Technique. The tooth is prepared, and a separating lubricant applied. Light or dual cure resin is placed in, but not bonded to, the preparation. The material is cured, removed from the preparation and cured again using heat. The restoration is cleaned, polished and cemented in position with dual cure resin cement just as with the completely indirect technique.

This technique does not require that a model be taken or poured. The restoration is fabricated directly in the tooth, cured well enough to be handled, then heat cured indirectly as well to increase its strength, surface smoothness and hardness.

Clinical Considerations

Appointment Scheduling. Completely indirect fabrication of a resin inlay requires two appointments: an initial appointment to prepare the tooth, take the impression and place a temporary restoration; and a second to deliver the restoration and educate the patient. Combination direct–indirect inlay fabrication requires only one appointment. An impression, model and temporary restoration are not needed. Dentist and staff can form, cure and place the restoration within a single patient visit.

Examination. Resin is more flexible than other indirect restorative materials and, except for metal alloys, less prone to fracture. It is subject to continued curing shrinkage, wear and discoloration. Margin integrity, occlusion, contacts and color should be assessed during each examination. At the dentist's discretion, margins may be sealed, or the restoration recontoured, built up or replaced.

Polishing. Resin inlays should be polished with fine abrasives to maintain their smooth surface. As discussed in Chapter 5, abrasives preferentially wear away the resin matrix. Coarse abrasives cut deeper into the resin and expose larger portions of the surface particles, leaving the surface rough and the particles subject to loss.

Fluoride Treatment. There is some controversy regarding appropriate fluoride treatment for resin restorations. Some operators believe acidulated phosphate fluorides should be avoided because resin contains *glass reinforcing beads,* which could be etched. Others believe the possibility is sufficiently remote that it is not necessary to use only neutral fluorides.

KEY POINTS

✓ Permanent indirect restorations are made outside the mouth, cemented or bonded in place and expected to last for a long time.
  • They are made of ceramic, metal alloy, ceramic–metal combinations or resin
✓ Ceramic and porcelain are both types of glass
  • Porcelain is fired; ceramic is cast or cut using a CAD-CAM technique
    • Porcelain is highly esthetic and translucent, but subject to brittle fracture
    • It is used for jacket crowns, veneers for natural teeth or metal substructures, and Class III or V inlays
    • Ceramic is opaque, therefore less esthetic, but stronger
    • It is most commonly used for veneering metal substructures
  • Only fine abrasives and neutral fluorides should be used on glass restorations
✓ Metal alloys are chemically combined metal solids
  • Gold-based high noble and palladium–silver based noble alloys are used for crowns, bridges, inlays, onlays and metal substructures
  • Base metal alloys are used to make strong substructures for crowns and bridges that will be veneered for esthetics
  • Metal alloy restorations should be polished routinely to reduce tarnish and corrosion
✓ Resin inlay material is another form of the acrylic resin used for sealants and composite
  • It is used for posterior inlays
  • Resin inlays are made using either a completely indirect light, heat, or heat and light cured technique, *or* a combination technique that combines light or dual curing in the mouth with heat curing outside of it
    • Resin inlays are stronger, smoother and harder than composite direct restorations
    • Resin inlays are the least expensive type of inlay
✓ Indirect restorations tend to be more costly than direct restorations because of the materials and complex fabrication techniques used to make them
✓ All indirect restorations should be examined carefully for surface defects and open margins

Questions 1–3: *Identify and state the use of the illustrated item.*

1.

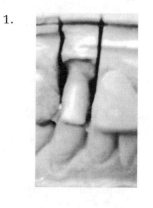

2.

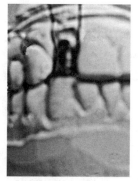

3.

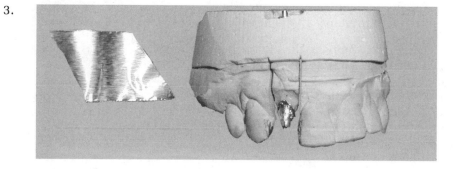

Questions 4–8: *Describe the following procedures.*

4. Firing porcelain

5. Casting using the lost wax technique

6. Veneering metal substructures

7. Using CAD-CAM technique to make a ceramic crown

8. Fabricating a resin inlay using the combination technique.

Questions 9–15: *Select the letter preceding the best answer.*

9. This jacket crown material is highly esthetic but subject to brittle fracture.
   a. Acrylic resin
   b. Gold-based high noble alloy
   c. Porcelain
   d. Silver–palladium-based noble alloy
   e. Base metal alloy
   f. Ceramic

10. Ceramming cast glass
    a. Increases its hardness and strength
    b. Allows metal–ceramic bonding to occur
    c. Forms a protective surface film on the glass
    d. Smooths and colors the glass

11. What functions does kaolin perform in porcelain and ceramic materials?
    a. Makes material cohesive when wet
    b. Fuses material ingredients together
    c. Adds opacity to the material
    d. Both a and c
    e. All of the above

12. High noble gold-based alloys are used for
    a. Crowns
    b. Bridges
    c. Metal substructures
    d. Both a and c
    e. All of the above

13. Which of the following is *not* a reason for including a metal in an alloy?
    a. Planned clinical use of the alloy
    b. Toxicity of the metal in its pure state
    c. Relative importance of the metal's characteristics to clinical success
    d. Ability of the metal to counteract undesirable characteristics of another metal

14. What does silver bring to an alloy?
    a. Hardness
    b. Whitening
    c. Ability to remove impurities from the alloy
    d. A higher melting point than most other metals
    e. a and b
    f. b and c

15. Indirect resin inlay techniques were developed in an attempt to solve this problem with direct composite restorations.
    a. Discoloration
    b. Thermal conductivity
    c. Margin integrity
    d. Shearing strength

.17.

CEMENTS

OBJECTIVES

After studying this chapter, you should be able to:

1. Define and state the use of luting cements.
2. Discuss how joints are formed between teeth and material.
3. Differentiate zinc oxide and polymer cements.
4. List and describe clinical concerns related to the use of cements.
5. List specific materials used as cements.
6. Discuss cement selection.
7. Describe the characteristics and handling of each zinc oxide, polymer and combination cement.

▼ DEFINITION AND USE ▼

Cements are a family of intermediary materials. As discussed in Chapter 10, different members of the family protectively coat or seal a tooth, fill the space between a tooth and material, or attach materials to teeth.

Dental personnel define different family members by their use. Cements that protectively coat a tooth preparation are *bases;* those that seal the teeth are *liners,* and those that attach materials to teeth are referred to by their family name, *cements,* or as *luting agents.* This chapter discusses only the subgroup of cements that attach materials to teeth. Liners and bases were covered in Chapter 10.

▼ MECHANISM OF ACTION—PROCEDURE LEVEL ▼

Cements attach indirect restorations and orthodontic appliances to teeth in two ways: luting and bonding. For *luting,* a layer of cement is spread on the surface of the item to be attached, then the item pressed onto the tooth. The cement fills in the defects on both surfaces and excess cement is forced out at the material margin (Figure 17-1). A thin film of cement that is slightly interlocked with both surfaces remains to form the joint (Figure 17-2).

Some cements bond to the tooth surface. The glass ionomers, which bond chemically, and the resins, which bond mechanically, are like their cousins used for direct restorations. They require preparing the tooth surface prior to placing them.

▼ MATERIALS USED AND MECHANISM OF ACTION ▼

Metal oxide powders with acid liquids—fill surface defects
    Zinc phosphate
    Zinc oxide and eugenol
Polymer powders with acid liquids—fill surface defects; also bond
    Glass ionomer—bonds chemically
    Resin—bonds mechanically
    Resin–ionomer—combines both resin and glass ionomer properties
Metal oxide powders with acidic polymer liquids—contains both zinc oxide and polymer
    Zinc polycarboxylate—fills surface defects; also bonds chemically

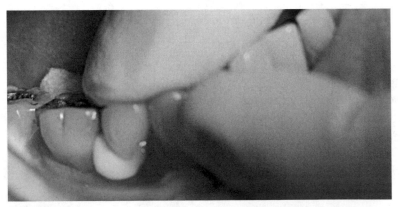

FIGURE 17-1 Cementing a crown. The cement must be cleaned up quickly because once hardened it is very difficult to remove.

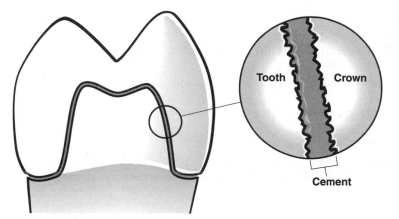

FIGURE 17-2 Cement joint. You can see how the cement can mechanically interlock in the slightly uneven tooth and crown surfaces.

▼ GENERAL COMPOSITION AND USE OF SPECIFIC MATERIALS ▼

Metal oxide cements

1. Zinc oxide and eugenol—temporary cementation of indirect restorations
2. Zinc phosphate—permanent cementation of indirect restorations and orthodontic bands
3. Zinc polycarboxylate—permanent bonding of indirect restorations and orthodontic brackets

Polymer cements

1. *Glass ionomer*—permanent bonding of porcelain fused to metal indirect restorations and direct bonding of orthodontic brackets
2. *Resin*—permanent bonding of all types of indirect restorations and direct bonding of orthodontic brackets
3. *Resin–ionomer*—permanent bonding of all types of indirect restorations and direct bonding of orthodontic brackets

It is important to note that material selection is subject to the operator's discretion. A cement may be suitable for more than one use, and more than one cement may be appropriate for a specific procedure. Zinc oxide and eugenol cement is not strong enough to be used for permanent cementation, thus is used only for temporary applications. Only resin cement is translucent, so resin is the material of choice for bonding translucent materials: porcelain jacket crowns, porcelain inlays, and polymer or ceramic orthodontic brackets. Glass ionomer cement expands when setting and will cause failure of porcelain jacket crowns, due to the increase in internal pressure on the crown, so cannot be used to cement them. In other cases, cements are interchangeable. The operator chooses to use a particular cement on the basis of an assessment of its characteristics in relation to the task to be accomplished, its record of success for similar applications, conditions in the patient's mouth, and personal preference.

▼ CLINICAL CONCERNS ▼

Clinical concerns include film thickness; cement acidity, strength, and solubility; and development of secondary decay. A thick cement layer between a tooth and restoration can alter restoration fit, proximal contact and occlusion; a thin film will not interfere. Acid cements may leach acids and damage the pulp, especially if they are placed in deep preparations.

Even a thin film of cement or bonding agent must form a joint strong enough to resist chewing forces. Permanent cements should not dissolve in oral fluids, as an open margin exposes the underlying tooth preparation, thereby increasing the possibility of secondary decay.

▼ MATERIAL CHARACTERISTICS ▼

All Cements

Form thin film
Brittle

All Cements Except Resin

Acid when placed
pH rises following set
Opaque

Metal Oxide Cements

Inexpensive
Long history of good service
Slightly soluble in oral fluids
Relatively long working time

1. Zinc oxide and eugenol
   Lowest strength
   Most soluble
2. Zinc phosphate
   High strength
   pH rise is slow
   Less soluble than Z-O-E, more soluble than polymers
3. Zinc polycarboxylate
   Acidity lessens quickly following set
   Low to moderate strength

Polymer Cements

Newer materials
More expensive
Short mixing and working time
Nearly insoluble in oral fluids

1. Glass ionomer
   Moderate to high strength
   pH rises moderately slowly
   Bonds to calcium in tooth structure
   Leaches fluoride
2. Resin
   Translucent
   Strongest
   Not soluble but does wear
   Time-consuming; must be mechanically bonded although some are appearing on the market that are self-etching

▼ HANDLING ▼

Cements are technique sensitive; the acidity, film thickness, strength and solubility of any cement is affected by the mixing procedure. As a general rule, incorporating more powder in a mix increases strength, film thickness and pH, and decreases solubility. This remains true within limits; too much powder decreases strength and increases solubility. The key when mixing is to ensure maximum reaction of powder and liquid, and to incorporate the greatest amount of powder possible without unduly increasing the viscosity of the mix. A number of steps can be taken to do this.

1. Proportion powder first. Liquids evaporate quickly, and the quantity of liquid used in cement mixing is so small that evaporation of even small amounts can seriously affect the mix.

2. Fluff powder particles before proportioning to separate them. Reactions occur on the surface; more surface means more area for reaction.

3. For the same reason, use your mixing spatula to break up any remaining powder clumps before mixing.

4. Recap powder and liquid containers immediately after proportioning to protect the powder from environmental humidity and the liquid from evaporation.

5. Mix polymer cements by quickly incorporating large increments of powder and spatulating only until the mix is homogenous in color and consistency, but still glossy. Once begun, polymerization quickly proceeds to completion. Loss of gloss signals working time has passed. At that point, the mix is too tacky to use and no more free acid is available to bond to the tooth.

6. Mix zinc oxide cements more slowly, using smaller increments of powder. Crush the powder particles well to increase surface reaction area. Ensure the mix is homogenous in color and consistency before adding a new powder increment.

7. Cement that has been properly mixed sticks to the spatula and flows evenly. If it sticks to the spatula and doesn't flow, it is too thick for cementation. If it drips, it is too thin.

8. In preparation for cementation, the inside of a metal item is roughened with a bur microetcher or sharp hand instrument, the powder from the resulting scratches is blown away with compressed air, and the item is washed and dried. This increases the number of internal surface defects on the tissue side of the metal and promotes solid adhesion.

9. Cement is placed in a dry environment to enable contact between the cement and both materials. A solid joint will not be formed if other substances, such as oral fluids, are interposed.

Handling of Specific Cements

The composition and characteristics of zinc oxide and eugenol, glass ionomer and resin were discussed previously. Different forms of the same materials are used for cementation.

Metal Oxides

Zinc Phosphate

Composition and Reaction

Zinc phosphate powder contains zinc and magnesium oxide particles. The liquid is a solution of phosphoric acid and water. When mixed, the acid dissolves the outer layer of the particles. The resulting ions react with the phosphoric acid to from a zinc orthophosphate matrix. The remaining portions of the particles are scattered throughout as reinforcers. Heat is given off as a reaction byproduct.

Mixing

Zinc phosphate is packaged as a powder and liquid. Type I powder, which has small particles, is used for cementation procedures. Use a clean, dry glass slab and a flexible cement spatula for mixing. Set cement that is encrusted on the slab interferes with mixing motions. Water accelerates zinc phosphate set, and even a drop of water quickly hardens the mix. Glass dissipates heat, another accelerator. Some operators chill the slab in a refrigerator or freezer, then wipe it dry before use, to enable it to dissipate even more heat.

- Proportion powder and liquid carefully and recap containers immediately.
- Divide the powder into small portions.
- Incorporate small increments of powder into the liquid and mix over a large part of the slab. As noted, zinc phosphate has an exothermic set; it liberates heat as it hardens. Small increments of powder generate less heat, which can be dissipated more easily before the next increment is incorporated.
- Crush the powder particles well as you mix. Crushed particles react with the liquid more quickly and more thoroughly. This allows more powder to be incorporated more quickly while maintaining an appropriate viscosity.

Test for Completion

Zinc phosphate has reached cementing consistency when it sticks to the spatula and forms a string down to the slab when the spatula is lifted 1" off the slab.

Like all cements, zinc phosphate is applied to the tooth and inside of the item to be cemented with the operator's choice of hand instrument. A wide variety of instruments is used.

Cleanup

Zinc phosphate cement is most easily cleaned from mixing implements if it is removed with a gauze square or tissue immediately following use. When not immediately cleaned, it sets to a hard, brittle, flaky consistency that can sometimes be flicked off. Recalcitrant cement can be softened by running the slab and spatula through an ultrasonic cleaner cycle or soaking them in baking soda solution, then scrubbing them with a brush. Once cleaned, glass slabs and metal cement spatulas can be sterilized.

Zinc Oxide and Eugenol

Z-O-E cement is available as a powder and liquid, as base and catalyst pastes in two tubes, and in preloaded unit dose capsules.

Powder and Liquid System

- Use a fluid-impervious paper pad and flexible cement spatula. Pad paper that is not coated absorbs liquid quickly, thereby increasing the ratio of powder to liquid.
- Ensure powder is well fluffed, and particles are separated with the spatula if needed, as zinc oxide powder tends to clump easily. Proportions are less critical than for zinc phosphate, but it is common for one scoop of powder to be used for each two drops of liquid.
- Recap powder and liquid containers immediately after proportioning each material.
- Divide the powder in halves or quarters and incorporate each separately.
- Crush the particles well to ensure thorough mixing to homogenous color and consistency. Z-O-E never sets completely. This, combined with its weakness, solubility and tendency to form relatively thick films, makes it ideal for temporary applications. Some operators add a small amount of lubricant to the mix to further decrease completeness of set.

- Temporary restorations luted with a Z-O-E plus lubricant cement can be removed easily. Zinc oxide and eugenol cement can be removed by scrubbing the spatula and slab with soap and water. Both can be sterilized. The mixing paper is discarded.

Two Tubes of Paste

- Use a fluid-impervious paper pad and flexible cement spatula for mixing.
- Proportion equal lengths of material, and recap each tube immediately after use.
- Place all catalyst on the base at once and spatulate with a rotary or figure-eight motion to homogenous color and consistency.
- This form of Z-O-E cement mixes quickly and easily and is extremely popular.

Preloaded Capsules

- Hold the capsule upright, and activate it using a twisting motion and pressure.
- Place capsule in the triturator and shake for the required number of seconds.
- This form of Z-O-E is more expensive, but is convenient and provides a consistent mix.

Glass Ionomer

Glass ionomer cement is another form of the same material used as a base, liner, restorative and core buildup material. The cement form is supplied as a powder and liquid, and in preloaded unit dose capsules and tips.

Powder and Liquid

- Use a fluid-impervious paper pad, Type I cement and a flexible cement spatula for mixing.
- Fluff and proportion powder carefully.
- Drop liquid on pad.
- Divide powder in 2–3 large increments, then incorporate each quickly and thoroughly. The glass-based powder is light and initially it seems as if there is too much powder for the liquid. However, if the powder increment is pulled to the center of the mix and rapidly and thoroughly spatulated, it rapidly reacts with the liquid to form a homogenous mass of cementation consistency.

Preloaded Capsules

- The capsule is activated, placed in the triturator, and shaken at the recommended speed for the required number of seconds.
- The mixed material is applied with a hand instrument.

Preloaded Tips

- Tips do not need to be activated.
- They are placed in the triturator, shaken at the recommended speed for the prescribed number of seconds, fitted into a small hand-held gun-type applicator, and squeezed directly onto the area of interest.

Characteristics

Glass ionomer cement requires almost 24 hours to set completely. During that time it is highly soluble and susceptible to drying, cracking and crazing. Many operators place a layer of bonding resin over new glass ionomer cement to protect it during set. Once set, glass ionomer is less soluble than any other cement except resin. It remains acidic enough to irritate the pulp, but at a lesser level than zinc phosphate.

Cleanup

Glass ionomer is easily removed from mixing implements by washing them in soap and water or running them through the ultrasonic cleaner cycle. The spatula and placement instrument can be sterilized. The pad paper is discarded.

Resin

Composition and Characteristics

Resin cement is another form of the acrylic resin that is used for sealants, composite restorative material, and as a bonding agent. The cement form is lightly filled for strength without undue increase in viscosity. Because it is translucent, resin is the cement of choice for porcelain, resin and ceramic restorations, especially inlays and onlays. Resin cements are light or dual cured, and metal does not transmit light. Although dual cure resin cements may be used to bond metals to teeth, all-metal items are usually attached with another material because the bonding strengths to metal are lower than to enamel and dentin.

Resin does not bond chemically to calcium in tooth structure; it must be bonded mechanically. To facilitate such bonding, the restoration or bracket may have mechanical retention incorporated in its design. Additionally, different cement formulations require use of various combinations of the etch–prime–link–cement steps that create bonded joints. The tooth and inside surface of an indirect restoration may be etched. Exposed dentin may be coated with an adhesive primer. Silane linking agent may be painted on porcelain or ceramic items to link them chemically to the cement. Whatever brand of resin cement you use, if you remember the etch–prime–link–cement steps (mnemonic: Every person likes candy.) and what each step accomplishes, you will be able to easily adapt your knowledge to a specific material.

Zinc Polycarboxylate

Composition and Reaction

Zinc polycarboxylate cement (termed *polycarboxylate* or *polyacrylate* by dental personnel) is both a metal oxide and a polymer. It is handled like a polymer and has the strength of a metal oxide.

The powder is glass based. It consists of zinc oxide; other oxides of such metals as magnesium, bismuth and aluminum; and sometimes fluoride; to be combined with water and polyacrylic acid. The acid may be freeze-dried and incorporated in the powder or it may be in the catalyst solution. Distilled water is the catalyst when the acid is in the powder.

When the powder and liquid are mixed, the acid attacks the metal oxide particle surfaces, liberating zinc, magnesium and other metal ions. These ions combine with the acid to form a polycarboxylate matrix with open acids that bond to the calcium in tooth structure. Unreacted particle cores are scattered throughout the matrix and serve as reinforcers. Following set, the pH of polycarboxylate cement rises relatively rapidly. Accordingly, it does not irritate the pulp and is considered to be kind to the tooth.

Mixing

Polycarboxylate cement is supplied in powder and liquid form. The highly viscous liquid must be, but is difficult to, proportion precisely. To simplify measurement, a syringe dispenser is now available in addition to the bottle form. The liquid should not be exposed to air any longer than necessary; always replace its container cap immediately. The liquid also thickens with age. Purchase small bottles more frequently or use a syringe dispenser of liquid. Note expiration dates, place new material in the rear of the storage area, and ensure that the oldest liquid is used first.

To simplify cleanup, polycarboxylate is prepared on a coated paper pad with a flexible cement spatula. It is mixed like a polymer; large increments of powder are spatulated into the liquid quickly and thoroughly. It is ready for use when it is homogenous in color and consistency, flows off the spatula and is still glossy. Glossiness indicates free polyacrylic acid is still available to bond with the tooth. Mixing should be completed within 30 seconds to leave adequate time for placement with a hand instrument before viscosity increases to the point the cement is no longer workable.

Cleanup

The assistant should clean excess cement from the spatula with a gauze square while the operator is placing the cement. Removal becomes annoyingly difficult if it is allowed to set before cleanup is attempted. If working alone, the operator can spray a cotton roll lightly with silicone release spray, then rub the cotton roll over the spatula before beginning to mix. Alternatively, a whisper-thin layer of lubricant can be used. Either will facilitate cleanup later without interfering with the cementing action of the material. The spatula and hand instrument can be disinfected or sterilized. The pad paper is discarded.

KEY POINTS

✓ Cements, also termed *luting agents,* are used to attach indirect restorations and orthodontic appliances to teeth
✓ All cements form joints by filling in surface defects on the two materials; some cements also bond materials together
  • Metal oxide cements do not bond; polymer and combination cements do
  • Glass ionomer and polycarboxylate bond chemically; resin bonds mechanically
✓ Metal oxide cements are inexpensive and have a long record of good service, but are soluble in fluids over time
  • Z-O-E is weak, dissolves easily and is used for temporary applications
  • Zinc phosphate is strong and dissolves more slowly, but retains its acidity after set; it is used for permanent cementation of metal restorations and orthodontic bands
✓ Polymer cements are new, strong and nearly insoluble in oral fluids, but more expensive
  • Glass ionomer bonds to calcium in tooth structure and leaches fluoride, but may irritate the pulp from residual acidity following set
    • It is used for bonding indirect restorations and orthodontic brackets
  • Resin is strong, insoluble and translucent, but must be bonded mechanically
    • It is used for bonding porcelain and ceramic restorations, and direct bonding of polymer and ceramic orthodontic brackets
✓ Zinc polycarboxylate combines the handling ease and chemical bonding of a polymer with the moderate strength supplied by zinc oxide reinforcement
  • It is used for bonding restorations and orthodontic brackets
✓ Material readiness for cementation is indicated by homogenous color and consistency, flow, and for polymers, a glossy surface
✓ Cements are technique sensitive; mixing and handling procedures for each material should be followed precisely

Questions 1–5: *Provide the short answers requested.*

1. How do cements attach materials to teeth?

2. Why is cement solubility important to restoration success or failure?

3. Which cements bond materials to teeth?

4. How does an operator select a specific cement for use?

5. Why is zinc oxide and eugenol cement used for temporary luting?

Questions 6–12: *Select the letter preceding the best answer.*

6. A cement slab used for mixing zinc phosphate should be dry to prevent
   a. Premature set
   b. Excess acidity
   c. Discoloration
   d. All of the above

7. Zinc polycarboxylate is a combination metal oxide–polymer cement that is mixed and handled like a
   a. Metal oxide
   b. Polymer

8. Select the material of choice for bonding porcelain and ceramic restorations.
   a. Glass ionomer
   b. Zinc phosphate
   c. Zinc polycarboxylate
   d. Resin
   e. Zinc oxide and eugenol

9. All cements are
   a. Brittle
   b. Opaque
   c. Slow to set
   d. Fully set within 24 hours following placement

10. Calcium hydroxide may need to be placed under these two cements to protect the pulp from acid leakage.
    a. Z-O-E and zinc phosphate
    b. Glass ionomer and resin
    c. Resin and zinc polycarboxylate
    d. Zinc phosphate and glass ionomer
    e. Only resin requires a calcium hydroxide liner

11. Which cement leaches fluoride into adjacent tooth structure?
    a. Zinc polycarboxylate
    b. Resin
    c. Glass ionomer
    d. Zinc phosphate

12. A glossy surface on a polymer cement indicates
    a. Incomplete mixing
    b. Free acid is present
    c. More powder is needed
    d. The liquid was too old to use

Materials for Tooth Replacements

When a tooth is completely lost, it must be replaced to maintain the integrity of the arch. An indirect restoration, a pontic on a fixed bridge, is one replacement option. However, bridge placement requires substantial financial investment as well as adequate support from, and cutting of, adjacent teeth.

Other options exist. Implants can be anchored in or on the bone, if enough bone exists or can be built up to provide adequate support, and a replacement tooth attached. Implants require a substantial investment of time, money and patience, plus a strong commitment to oral hygiene care, but they can be placed without cutting down adjacent teeth or where no adjacent teeth are present. They appear natural and feel comfortable. Improvements in materials and techniques are making this option quicker, more predictable and more versatile

Additionally, full and partial dentures can replace all or some of the teeth in an arch, often less expensively than a fixed bridge. Partial dentures require adjacent teeth for support but full dentures do not. Less time is required for fabrication. They are removable and easily cleaned. On the other hand, any type of denture may not appear as natural or feel as comfortable as other options. Partial dentures also place stress on supporting teeth. Partial denture connectors trap food and if not cleaned well contribute to decay and periodontal problems.

After considering replacement options, the patient may select a bridge, an implant, or a full or partial denture. This section discusses the materials used to construct them.

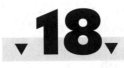

MATERIALS FOR DENTAL IMPLANTS

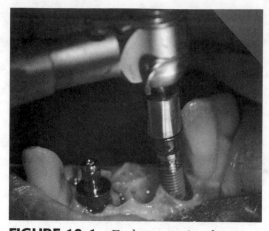

FIGURE 18-1 Endosseous implant. This implant is being driven into the pilot hole drilled by the surgeon. Notice the implant to the left already in place. The top will be removed and replaced with a healing cap.

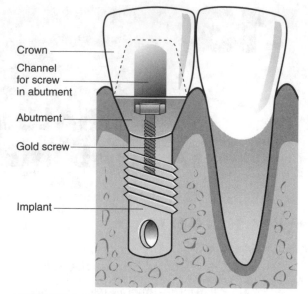

Crown
Channel for screw in abutment
Abutment
Gold screw
Implant

FIGURE 18-2 Implant parts. This shows a common method of attaching the prosthesis to the implant. A gold screw is placed through a channel in the abutment and tightened. The crown is then cemented to the abutment.

▼ DEFINITION AND USE ▼

Implants are tooth replacements that are either anchored in bone or attached to a frame that is placed on the bone surface. This implant will then support a dental prosthesis.

Two types of implants are in common use, both named for their relationship to the bone: *endosseous* and *subperiosteal. End* means "in" and *osseous* refers to "bone." Endosseous implants (Figure 18-1) have metal screw or cylinder fixtures anchored in the bone. This implant often has three parts (Figure 18-2): the *fixture,* the substructure that serves as an anchor or frame; an *abutment,* a connector between the fixture and the prosthesis; and the *prosthesis,* which may be a crown, bridge, or full or partial denture. On occasion the abutment is left out and the prosthesis is attached directly to the implant.

Sub means "below" and the *periosteum* is the soft tissue covering the bone. Subperiosteal implant fixtures are saddle-shaped frames placed below the periosteum. They are positioned on the bone surface and are held in place by the connective tissue. With the success of endosseous implants and increased versatility due to new designs, subperiosteal implants are rare today.

▼ MATERIALS USED ▼

Titanium—pure titanium and titanium alloy
Major alloying metals are aluminum and vanadium
Ceramics
Bioactive—porous hydroxyls and dense ceramics
Inert—aluminum oxide ceramics

▼ MECHANISMS OF ACTION ▼

The dentist has four objectives for an implant:

1. Avoidance of foreign body rejection
2. Development and maintenance of:
   a. osseointegration
   b. a perimucosal seal
3. Esthetics
4. Successful function in occlusion.

Avoidance of Foreign Body Rejection

The body will activate its inflammation and immune systems to reject an internalized foreign body, such as an implant fixture, unless it is made of an inert or compatible material. *Inert* materials do not react chemically. *Compatible* materials react in a nonharmful, and sometimes beneficial, way.

Titanium is a reactive metal but becomes inert in the body through development of *passivity.* It reacts with oxygen in the tissues to form a tough, adherent, nonreactive (passive) surface film. It does leach titanium ions into the tissues but these ions have not been shown to be harmful. Often the titanium is coated with ceramic to promote osseointegration. However, implants without such a coating have proven to be very dependable.

Aluminum oxide ceramics are biocompatible but not bioactive. They are dense, strong, hard ceramics that function well in occlusion and do not react with the bone.

Development of Osseointegration

Bioactive ceramics actively participate in osseointegration. There are two types: *hydroxyl* and *dense ceramic.* Both are calcium–phosphate based and attach to bone. Hydroxyl is a porous ceramic bone substitute. It is used for augmentation of skimpy ridges, filling in bone defects and as a coating for metal substructures. Because it is porous, hydroxyl forms a supporting framework into which new bone can grow. Dense ceramic is used to coat metal implant fixtures or as abutments in partially edentulous patients. It forms surface bonds with bone.

Chemically, bone is also a calcium phosphate so it treats the ceramic as bone and grows into the surface of bioactive ceramics. This provides a seamless link between the two substances.

Development of a Perimucosal Seal

Natural teeth are attached to bone by a periodontal ligament that provides vertical and horizontal support. The gingiva is closely adapted to natural teeth by circular fibers in the gingival portion of the ligament and is attached to tooth structure with epithelial cells (Figure 18-3). When the tooth is gone, the periodontal ligament resorbs, but circular fibers in the gingiva continue to surround the implant. Cells from the sulcus epithelium will attach themselves to the implant but the connection is not as strong as the bond with the natural tooth. The *perimucosal seal* thus formed is a critical factor in preventing microbial invasion adjacent to the implant.

Esthetics

As in every procedure, the esthetics of an implant prosthesis are dependent on the architecture of the intraoral tissues, the knowledge and skill of the dentist and laboratory technician, and the characteristics of the materials used to make it. Refer to Chapter 16 for a discussion of the materials used to fabricate crowns and bridges, and Chapter 19 for a description of materials for full and partial dentures.

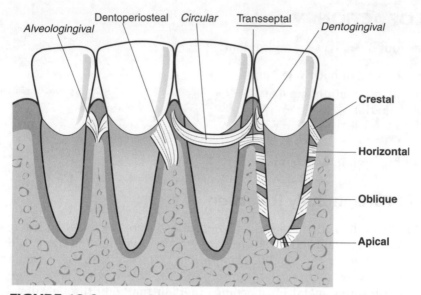

Alveologingival Dentoperiosteal *Circular* Transseptal *Dentogingival*

Crestal

Horizontal

Oblique

Apical

FIGURE 18-3 Periodontal attachment fibers. This shows the gingival fiber groups (italics), principal ligament fibers (bold) and interdental ligament fibers (underlined) on the anterior teeth. This will be changed significantly if an implant takes the place of the tooth root.

Occlusal Function

Successful function in occlusion depends on restoration design and position and material resistance to biting forces. Titanium is a strong, lightweight material that rarely fractures in occlusion. Therefore, the implant is the strongest part of the system. Failure is often seen at the screws that hold the prosthesis to the abutment or implant, at the bone implant interface, or at the ceramic–titanium interface. Titanium also has low susceptibility to corrosion, an advantage in the saline internal body environment. Its principal disadvantage is that it scratches easily, an important factor to consider when developing appropriate oral hygiene procedures for patients with implants.

Ceramic materials are more brittle and can fracture from biting forces; dense ceramics are stronger than hydroxyls. The ceramic–titanium interface on coated implants is a weak point susceptible to fracture.

▼ IMPLANT PROCEDURES ▼

The first step, as always, is patient evaluation. The dentist is concerned that adequate bone and adjacent dental support be available, as well as strong oral hygiene commitment, adequate financial resources and no medical contraindications. Radiographs and models are made to facilitate the diagnostic process.

Once the decision is made to proceed, one of two basic processes is followed, depending on whether the implant will be endosseous or subperiosteal. Endosseous implants are used for crowns, bridges or attachment points for *overdentures;* subperiosteal implants are used only for overdentures. Overdentures are full and partial dentures supported by implants or retained natural tooth roots.

Endosseous procedures begin with surgery to prepare the bone and place the implant fixture and cover. The site is then closed and the fixture is left unloaded (immobile and out of occlusion) for 2–6 months to allow osseointegration to occur. Newer design implants that can be loaded immediately are starting to be used more often.

Once osseointegration is present, the site is reopened. The cover is removed and replaced with an abutment if one is to be used. A healing cap extending into the oral cavity is screwed onto the abutment or if no abutment is used, right down onto the implant itself. The cap is placed to allow formation of a perimucosal seal and to shape the gingiva for an esthetic result.

Tissues surrounding an implant heal at different rates. Because osseointegration takes longer than epithelial attachment, the dentist may place a small piece of membrane between the implant–bone complex and the sulcus epithelium to permit osseointegration to occur without epithelial interference. Such membranes may be self-resorbing but others need to be removed in a separate surgery.

Following healing, implant osseointegration and development of a perimucosal seal, the prosthesis is made and attached. The healing cap is removed. An impression coping is screwed to the abutment and a precisely fitted cylinder is placed over the implant. An impression of the cylinder is taken and used to pour a model on which the crown or bridge will be fabricated. The completed prosthesis is screwed or cemented to the abutment. The entire endosteal implant process may require 6–9 months to complete.

Subperiosteal procedures begin with surgery to expose and take an impression of the alveolar bone. The site is closed and the impression sent to a laboratory for fabrication of a metal, saddle-shaped frame that will fit over the bone. Posts that will serve as abutments protrude from the frame. The site is again entered surgically to position the frame on the bone. The posts are left protruding above the gingiva, a membrane may be placed, and the site is closed and left to heal. As with an endosseous implant, the prosthesis is made and attached following healing and development of a perimucosal seal.

▼ CLINICAL CONCERNS ▼

Clinical concerns include mobility, microbial invasion, mechanical overload and scratching of the implant surface. The concerns are interrelated. Mobility may indicate loss of osseointegration, microbial invasion and inflammation or infection, or loosening of the screw connecting the prosthesis to the abutment. Microbial invasion may result from loss of the perimucosal seal and resulting inflammation, infection, tissue destruction and mobility. Mechanical overload may result in inflammation, tissue destruction and mobility, or implant fracture.

Scratched implant surfaces may aid microbial invasion. Scratching is most likely to result from oral hygiene procedures. As with natural teeth, plaque and calculus form on implants. Toothbrushes, oral hygiene aids, periodontal probes, scalers and polishing procedures can scratch implants if improperly chosen or used. Soft toothbrushes, resin plastic probes and hand scalers, special covers for ultrasonic scaler tips, and mild abrasives are suggested for the patient with implants. Other oral hygiene aids can be used but procedures must be individualized.

Periodontal probing may break the weak perimucosal seal surrounding the implant. Operators disagree about whether implants should be probed. All agree that if implants are probed, careful technique is essential.

The patient with implants needs frequent, thorough professional examination; frequent, conscientious professional prophylaxis; and an individualized home care plan. When problems are found, the cause must be located and corrected. Current titanium implants enjoy a high success rate and are an important component of professional treatment.

KEY POINTS

✓ Implants are tooth replacements that are anchored in bone or attached to a frame that is positioned on the bone
  • Endosseous implants are anchored in bone; subperiosteal implants are attached to frames placed on the bone

✓ The screws, cylinders and frames that anchor implants are made of titanium, a strong, lightweight metal that becomes passive in the tissues
  • Titanium can be coated with bioactive ceramics to enable osseointegration and formation of a perimucosal seal
✓ Aluminum oxide ceramics are biocompatible but not bioactive; they may be used as nonreactive implant components
✓ Fabrication and placement of implants is a complex process that requires months to complete
✓ The patient with implants requires frequent, conscientious, thorough professional examination and prophylaxis and an individualized program of home care

SELF TEST

Questions 1–5: *Describe each process listed below.*

1. Osseointegration

2. Formation of a perimucosal seal

3. Development of titanium passivity

4. Placement of a subperiosteal impant

5. Placement of an endosseous implant

Questions 6–10: *Select the letter preceding the best answer.*

6. Which implant materials are bioactive?
   a. Calcium–phosphate ceramics
   b. Aluminum oxide ceramics
   c. Titanium
   d. Titanium alloys

7. Which reactive material forms a nonreactive surface in the tissues?
   a. Hydroxyl
   b. Dense ceramic
   c. Aluminum oxide ceramic
   d. Titanium

8. How is an implant prosthesis attached to an abutment?
   a. Cemented
   b. Fired
   c. Screwed
   d. Both a and c
   e. All of the above

9. Resin scalers and periodontal probes are used on implants to
   a. Enhance fixture passivity
   b. Improve the operator's tactile sense
   c. Prevent implant scratching
   d. Minimize implant mobility

10. Implant fracture is most likely to occur
    a. When titanium alloy is used
    b. At the titanium–ceramic interface
    c. If titanium is not alloyed with aluminum
    d. If commercially pure titanium cannot be obtained

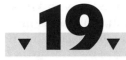

DENTURE MATERIALS

In order to understand the materials used to make dentures, it is necessary to know something about denture types, parts, and clinical procedures. A basic introduction is provided here, but the reader is referred to a clinical text for a more complete discussion of clinical procedures.

▼ TYPES OF DENTURES ▼

Dentures are classified on the basis of number of teeth replaced and time of delivery in relation to completion of preliminary surgery. A *full denture* (Figure 19-1) is a replacement for all the teeth and associated structures in one arch. A *partial denture* (Figure 19-2) replaces some of the teeth and associated structures. A *conventional denture* is not constructed until any necessary surgery has been completed and the tissues have healed. An *immediate denture* is constructed prior to completion of surgery and delivered at the final surgical appointment. The classification categories are not mutually exclusive. For example, an immediate full or partial denture may be constructed.

▼ COMPONENTS ▼

Parts of a Full Denture (Figure 19-3)

Base—portion that mimics the soft tissue and fits over the alveolar ridge. A base restores soft tissue contour, supports the artificial teeth and holds the denture in position.

Flange—portion of the base that extends vertically from the cervices of the teeth toward the mucobuccal fold

Periphery (also termed *border*)—encircling edge located at the deepest part of the flange

Parts of a Partial Denture (Figure 19-4)

Framework—supporting skeleton

Connector (also termed *bar*)—link between parts of the framework

Saddle—portion that overlies soft tissue and supports the artificial teeth

Clasp (also termed *retainer*)—extension that partly encircles an abutment tooth. A clasp provides horizontal stability and support. It consists of two arms. The *reciprocating arm* provides a guide and resistance to the *retention arm* that holds the denture to the tooth.

Rest—small, metal extension near a clasp that fits into a prepared depression on an abutment tooth. Rests provide vertical support and prevent the denture from putting

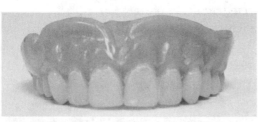

FIGURE 19-1 Full denture. This is an example of a full denture. Note the amount of soft tissue replaced by these restorations.

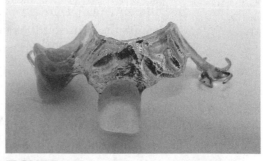

FIGURE 19-2 Removable partial denture. This is an upper partial denture with just two teeth on it.

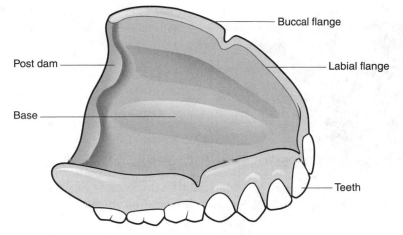

FIGURE 19-3 Full denture. The parts of an upper full denture.

excessive pressure on the ridge. Constant overloading of the ridge will cause bone re-sorption and the loss of bone under the prosthesis will result in improper fit and pa-tient discomfort.

▼ CLINICAL PROCEDURES FOR FULL DENTURE FABRICATION ▼

Appointment 1: Preliminary alginate impressions are taken.

Between appointments 1 and 2: Models are poured and custom trays made.

Appointment 2 Final impressions are taken.

Between appointments 2 and 3: The impressions are sent to a laboratory, which pours working casts, constructs baseplates and occlusal rims (Figure 19-5), and mounts the casts on an articulator. *Baseplates* are temporary denture bases. They are formed of shellac or resin and covered with baseplate wax. They will position and support the occlusal rims when the dentist tries the denture in the patient's mouth to record jaw relationships. *Occlusal rims* (also termed *bite rims*) are arch-shaped blocks of wax attached to the base plates. They occupy the space where teeth will be in the completed denture. An occlusal rim serves to maintain the patient's *vertical dimen-*

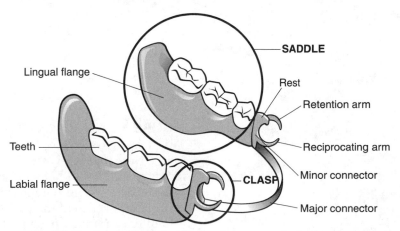

FIGURE 19-4 Partial denture. The parts of a lower partial denture. Note that the lower denture has a lingual flange that upper dentures lack.

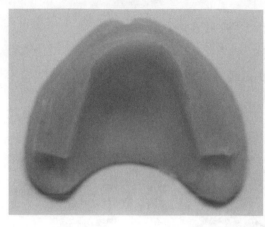

FIGURE 19-5 Occlusal rim. The wax rim is easily changed to find the proper location for the teeth so that the patient has the proper bite and phonetics.

sion, that is, the distance between his or her nose tip and chin center when teeth are present. Together, the baseplate and bite rim form a temporary pattern for the denture.

Appointment 3: The baseplates with occlusal rims attached are tried in the patient's mouth to assess fit and record jaw relationships. Any indicated adjustments are made, the patterns are replaced on the casts and a warm hand instrument is used to lute the rims together at the anterior center to ensure they are stabilized in correct relationship. The dentist also selects the type of material, shade (color) and *mold* (shape; Figure 19-6) to be used for the teeth in the final denture.

Between appointments 3 and 4: The entire assembly is returned to the laboratory, where a technician sets teeth of the prescribed type in correct positions in the wax. The assembly now consists of the baseplate plus the artificial teeth that will be present in the finished denture, and is termed a *wax-up* (Figure 19-7).

Appointment 4: The wax-up is inserted in the patient's mouth, again assessed for fit and function and any indicated adjustments made.

Between appointments 4 and 5: The wax-up is returned to the laboratory, where the permanent denture is constructed, finished, and polished.

Appointment 5: The completed denture is delivered to the patient. He or she is also taught how to insert, remove, and care for it, and may participate in supervised speaking practice.

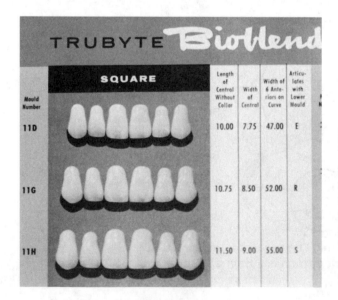

FIGURE 19-6 Mold guide. This is a small portion of a mold guide. Note that it gives measurements of width and height of the central incisors and the measurement of all of the anterior teeth. It also offers a number of shapes. This will guide the dentist in choosing an esthetically pleasing tooth for that patient.

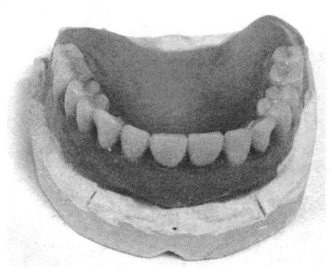

FIGURE 19-7 Wax-up. The wax-up looks like the final denture. It is used to check the esthetics, bite, and fit in the patient's mouth prior to finishing. However, unlike the final denture, the teeth are set in pink baseplate wax.

Appointment 6 and subsequent: The underlying soft tissue is checked and minor adjustments are made to the denture as the patient's tissues adapt in size and shape to daily denture use.

▼ CLINICAL PROCEDURES FOR PARTIAL DENTURE FABRICATION ▼

Appointment 1: Preliminary impressions are taken and models poured.

Between appointments 1 and 2: If custom trays will be needed, they are made. The casts are surveyed to make sure the connectors and clasps will fit the mouth. Any adjustments that will need to be made are marked on the model.

Appointment 2: Any adjustments needed on the teeth are made and final impressions are taken.

Between appointments 2 and 3: A wax pattern is made for the framework and cast using the lost wax technique. Occlusal rims are constructed on the framework.

Appointment 3: The framework is tried in and assessed for fit. An occlusal registration is made. The shade and mold of replacement teeth are selected.

Between appointments 3 and 4: The selected teeth are set in the prescribed positions and the partial is finished and polished.

Appointment 4: The partial denture is delivered. The patient is taught how to insert, remove, and care for the new prosthesis, and may undergo supervised speech practice.

Appointment 5 and subsequent: The denture is checked for continued fit and function, the underlying soft tissue is assessed, and adjustments are made when indicated.

▼ MECHANISMS OF DENTURE ACTION—PROCEDURE LEVEL ▼

Dentures maintain facial contour and esthetics, enable chewing and assist speech, particularly formation of consonants.

▼ MATERIALS USED IN DENTURE CONSTRUCTION ▼

For bases and saddles: Acrylic sometimes with metal palate for added strength
For teeth: Acrylic or porcelain

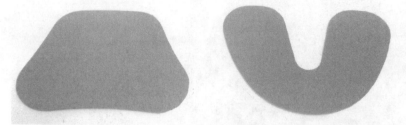

FIGURE 19-8 Shellac. These are shellac baseplate forms. They are rarely used today but were used for final impression trays and baseplates.

For frameworks, connectors, clasps, and rests: Cobalt–chromium, nickel–chromium, or gold alloy
For baseplates: Shellac or resin (Figure 19-8)
For occlusal rims: Baseplate wax (Figure 19-9)

▼ TYPE OF MATERIAL ▼

Acrylic—methyl methacrylate polymer
Porcelain—ceramic
Metal alloys—combinations of metals
Shellac—resinous substance formed of lacquer in alcohol or acetone
Baseplate wax—compound of natural and synthetic waxes

▼ SPECIFIC MATERIALS ▼

Acrylic

The acrylic used in dentures is polymethyl methacrylate, a different member of the acrylic acid polymer family used in varying formulations for sealants, composite restorations, temporary crowns and bridges, direct bonded veneers and implant prostheses.

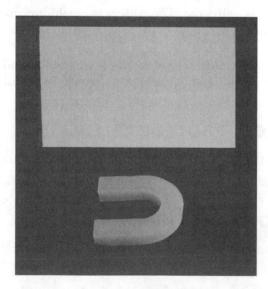

FIGURE 19-9 Baseplate wax. The picture shows two different forms of baseplate wax but cannot show that the waxes also come in different hardnesses.

Composition

A liquid *monomer* is commonly combined with a *polymer* powder to make denture base acrylics. As you are aware from earlier chapters, polymers are formed of repeating molecule units. The repeating unit of denture acrylic is methacrylic acid. The liquid monomer contains separate molecules that are small enough to flow over each other, and hydroquinone as an inhibitor. The powder consists of set polymer that has been ground into small particles, and an initiator, usually benzoyl peroxide. When the powder and liquid are mixed, the particles provide body and the initiator begins the molecule chaining process.

Additional ingredients are included to meet specific needs. Copolymers may be added: vinyl for softening, styrene for hardening, or glycol dimethacrylate for strengthening. Plasticizers make the material more pliable. Colored pigments and inert fibers may be added to create a more natural appearance.

Reaction

Denture base acrylic is formed by polymerization of methacrylic acid molecules. The most complete polymerization of these molecules is initiated by heat rather than by chemical or light. Therefore, since dentures are made out of the mouth, the laboratory usually uses heat as the initiator. Otherwise, it is the same process we have seen in all-acrylic-based materials such as sealants and composites. Of course, shrinkage is a great concern because of the size of the denture base and the necessity of having a tight fit for retention of the prosthesis in the mouth.

Denture Construction

Several techniques are available. *Compression molding* of heat-activated resin is most commonly used.

1. Plaster is placed in the bottom part of an open metal flask. The denture pattern is positioned on it and the assembly set aside to let the plaster harden (Figure 19-10).
2. A separating medium such as petrolatum or alginate solution is painted on all parts of the pattern except the teeth.
3. The pattern is invested. The top part of the flask is attached. Additional plaster is poured around the pattern until the flask is filled, and left to harden (Figure 19-11).

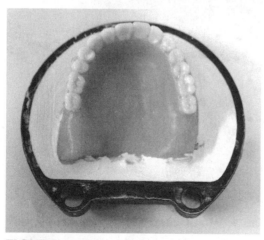

FIGURE 19-10 Flasking. The model is set into the flask and plaster added to secure it in place. No undercuts are allowed to remain in the model.

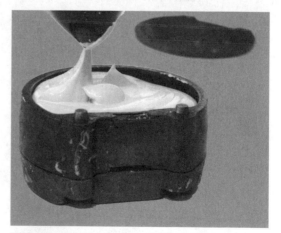

FIGURE 19-11 Flasking. The plaster in the lower section is coated with a releasing agent, the next section of the flask is put on and filled with plaster. The top of the flask can be seen in the background.

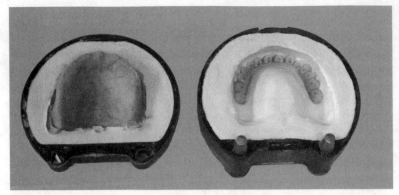

FIGURE 19-12 Boil out. After boiling out the wax the teeth will remain in the upper portion of the flask and the final cast will remain in the lower section.

4. The lid is placed on the flask, which is then placed in simmering water for 10–15 minutes to soften the wax denture base.
5. The parts of the flask are separated and the wax is removed. The teeth do not fall out because they are held in place by the hard plaster. The space formerly occupied by the wax will serve as a mold for the denture base (Figure 19-12).
6. Acrylic resin dough is prepared and placed in the space.
7. The flask is carefully closed to pack the dough into the mold.
8. Pressure is applied to the flask to force excess dough out (Figure 19-13).
9. Excess dough is removed and the flask is subjected to pressure again.
10. When all excess dough has been removed, pressure is again applied; the flask is immersed in a hot water bath and maintained at a controlled temperature for several hours to polymerize the resin.
11. The flask is gradually cooled.
12. The finished denture is removed from the mold, cleaned and polished (Figure 19-14).

A *microwave technique* can also used to polymerize heat-sensitive resin. In that case, the fabrication steps are similar but the flask is nonmetallic and polymerization time is greatly reduced.

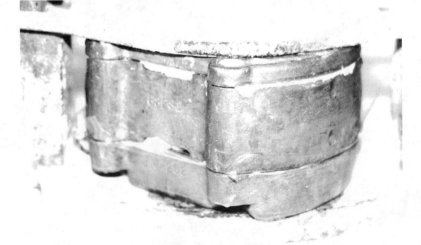

FIGURE 19-13 Compressing material. The flask is put into a vise and the acrylic compressed to make sure it is very dense.

A *pour technique* is used. In that case, the fabrication steps are similar but a special small-particle resin is used and the investing material is reversible hydrocolloid. Vents and sprues are cut into the hydrocolloid and low-viscosity resin is poured into the mold through the sprues. The resin is chemically activated and does not require heat processing.

A *light-activated resin technique* is different. The material is a urethane dimethacrylate with a camphoroquinone initiator. When exposed to visible light, the camphoroquinone decomposes, forming free radicals that initiate polymerization. The material is available in sheets and ropes packaged in lightproof pouches.

For this technique, the teeth are positioned on the cast and the denture base material is sculpted by hand. When the base is complete, the assembly is placed in a light box and exposed for the recommended time. Following polymerization, the denture is smoothed and polished as for the other techniques.

Clinical Concerns

Esthetics. Acrylic is colorless and transparent. It can be modified to simulate a nearly infinite variety of patient tissue shades. Fibers can be inserted to look like blood vessels in the denture base.

Tissue Irritation. Residual monomer in the acrylic resin of a new denture leaches into the oral cavity and may irritate adjacent soft tissue. This is a temporary process that ends when the free monomer has been exhausted. It must be distinguished from tissue irritation caused by poor denture fit, which will worsen if not corrected. Irritated tissue should be professionally evaluated and the denture fit adjusted when indicated.

Fracture. Similar to other polymers, acrylic has better tensile than compressive strength. Accordingly, it flexes well but can fracture when dropped on a hard surface such as a bathroom floor or sink. Patients should be educated to place a paper towel and a few inches of water in the bottom of a sink before cleaning their dentures. If the denture is dropped, the towel and water will cushion its fall.

Acrylic resin is used to repair a fractured denture base or tooth (Figure 19-15). The pieces of a base are anchored in correct position with sticky wax. The inside of the denture is coated with petrolatum or lined with a metal foil separator. A stone gypsum mix is prepared, poured into the tissue side of the denture and set aside to harden. The wax is removed, replaced with resin and set aside to allow the resin to cure. The denture is removed from the model and the resin is finished and polished.

A fractured tooth is cut out of the base with a lab bur, and the dust is blown away. An acrylic mix is made, a new tooth anchored in position with acrylic and the denture set aside to allow the material to polymerize. The area is then finished and the denture polished.

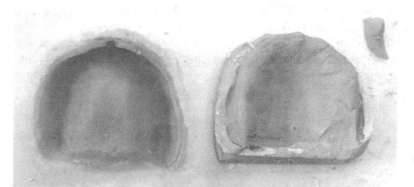

FIGURE 19-14 Removing denture. The model has to be broken out of the denture undercuts. Note the big broken piece in the picture.

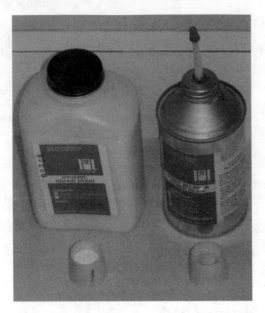

FIGURE 19-15 Repair acrylic. Some repair acrylic has red fibers that are supposed to mimic the blood vessels in the gingiva.

Dimensional Stability. As noted, acrylic shrinks as it cures. To compensate for the shrinkage of the base, a post dam is placed along the posterior border of the upper denture. This is done by carving the model with a sharp instrument prior to flasking. This bulk of material along the back edge helps produce a vacuum seal under the denture and also keeps the denture from warping as it sets. Once in the mouth set acrylic sorbs fluids into the spaces between the tumbled polymer strands. This also expands the acrylic to compensate for shrinkage. The fluid will evaporate from the denture if left out in the air, so patients must be instructed to place the dentures in water when not in the mouth to avoid shrinkage.

Discoloration. Fluids may carry microorganisms and dissolved coloring agents into a denture. Although acrylic dentures can discolor and acquire odors through this mechanism, good oral hygiene practices normally prevent both problems.

Material Stability. Material components, particularly plasticizers and coloring agents, may leach out of a denture. This is a more serious problem that can result in brittleness and discoloration.

Some patients soak their dentures in bleach solution to clean them and remove odors. Bleach is safe for acrylic but removes color from the inert fibers added to simulate blood vessels and attacks the metal of partial denture frameworks. Patients with fiber-enhanced dentures or partial dentures should be educated to avoid soaking them in bleach solutions.

Brittleness and discoloration that result from leaching or bleaching cannot be rectified short of replacing the base material.

Distortion. Acrylic is subject to softening and distortion at temperatures as low as 180°F. Thermostats in homes and public buildings are often set for hot water to emerge from the faucet at not too far below that temperature. Patients should be educated to avoid cleaning their dentures with hot water.

Wear. Both natural and porcelain teeth wear opposing acrylic teeth. Acrylic also roughens and wears readily when subjected to abrasive agents. Therefore, anything used to clean dentures must be nonabrasive. Many suitable commercial cleaners are available. Ordinary soap also works well.

Porcelain

Porcelain is no longer the material of choice for the majority of denture teeth. It is an esthetic ceramic that is dimensionally stable and does not discolor, but is subject to brittle fracture and wears opposing natural or acrylic teeth. Porcelain denture teeth can also click annoyingly when in use.

Porcelain teeth are now selected primarily for the anterior where appearance is a paramount consideration, biting forces are low, clicking is unlikely to occur, and opposing teeth will not be harmed.

Metal Alloys

Cobalt–Chromium

Cobalt–chromium is a base metal casting alloy that typically also includes molybdenum and small amounts of other metals. It is used for denture frameworks and orthodontic wires. Cobalt–chromium alloys offer low cost, strength, light weight, good sag and corrosion resistance, hardness, biocompatibility, and an ability to bond to ceramic.

All three metals bring low weight, hardness, strength and a white metal color to the alloy. Cobalt also brings ductility, but is brittle. Chromium adds corrosion resistance, the ability to take a high polish and passivity in oral fluids, but is susceptible to pitting when exposed to chlorine. Molybdenum counteracts brittleness with its ductility and malleability, and resists corrosion.

Gold

Gold is a soft metal that is ductile, malleable, chemically inactive and unaffected by moisture, but susceptible to attack by halogens such as fluorine and chlorine.

Gold alloys are no longer widely used for denture components because of their cost and relative softness. They are flexible and are occasionally used to form metal stress relievers embedded in the palatal portion of full maxillary dentures.

Older patients may have partial dentures with gold alloy components. Gold clasps are easily adjusted because of their ductility. Partials with exposed gold alloy components should not be soaked in bleach solutions.

KEY POINTS

- ✓ Denture acrylic is polymethyl methacrylate
  - • Methyl methacrylate is another member of the acrylic polymer family of materials with varying formulations used for sealants, composite restorations, resin inlays, veneers, implant prostheses and resin cement
- ✓ Monomer (liquid) and polymer (powder) are mixed to form acrylic dough
- ✓ Compression molding is used to construct the vast majority of acrylic dentures
- ✓ Following polymerization, free monomer remains in acrylic; it may leach from new dentures and irritate the tissues
- ✓ Dentures are dimensionally stable if kept moist and protected from hot water
- ✓ Denture acrylic flexes well but is subject to brittle fracture
- ✓ Bleach solutions can pit metal alloy partial denture parts and remove color from the inert fibers used in acrylic to simulate blood vessels
- ✓ Acrylic denture bases and teeth are subject to wear from abrasive agents
- ✓ Porcelain denture teeth wear opposing natural and acrylic teeth
- ✓ Cobalt–chromium alloy is used for casting metal partial denture parts; it is strong, light-weight, biocompatible and resistant to tarnish and corrosion

Questions 1–10: *Select the letter preceding the best answer.*

1. The framework of a partial denture is cast in
   a. Methyl methacrylate
   b. Cobalt–chromium alloy
   c. Plasticized methacrylate
   d. Gold alloy

2. A denture base
   1. Restores soft tissue contour
   2. Covers the alveolar ridge
   3. Supports the artificial teeth
   4. Overlies and mimics soft tissue
   a. 1 and 3
   b. 2 and 4
   c. 1, 2, and 3
   d. 4 only
   e. All of the above

3. Partial denture clasps provide _____ support; rests provide _____ support.
   a. Vertical; horizontal
   b. Vertical; vertical
   c. Horizontal; vertical
   d. Horizontal; horizontal

4. Baseplate is a thermoplastic material comprised of _____ in alcohol or acetone.
   a. Polymer
   b. Shellac
   c. Conditioner
   d. Acrylic

5. Occlusal rims maintain _____ while the dentist records _____.
   a. Vertical dimension; jaw relationships
   b. Jaw relationships; vertical dimension
   c. Occlusal stability; bite relationships
   d. Bite relationships; occlusal stability

6. Polymers formed by condensation reactions are usually _____ polymers that _____.
   a. Thermosetting; are dimensionally stable
   b. Thermosetting; shrink as they cure
   c. Thermoplastic; are dimensionally stable
   d. Thermoplastic; shrink as they cure

7. Which of the following is used to initiate polymerization?
   a. Hydroquinone
   b. Vinyl
   c. Styrene
   d. Benzoyl peroxide

8. The patient with a new denture may experience tissue irritation because ceramic fibers have leached from the denture material and abraded the tissue.
   a. Both statement and reason are correct and related.
   b. Both statement and reason are correct but not related.
   c. The statement is correct but the reason is not accurate.
   d. Neither statement nor reason is accurate.

9. Bleach solutions may damage
   a. Cobalt–chromium alloy
   b. Denture acrylic
   c. Inert colored fibers
   d. Both *a* and *c*
   e. All of the above

10. Adding a styrene copolymer to acrylic resin _____ the material.
    a. Hardens
    b. Softens
    c. Strengthens
    d. Cross-links

Questions 11–14: *Identify the indicated denture parts in the illustrations below.*

11–12.

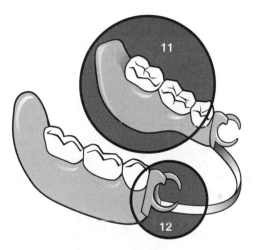

13–14.

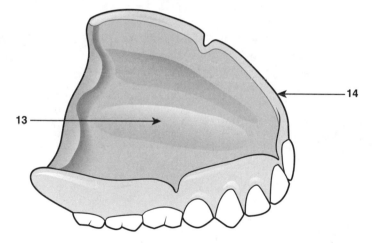

VI

Materials for Pulp Therapy

Badly injured, infected or broken down teeth that will be restored using dental materials often also undergo endodontic treatment. This section discusses the materials used in pulp therapy procedures.

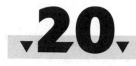

ENDODONTIC MATERIALS

OBJECTIVES

After studying this chapter, you should be able to:

1. Recognize procedures in which endodontic materials will be used.
2. Define and describe the general functions of endodontic irrigants, medicaments, sealers and fillers.
3. List materials used for each of the four types of endodontic tasks, and state why the dentist may select a specified material for use.

▼ DEFINITION ▼

Endodontic materials are materials used during procedures to remove pulp tissue and fill the resulting space within the tooth.

▼ USE ▼

Endodontic materials are used in pulp therapy procedures. When tooth pulp is irreversibly damaged through infection or other injury, several distinct steps are followed for its removal and replacement with a filling material. First, the tooth is isolated through placement of a dental dam. Next, access to the pulp is gained by entering the tooth with a bur and sometimes a hand instrument. Third, the pulp is removed. When the tooth is nonvital and all of the pulp is removed, the procedure is termed pulp *extirpation*. If the tooth is vital and all of the pulp is removed, it is a *pulpectomy*. If it is vital and only the coronal pulp is removed, the procedure is a *pulpotomy*. When the tooth is vital but immature, therefore has no root apex, special procedures are followed to stimulate the production of an apex and its covering with cementum. This process is termed *apexification*.

Following pulp removal, debris is flushed from the space, it is shaped to receive a filling material, sealed and filled. Materials are used at each therapeutic step. The dentist chooses specific materials from among those available based on the goals of the therapy and the specific characteristics of each material. None are perfect, but all have long records of good service and some have been used successfully for over 200 years. This description of endodontic procedures is necessarily brief, and the interested reader is referred to a clinical text for a fuller discussion.

Materials Used—Function

Irrigating agents—cleanse the cavity by flushing away debris and tissue fluid, and provide lubrication for instruments entering the area. Some also have a disinfectant action.

Sodium hypochlorite
Sterile saline solution
Sterile water
EDTA

Medicaments—used to sterilize or disinfect the area. Some also stimulate the production of dentin and cementum.

Calcium hydroxide
Formocresol
Camphorated parachlorophenol
Metacresyl acetate
Beechwood creosote
Eugenol

Sealers—seal the microspace between the tooth and the filling material to prevent entrance of fluids and microorganisms

Zinc oxide and eugenol cements
Non-eugenol materials
Therapeutic sealers

Fillers—obturate the space

Gutta percha
Sargenti paste
Silver points

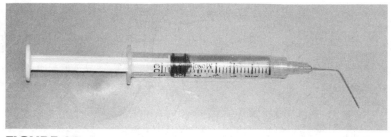

FIGURE 20-1 Irrigating syringe. This is an endo irrigating syringe ready for use. The tip of the cannula is flat-ended and has an open section on the side near the tip. They do not come bent but to make it easier to insert into the canal they are easily bent to any angle desired.

▼ SPECIFIC MATERIALS ▼

Irrigating Agents

Irrigating agents are liquids that are placed in a small glass or plastic syringe and injected into the space within the tooth that remains following pulp removal (Figure 20-1).

Sodium Hypochlorite

Sodium hypochlorite is more familiar as household bleach, which is a solution of 5.25% sodium hypochlorite in water. It is an excellent tissue solvent so it is useful for dissolving tiny tissue tags that can be difficult to remove. It also serves as a lubricant, and because of its chlorine content is a disinfectant. Additionally, because many of the bacteria that infect the periapical tissues are anorobic, meaning they can survive only in areas without oxygen, the oxygen in sodium hypochlorite solution aids in providing a hostile environment for them. Sodium hypochlorite solution may be used at full strength, but is often diluted with 1–2 parts water to lessen its chlorine odor and its ability to damage the soft tissue or bleach fabric if it is spilled.

Sterile Saline Solution

Water is mixed with sodium chloride, more familiar as common table salt, in a ratio of 0.9 grams salt to 100 milliliters water, and sterilized to form a sterile physiologic saline solution. It provides mild disinfection, some dissolution of tissue and irrigation of the area.

Sterile Water

Sterile water can be used as an irrigant. It decreases the bacterial count by flushing organisms away, but in itself is not a disinfectant and does not decrease microorganism numbers sufficiently well to obtain a negative culture. It does serve as a lubricant for instruments entering the canal.

Hydrogen Peroxide

Hydrogen peroxide releases oxygen in the canal to kill anaerobic bacteria and if used alternately with sodium hypochlorite will bubble, helping to loosen and bring debris to the access opening in the tooth.

EDTA (Ethylenediaminetetraacetic Acid)

This chemical is used to dissolve debris and the smear layer of tooth shavings within the canal. This allows the sealer to work more effectively to coat the entire inner tooth surface. It also acts to disinfect the area and in paste form is an excellent lubricant.

▼ MEDICAMENTS ▼

Medicaments may be disinfectants, sterilants, caustics, or may stimulate the formation of new hard or soft tissue.

Calcium Hydroxide

Calcium hydroxide is a biologically active disinfectant. It was discussed at some length in Chapter 11 because it is used as a liner in cavity preparations for direct restorations. The same material is used in endodontic therapy procedures, where its high pH, relatively slow release of hydroxyl ions, and ability to irritate the pulp can be used to good advantage in disinfecting the pulp cavity and stimulating formation of new dentin and cementum.

As a water-soluble compound with a high pH (11–12), calcium hydroxide provides a hostile environment for bacterial growth. Also, when vital pulp is present (during a pulpotomy or apexification procedure), calcium hydroxide acts as a tissue irritant. Immediately subjacent to (underneath) the hydroxide layer, a layer of coagulation necrosis is formed. Subjacent to that, a zone of inflammation appears. Subjacent to the inflammation, the tissue remains vital. Within four weeks following placement, odontoblasts (dentin forming cells) have differentiated in response to the inflammation and a new dentin matrix is beginning to be secreted. Because calcium hydroxide continues to release hydroxyl ions into the immediate environment for several weeks following placement, keeping the pH high, the enzyme phosphatase, which releases inorganic phosphate from the blood, becomes active. Phosphatase release causes calcium phosphate to precipitate in the area, and this precipitation aids in repair of the dentin forming the cavity walls. If calcium hydroxide is left in place for several months to a year and covered with a temporary restoration, cementum will also form. This is useful in cases where an immature tooth has no apex and one must be created (Figure 20-2), or where a small area of cementum on a tooth has been lost because of disease or other injury and needs to be replaced. When calcium hydroxide is placed for the long term, it may be mixed with camphorated parachlorophenol, a stronger disinfec-

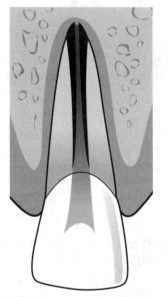

FIGURE 20-2 Apexification. The dark area shows the pulp of an immature tooth and the light line the pulp that results after apexification.

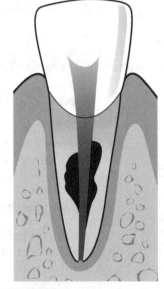

FIGURE 20-3 Internal resorption. The light area shows a normal pulp and the dark area a pulp undergoing internal resorption.

tant, to make a paste that is placed as a temporary filling material which performs all of the functions of calcium hydroxide and also helps to prevent infection.

Calcium hydroxide is a very helpful, commonly used agent, but it is not an unalloyed good. Sometimes vital pulp in a tooth in which it was placed undergoes metaplasia (cell change), and the tooth experiences internal resorption (resorption from the inside out—Figure 20-3) rather than repair. Placement of calcium hydroxide in a tooth may also result in hypermineralization of dentin.

Currently calcium hydroxide is the only medicament used and it is confined mainly to apexification procedures. The following medicaments are rarely used although they still have a role in pulpotomy procedures. As the instrumentation for endodontics has improved, most root canal therapy is done in one visit, ending the necessity of keeping bacteria out of the canal between visits.

Formocresol

Formocresol is a combination of tricresol, aqueous formaldehyde, glycerin and water that is used to cauterize small tags of tissue that stubbornly remain and continue to bleed following pulp removal. The canal is dried with a paper point (Figure 20-4), then a paper point or cotton pellet is dipped in the formocresol and placed in the canal for 3–4 minutes. If a formocresol pellet is to be left in place until the next visit, open space is left in the cavity as an area for accumulation of exudates. The formocresol pellet may then be covered with a dry cotton pellet and the whole covered with a zinc oxide and eugenol temporary restoration.

Formocresol is also used as a bactericide and moderate to strong pulp irritant in pulpotomy procedures. Application of formocresol results in fixation of the surface pulp tissue, under which a zone of inflamed tissue develops. That in turn overlies a zone of normal tissue. Formocresol works by diffusion and volatization to affect the entire pulp cavity and the periapical tissues. Approximately seven weeks after application, an ingrowth of apical granulation tissue begins. By six months, vital pulp tissue and deposition of new dentin are seen throughout the area, extending to the crown.

Metacresylacetate (Cresatin)

Cresatin is another phenol derivative; it provides mild disinfection and pulp irritation. It too is placed in the canal on a paper point or cotton pellet, and works by diffusion and volatization. *Beechwood creosote* is also a phenol derivative that works by diffusion and volatization. It is less irritating to the pulp than formocresol, and more irritating than methylcresylacetate.

Eugenol

Eugenol, or oil of cloves, is an acidic essential oil that is also used as a pulp irritant and mild antiseptic when canal finishing and filling must be delayed. A cotton pellet is

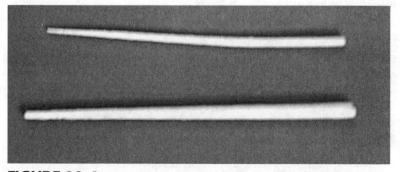

FIGURE 20-4   Paper points. You can see that they are tapered to fit into the canal and come in different sizes.

soaked in eugenol and sealed in the canal until all bleeding is stopped, all pulp tissue tags are removed, all infection is gone and permanent obturation of the canal can be completed.

Camphorated Parachlorophenol (Cresanol)

Cresanol is 35% parachlorophenol in camphor that functions as a bactericide and moderate pulp irritant. It is mixed with calcium hydroxide to form a paste that is placed in the canal to induce cementum formation, to cover any unwanted opening in the root cementum or to close the apex of an injured immature tooth with hard tissue.

Sealers

A sealer forms a fluid-tight seal at the apex of an endodontically-treated tooth by filling the microspace between a root canal filling and the tooth. It must adhere tightly to the tooth surface, be insoluble in oral fluids and should not escape from the pulp cavity to irritate the periapical tissues. Sealers may be placed by spinning them into position with a lentulo spiral (Figure 20-5), a thin instrument which fits into and rotates on the end of a handpiece, or spreading them in position with a hand instrument. Three types of sealers are used: zinc oxide and eugenol (Z.O.E.) sealers, non-eugenol sealers, and therapeutic sealers. Zinc oxide and eugenol sealers are by far the most commonly used.

Eugenol Sealers

Eugenol sealers are zinc oxide and eugenol cements which have a base of zinc oxide particles, a eugenol catalyst, and modifiers such as other essential oils, waxes, opacifiers and resins. They may be packaged as a powder and liquid or as two pastes. They are mixed on a sterile slab and placed with a sterile instrument.

Z.O.E. sets by a combination of chemical and physical processes that create a hard mass of zinc oxide in long sheath-like crystals of zinc eugenolate. There is always some unreacted eugenol left over and it serves to decrease the strength of the set material.

Although eugenol sealers are effective, eugenol is cytotoxic and should not escape into the periapical tissues. Additionally, a measurable segment of the population experiences an allergic response when exposed to it. Accordingly, manufacturers developed sealers which do not contain eugenol.

Non-Eugenol Sealers

Non-eugenol sealers are cements which have a base of powdered zinc oxide, gutta percha or silver. The catalyst may be chloroform, ether, caproic acid or vinyl copolymers. Modifiers such as rosin and metallic opaquers may be added. Such sealers may be packaged as powder and liquid, two pastes or as self-cured polymer formulations. They are effective, but are also cytotoxic and have more problems with shrinkage following placement than do the eugenol sealers. Where shrinkage occurs, leakage may follow, so they have not been embraced as well as eugenol-based materials.

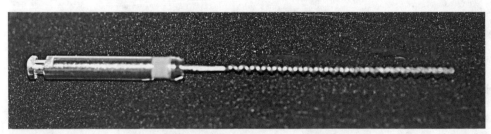

FIGURE 20-5 Lentulo-spiral. This drill uses a principle developed by Archimedes 2,500 years ago to propel cement down the canal.

Therapeutic Sealers

Therapeutic sealers are cements with a base of zinc oxide, iodophor or calcium hydroxide. Calcium hydroxide stimulates new hard tissue formation. Iodophor is an antiseptic; other antiseptics such as creosote, paraformaldehyde or essential oils may be incorporated as well. Modifiers such as opacifiers, corticosteroids to lessen post-operative pain, and self-polymerizing resin systems to prevent material dissolution may be included.

Fillers

Once the canal is cleaned, flushed, sterilized and sealed, it must be filled to obturate the space so that there is no area available for bacteria to live and reinfect the tooth. Gutta percha is most commonly used for this, but in the past silver points, special cements and Sargenti paste were used.

Gutta Percha

Gutta percha is a natural thermoplastic polymer that is both viscous and elastic. This makes it useful for compacting into root canal spaces. The monomer which polymerizes to form gutta percha is isoprene, the same monomer that forms natural rubber. They are two distinct materials, however. The bonds in natural rubber (the *alpha* form) are in a different position than they are in gutta percha (the *beta* form), so the two materials have different properties.

Gutta percha is a very old material that predates the requirement that manufacturers list the components of any material used in treatment procedures. Chemical analysis indicates it contains gutta percha, zinc oxide filler, radiopaquers, waxes, plasticizers, coloring agents, and antioxidizing agents. The synthetic form, which is used in dentistry, is crystalline, but tends to revert to its natural amorphous form when heated.

Dentists use gutta percha points and cones to fill root canal spaces (Figure 20-6). Generally the gutta percha is fitted into the canal and then heated to soften the material so it can be compacted into the canal. This allows the gutta percha to flow into small lateral canals and crevices in the main canal, thus filling the space completely. The heating can be done in an oven and the warm gutta percha taken to the tooth and pressed into place (Figure 20-7). Alternatively, gutta percha can be placed in the tooth, then heated and pressed with a suitable instrument. When endodontic procedures are completed, the patient may choose to have a post, core, and synthetic crown placed on the tooth to prevent later fracture. Endodontic treatment weakens the tooth substantially.

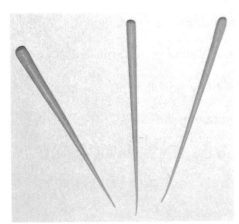

FIGURE 20-6 Gutta percha points. These try to approximate the taper of the root canal instruments and are compressed into the canal usually with heat to make them adapt better to the canal walls.

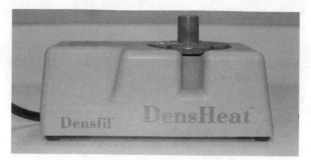

FIGURE 20-7 Oven. This oven warms gutta percha on special carriers so that it can be placed into the tooth when warm.

Sargenti Paste

Sargenti filling paste has never been well embraced in the United States, but was once used here by many practitioners. Very few use it now. It was more popular in Europe, where it originated. The material contains a zinc oxide base, corticosteroid anti-inflammatory agents, a formaldehyde antiseptic, metal opacifiers and other modifiers. Eugenol is used as a catalyst. The toxicity of the material is high. It is soluble in oral fluids so it leaches out of the tooth over time, severely compromising its performance. Problems such as transient parasthesia (temporary loss of sensation) and periapical cytotoxicity have been associated with its use.

Silver Points

Prior to the better instrumentation available now, which allows better shaping of canals and better compaction of gutta percha, silver points were often used by practitioners, especially in canals with severe curvatures. The points were made of a soft silver that would bend to follow the canal curvature. Copious amounts of sealer were needed to fill the crevices and non-round areas in the canal. Silver points can still be seen in some older patients' mouths, attesting to their sealing ability in the right environment. However, because canals filled with silver points relied on sealer for their sealing ability and sealer can dissolve over time, the open spaces that resulted enabled reinfection to occur more easily. Today, there is consensus that gutta percha gives the patient the best long-term prognosis.

KEY POINTS

✓ Endodontic materials are used during pulp therapy procedures to irrigate, medicate, seal or fill the pulp cavity.

✓ Irrigating agents flush debris from the canal and provide lubrication for instruments used in the canal.
  • Sodium hypochlorite, sterile saline solution and sterile water are used as irrigants.

✓ Medicaments soften the sides of the canal to enable its widening and shaping to receive a filling, and sterilize or disinfect the area. Some also stimulate the production of new hard or soft tissue.
  • Calcium hydroxide, camphorated parachlorophenol, formocresol and other phenol derivatives are used as medicaments.

✓ Sealers seal the microspace between the tooth and the filling material to prevent microleakage and contamination.
  • A variety of eugenol, non-eugenol and therapeutic sealers is available.

✓ Fillers obdurate the space and provide strength to the tooth.
  • Gutta percha, a viscoelastic polymer, is the preferred filling material at present.

1. Suggest several reasons why it makes a difference which endodontic procedure is being completed.

2. How can endodontic materials be used to cause formation of a tooth apex on an immature tooth or to repair damaged cementum?

3. Why are disinfectants routinely used in endodontic procedures?

4. Why are endodontic sealers used in addition to fillers?

5. Why is it important that an endodontic sealer or filler not shrink excessively once it is placed?

6. Why is formocresol used in endodontic procedures and how does it work?

GLOSSARY

Abrade: Wear away.

Abrasion: Resistance to wear.

Abrasive: Material composed of hard particles that is used to wear away a softer material.

Abutment: (1) A tooth that is used to anchor a bridge or removable partial in position; (2) connector between an implant fixture and prosthesis.

Acrylic: Also termed *resin*; a plastic material; a polymer that consists of repeating units of acrylic acid, methacrylic acid, or dimethacrylic acid that is used for sealants, direct restorations, inlays, denture bases and saddles, denture teeth and orthodontic appliances.

Activator: A material that adds energy to monomers to open some of their end bonds.

Adhesion: Means of attaching two solids together. Bonding may occur through mechanical interlocking or the sharing of outer shell electrons, to eliminate microleakage, or the filling in of defects on the surfaces of the two materials, to create a mechanical joint.

Adsorption: Attraction of a liquid to the surface of a solid.

Agar: Reversible hydrocolloid material; a suspension of polysaccharides in water that is used for final impressions for pouring accurate models in the indirect restoration fabrication process.

Alginate: Also termed *irreversible hydrocolloid*; a suspension of alginate and silica in water that is used to take impressions for pouring study models, models for custom trays and fabrication of some items that do not require precise accuracy of fit.

Aluminum: A silver-colored metal that is used in the form of prefabricated temporary crown shells.

Aluminum oxide: A reddish-brown or white natural mineral that is mined from the earth and made into a powder that is used as an abrasive in dentistry.

Amalgam: A nonesthetic material made of mercury and another metal. Silver alloy amalgam is used for direct restorations, core buildups and retrograde restorations.

Amorphous: Having an irregular arrangement of internal atoms, less regular melting and solidifying temperatures and sometimes the ability to flow in the solid state.

Apicoectomy: Surgical removal of the apical portion of a tooth root.

Appliance: Device used to replace or act on oral tissues.

Base: A relatively thick layer of cement under a restoration to protect the pulp from thermal, chemical or mechanical injury.

Bioactive: Capable of reacting with tissue.

Biocompatible: Nonharmful, and sometimes beneficial, to tissue.

Black's Cavity Classification: A system of categorizing prepared teeth according to their location and extent that was first proposed by Dr. G. V. Black. Class I—on occlusal surface or in occlusal two-thirds of a broad surface; Class II—includes a posterior proximal surface; Class III—includes an anterior proximal surface; Class IV—includes an incisal angle; Class V—in the cervical third of a broad surface; Class VI (added by others later)—abraded cuspal or incisal surface

Bonded bridge: A Maryland bridge; a bridge that is bonded to the adjacent tooth.

Bonding: The mechanical interlocking of two solids or the sharing of outer shell electrons by two solids.

Bridge: An indirect restoration that replaces one or more missing teeth and is cemented or bonded in position.

Cake: A pressed solid composed of abrasive particles in a binding material that is used in the laboratory.

Calcium hydroxide: A material with a very basic pH that is used as a liner in the deepest part of a cavity preparation.

Cantilevered bridge: A bridge that has a pontic on either or both ends.

Carbamide peroxide: A nitrogen peroxide oxygenating agent that serves as a tooth bleaching material.

Carbide: A type of steel supplied as burs, disks, and wheels that is used to cut natural teeth, and contour and smooth restoration materials.

Cartridge: A disposable, multidose container that contains two materials that will be mixed as they are expelled through a rotary mixing tip attached to a hand-held, gun-type syringe.

Catalyst: A trigger for setting.

Cement: (1) A member of the cement family of materials; various cements may be used as a base, liner, direct restoration, luting agent or wound dressing; (2) a luting agent.

Ceramic: A glass material that is a combination of kaolin, feldspar, and quartz, all of which are natural minerals, and is used for inlays, onlays, crowns, bridges and veneers.

Ceromer: An esthetic hybrid of ceramic and an acrylic polymer.

Chroma: Vividness (saturation) of a color.

Coarse: Large and irregular, therefore rough.

Color: Human perception of the light waves reflected by an object.

Compomer: A hybrid material composed of composite resin and glass ionomer.

Composite: Also termed *composite resin*; a dimethacrylic acid polymer material that is heavily filled and used for direct restorations, veneers, inlays, cementation and sealants. This is the same material as resin but is more heavily filled, therefore stronger.

Compression: Pushing load.

Compressive strength: The ability to resist pushing.

Compule: A unit dose packaged as a disposable syringe tip.

Condensation: The pushing of a material into a cavity preparation.

Conditioner: (1) Material used in an intermediary manner between a prepared tooth and a restoration; (2) etchant; (3) polymer used to promote tissue healing under a denture.

Conductivity: The ability of a material to move an electrical current or temperature change through itself.

Conventional bridge: An indirect restoration that replaces one or more missing teeth and is cemented to abutment teeth on both sides.

Corrosion: Pitting and disintegration of a material from electrochemical assault.

Creep: Flow after set.

Cross-linking agent: A copolymer added to a monomer material that will attach developing chains to one another during the polymerization process, thereby strengthening the resulting polymer.

Crown: A "cap"; an indirect restoration that replaces all or almost all of the natural tooth crown and is cemented or bonded in position.

Crystalline: Composed of crystals formed by solidification of a chemical element, compound, or mixture, and often external plane faces.

Cure: To polymerize; to harden a polymer material.

Custom tray: Tray made from a model of a specific patient's oral structures and used to take a very accurate final impression.

Deformation: A change in shape.

Denture: An appliance that replaces all of the lost teeth and associated structures in one arch.

Die: A very strong, accurate model of a single tooth.

Direct restoration: A "filling"; a restoration that is made in the tooth.

Disintegration: The breaking up of a solid in a liquid.

Disk: A thin, round piece of plastic or metal to which abrasive particles have been attached.

Ditching: Marginal breakdown of an amalgam restoration that creates a visible space around it.

Dry strength: The strength of a gypsum model after its excess water has evaporated; the full strength of a gypsum model.

Ductility: The ability of a metal to be drawn into a wire.

Elastic limit: The point beyond which a deformed material cannot regain its original size and shape.

Elastic modulus: Stiffness.

Elasticity: The ability to return to original size and shape following deformation.

Emery: Also termed *corundum*; an abrasive that appears similar to an emery board fingernail file and is used as an abrasive.

Endosseous implant: Tooth root replacement that is anchored in the bone.

Esthetic: Having a natural appearance; tooth-colored.

Etchant: An acid solution used to make small depressions on a tooth surface to prepare it for mechanical bonding.

Eugenol: Oil of cloves; used as a catalyst and pulp irritant in various zinc oxide and eugenol material formulations.

Excess water: Unreacted water in a recently poured gypsum model.

Fabricate: Construct; make.

Filler: An inert ingredient in a material that provides body and strength.

Fine: Small and rounded, therefore relatively smooth.

Finish: Cut and contour.

Flask: Container for holding materials in correct position while a denture is being constructed and allows pressure to be added to the material during setting.

Flow: The ability to move in a smooth, uninterrupted manner.

Fluorescence: The emission of previously absorbed energy as light at a different wavelength.

Formocresol: Material derived from phenol and containing formaldehyde that is used in pulp therapy procedures to cauterize small bleeding tissue tags left in the canal and as a bactericide and pulp irritant.

Fracture: Break.

Full denture: An appliance that replaces all of the teeth and associated structures in one arch.

Glass ionomer: A polymer cement that is used for sealants, direct restorations, cementation and as a liner that is also a bonding agent.

Grit: The particle size and smoothness of an abrasive material.

Gutta percha: Thermoplastic, viscous, elastic root canal filling material that is an isoprene polymer.

Gypsum: A family of calcium sulfate materials that consists of natural mineral mined from the earth, then processed and used to pour models and make molds for casting metals; plaster, stone, die stone and investment are all gypsum materials.

Healing cap: A cover for an implant abutment, or for the implant itself if no abutment is present, that extends into the oral cavity and permits formation of a perimucosal seal.

Homogenous: All the same; e.g., homogenous color and consistency.

Hue: The name of a color—e.g., red—that describes a human perception of light waves reflected from an object.

Hybrid: A mixture of two materials.

Hydrocolloid: Also termed *reversible hydrocolloid* or *agar*; an elastomeric agar natural polymer final impression material.

Hydrogen peroxide: An oxygenating agent that is used as a tooth bleaching material.

Hydrophilic: Water-loving; combines well with water; flows over a wet solid well.

Hydrophobic: Water-hating; does not combine well with water; does not flow over a wet solid well.

Hydroxyl: A porous, synthetic bone substitute that is used as an implant coating to assist in the development of osseointegration.

Imbibition: The absorption of water into a material from the surrounding environment, especially in relation to alginate, hydrocolloid or gypsum.

Impression: A mold of a patient's oral structures that will be used to pour a duplicate.

Indirect restoration: A restoration that is made outside the tooth and cemented or bonded in position.

Inert: Nonreactive.

Initiator: A substance that responds to an activator by opening some of its molecule bonds to begin the polymerization process.

Inlay: A restoration similar to a "filling" but made outside the tooth and cemented or bonded in place.

Intermediary material: A material used between a restoration and a cavity preparation; includes bases, liners, varnishes and bonding agents.

Invert: Turn over.

Irritation: Localized reddening, soreness, and sometimes blister formation on the soft tissue in response to contact with a material.

Liner: A thin layer of material on the walls or floor of a cavity preparation that seals the tooth from chemical or bacterial injury and may promote formation of new dentin.

Liquid: A substance that moves smoothly and in unrestrained fashion unless confined by a container.

Load: A force placed on a material.

Luting agent: A material used for cementation; a material used to attach two solids together by forming a mechanical joint.

Malleability: The ability of a metal to be made into a thin sheet.

Mandrel: A metal rod that fits into a handpiece or angle and is used to attach and carry an abrasive disk, point, stone, cup or wheel to the mouth.

Maryland bridge: A bonded bridge.

Metal alloy: A mixture of metals.

Microabrasion: The roughening of a tooth surface using a stream of aluminum oxide particles.

Microleakage: The flow of fluids and dissolved substances into the tiny space between a restoration and the tooth surface.

Model: A duplicate of a patient's oral structures.

Modifier: A substance added to a material to change its properties somewhat.

Monomer: A small organic molecule that can be chained to form a polymer.

Mouthguard: Also termed *athletic mouthguard*; a flexible plastic cover for the teeth of one arch, usually the maxillary, to protect them from trauma.

MSDS: Material Safety Data Sheet; legally required information supplied by a chemical manufacturer regarding the characteristics of a specific material, as well as safe storage, handling, and disposal procedures.

Occlusal registration: A bite; an impression of how the teeth in opposing arches fit together.

Occlusal rim: An arch-shaped block of wax that is placed on the baseplate that is being used to construct a denture. The rim serves as a guide for the laboratory to place the teeth in the correct position.

Onlay: A restoration of the occlusal or incisal portion of a tooth including a cusp that is made outside the mouth and cemented or bonded in position.

Opaque: Absorbs all entering light.

Osseointegration: Forming of surface bonds between an implant and bone.

Overdenture: A denture that replaces some or all of the teeth in an arch and is held in position by implants or retained tooth roots.

Overhang: An extension of restorative material beyond the tooth contour.

Partial denture: A denture that replaces some of the teeth and associated structures in one arch.

Passivity: The condition of being nonreactive in the tissue. In the case of titanium implants, it occurs through formation of a tough, adherent, nonreactive surface film by initial reaction of the titanium with oxygen in the tissue.

Paste: A thick mixture of abrasive particles in water or oil.

Pattern: A temporary model used as a form for making an indirect restoration or an appliance.

PEL: Permissible exposure limit; maximum amount of a hazardous chemical to which a person may safely and legally be exposed.

Perimucosal seal: Attachment of sulcus epithelium cells to the surface of an implant. Its preservation is very important in preventing microbial invasion.

Plaster: A natural material that consists of ground gypsum that is processed without pressure at a relatively low temperature.

Point: A pressed, relatively long and thin rotary instrument, composed of abrasive particles in a binder, that will be attached to a handpiece or angle and used in the mouth.

Polish: Smooth.

Polyacid modified glass ionomer (PMGI):   A hybrid esthetic material composed of a larger amount of glass ionomer and a smaller amount of composite resin.

Polycarbonate: A polymer material used in the form of prefabricated temporary crown shells.

Polycarboxylate: A polymer cement used for permanent bases and cementation.

Polyether: An elastomeric rubber base final impression material.

Polymer: A material composed of many repeating units termed *monomers*.

Polymerization: Combining monomers to form a polymer material; curing.

Polysulfide: Also termed *mercaptan* or *rubber base*; an elastomeric rubber base impression material that is used for final impressions.

Pontic: A replacement tooth on a bridge.

Porcelain: Fired (baked at high temperature) glass material used for crowns, veneers, inlays, onlays, and sometimes bridges or denture teeth.

Post: (1) Projection from the frame of a subperiosteal implant that serves as a connector between the frame and the prosthesis. (2) Rod that is anchored in the pulp canal area of the tooth root and extended coronally to support the restoration.

Precision attachment: A sliding mechanism that snaps into position to anchor a bridge to its abutment teeth.

Primer: A weak acid solution used as a dentin wetting agent prior to bonding.

Prosthesis: (1) Restoration that is attached to an implant. It may be a crown, bridge, or full or partial overdenture. (2) Any replacement part, e.g., a full or partial denture or bridge.

Pumice: Ground volcanic rock that is used as an abrasive.

Putty: A high-viscosity final rubber base impression material used to provide bulk for ease of handling the finished impression.

Quadrant: One quarter of the entire mouth; one half of a single arch.

Quartz: Also termed *sandpaper* and formerly termed *cuttle*; a beige abrasive used to finish acrylic, composite and gold.

Reinforce: Strengthen.

Relaxation: Attempt by a material to return to its original size and shape.

Resin: A plastic material; an acrylic acid polymer. This is the same material as composite, but is less heavily filled, therefore not as strong and less resistant to wear.

Retrograde restoration: A direct restoration that was placed from the root end of a tooth following an apicoectomy.

Sargenti paste: Root canal filler material comprised of zinc oxide and eugenol, formaldehyde, anti-inflammatory agents, opacifiers and modifiers that is toxic to periapical cells, soluble in oral fluids and has been associated with the development of transient parasthesia (temporary loss of sensation).

Sealant: A thin plastic coating placed on the pits, grooves, and fissures of a tooth to protect it from decay.

Sensitivity: General body allergy reaction to a foreign substance.

Set: As a verb, to harden; as an adjective, hardened.

Sextant: One sixth of the entire mouth; one third of a single arch. Premolars and molars in a single quadrant constitute a posterior sextant; incisors and canines of a single arch constitute an anterior sextant.

Shearing: A cutting load; pushing and pulling a material at the same time.

Shearing strength: Ability to resist tearing.

Shellac: A material composed of lacquer dissolved in alcohol.

Silicone: General term for *siloxane* and *condensation silicone,* both elastomeric rubber base final impression materials.

Slurry: A thin paste of abrasive particles in water or oil.

Sodium hypochlorite: Chlorine bleach solution used as an irrigant and antiseptic in root canal therapy procedures.

Soft liner: Soft polymer used to improve the fit of a denture or provide a more resilient surface.

Solid: A substance that has a definite shape and volume, appears firm and is comprised of tightly bonded molecules.

Solubility: The ability of a substance to dissolve in a liquid.

Solute: The substance that is dissolved in the liquid.

Solvent: A liquid used to dissolve a substance.

Sorption: The absorption of a liquid into a solid.

Specification: A standard; a description of what a dental material should contain to be labeled as that material.

Splint: A device used to connect teeth to distribute biting forces around the arch. An *occlusal splint* is a hard plastic cover that fits over the maxillary teeth and distributes biting forces around so as to prevent tooth, alveolar bone, or temporomandibular joint injury. A *periodontal splint* is a plastic or wire device bonded to adjacent teeth to distribute biting forces to adjacent teeth, thereby providing stabilization to mobile teeth while the periodontium heals.

Stainless steel: A metal alloy used to make prefabricated temporary crowns that are usually used to restore primary posterior teeth.

Stone: (1) A natural material that consists of ground gypsum processed at a relatively high temperature under pressure; (2) a pressed, rounded rotary instrument composed of abrasive particles in a binder that will be attached to a mandrel, inserted in a handpiece or angle and used in the mouth.

Strain: Rearrangement of the atoms in a material in response to stress.

Strength: The resistance of a material to load.

Stress: The amount of force placed on a given area of material.

Strip: A thin piece of paper or plastic to which abrasive particles have been attached.

Subperiosteal implant: Tooth root replacement that consists of a metal framework placed on the bone, below the periosteum.

Substrate: A softer material that is being worn away by a harder abrasive material.

Syneresis: The loss of water from a material to the surrounding environment, especially in relation to alginate, hydrocolloid or gypsum.

Syringe: (1) A disposable, multidose container that contains a single material; (2) a gun-type applicator that carries a material to the mouth.

Tarnish: Surface discoloration of a metal from electrochemical assault.

Tensile strength: The ability of a material to resist pulling.

Tension: A pulling load.

Thermoplastic: Able to be reversibly softened by heating and hardened by cooling.

Thermoset: Hardened by heating.

Thixotropic: Having the ability to flow under load.

Tin oxide: A white mineral mined from the earth and used as a mild abrasive.

Torsion: A twisting load.

Translucent: Having the ability to absorb some light and let some pass through.

Transparent: Having the ability to permit light to pass through.

Trituration: The mixing of amalgam by shaking a container holding alloy and mercury. By extension, this term has also come to mean the mixing of any powder and liquid by shaking them together.

Ultimate strength: The point just prior to fracture; the point at which a material is most resistant to load.

Unit: A single component of a bridge. Each pontic and each abutment is considered a unit.

Value: A shade of a color; e.g., rose.

Varnish: As a verb, to seal cut ends of dentin tubules to bar fluid entry; as a noun, a material which seals the cut ends of dentin tubules.

Vehicle: A material used to hold abrasive particles and carry them to the site of interest, normally water, oil, paper or plastic.

Veneer: A thin layer of tooth-colored material cemented or bonded to the facial surface of a natural or replacement tooth to improve its appearance.

Vinyl polysiloxane: Also termed *polyvinyl siloxane*, *vinyl*, or *addition silicone*; a highly accurate, elastomeric, rubber base final impression material.

Viscosity: Resistance to flow.

Void: A space filled with air in a material.

Wash: A thin layer of low-viscosity final impression material used to record fine detail.

Wax-up: (1) A baseplate denture pattern into which the artificial teeth that will be used in the finished denture have been placed in correct position. (2) The wax form used as a base for a lost wax casting.

Wear: As a verb, rub; as a noun, loss of structure from abrasion.

Wet: To flow a liquid over a solid.

Wet strength: The strength of a gypsum model before its excess water has evaporated. Wet strength is much lower than dry strength.

Wheel: A relatively thick, round piece of paper, rubber, plastic or metal to which abrasive particles have been attached.

Whitening: Bleaching.

Working cast: Model on which a dental item is made.

Yield strength: The point beyond which a material starts to deform.

Zinc oxide and eugenol (Z-O-E): A weak metal oxide cement that is used for temporary cementation and as a base, liner, wound dressing and temporary direct restoration material.

Zinc phosphate: A relatively strong metal oxide cement that is used as a permanent base and for permanent cementation, especially of metal castings and orthodontic bands.

Zinc polycarboxylate: A combination polymer–metal oxide cement that is used as a permanent base and luting agent.

ANSWERS TO SELF TEST QUESTIONS

▼ Chapter 1 ▼

1. Direct restoration. It is used to restore a tooth to form and function directly in the mouth relatively easily and inexpensively.

2. Crown. It is used to replace all the surfaces of the crown of a natural tooth that is severely decayed, injured or unsightly.

3. Removable partial denture. It replaces one or more, but not all, of the teeth in an arch.

4. Impression. It is used as a mold of the patient's oral tissues. Material will be poured into the mold to create a model, or duplicate, of the tissues.

5. Endosseous implant. It is surgically placed into the patient's jawbone and used to support a superstructure, such as a crown, bridge or denture, to replace a lost tooth.

6. d. Mouthguard. Mouthguards protect oral and facial tissues against athletic injury.

7. d. Both bonded bridge and partial denture. It is unlikely an implant would be used because surgery would be required and the patient is frail.

8. b. Sealants. A 6-year-old child probably has newly erupted first permanent molars that should be protected from decay. In the case of a 6-year-old, the target of your educational message would be the father, although you would also want to create enthusiasm for the procedure on the part of the child.

9. b. Esthetic veneers. The concern here is with appearance and esthetic veneers could be used to cover the unsightly areas with a thin layer of natural-appearing material.

10. c. Indirect restorations. You would want to make the patient aware that options for treatment of her condition include various types of crowns, bridges or implants, and that the dentist will suggest a particular type to choose based on a professional assessment of the conditions in her mouth.

▼ Chapter 2 ▼

1. c. Microleakage. Note the open tooth-restoration interface, which allows fluids and dis-

solved substances to enter and percolate toward the pulp.

2. a. Etched surface. Note the roughened nature of the surface ready for the bonding material.

3. b. Shade guides. Remember that a shade guide is useful only for the type and brand of material for which it was designed.

4. d. Pitted restoration. Note the discoloration and pitting on the restoration surface.

5. d. Molecular solid. Note the regular, stacked arrangement of the atoms.

6. a. Bonded. Two solids may be caused to adhere to each other through the use of bonding procedures.

7. c. Viscosity. Viscosity is resistance to flow, so a material that does not flow well has high resistance to flow, that is, high viscosity.

8. b. Dual cured. This material requires the use of two procedures, mixing and light curing, to set properly. The term *dual cured* includes both procedures.

9. a. Soluble. Solids that dissolve in liquids are soluble in the liquids.

10. d. Cure. Polymer materials harden when exposed to light. Polymer hardening is termed *cure*.

▼ Chapter 3 ▼

1. Gloves are worn to prevent transfer of chemicals and infectious microorganisms through the skin to the inside of the body.

2. A mask is worn to prevent entry of chemicals or microorganisms into the body through the nose or mouth.

3. Safety glasses are worn to prevent chemical splash or microorganism splatter into the eye.

4. A lab coat is worn to protect exposed skin from chemical injury or microbial contamination. It also protects clothing from staining and chemical attack.

5. Visit the OSHA website at *www.osha.gov.*

6. Chronic chemical exposure means repeated contact with a small amount of a chemical over

a long period of time. It can lead to chemical injury but the results may not be manifest for months or years.

7. The tooth is considered potentially infectious, therefore biohazardous. You should place it in a leakproof container, normally a red biohazard bag, label it *Biohazard*, close the container and dispose of it using proper infection control procedure.

8. The MSDS sheet for the bonding material should be consulted and the manufacturer's recommended procedures followed.

9. You know the material was evaluated by the American Dental Association's Council on Scientific Affairs and found to be safe and effective.

10. The shelf life of a material is the time preceding its expiration date. This is the time the chemical is at useful strength, provided it has been transported and stored correctly.

▼ Chapter 4 ▼

1. Model trimmer. It cuts models to esthetic proportions.

2. Capsule. It contains premeasured powder and liquid to be mixed in an amalgamator.

3. Cartridge and automix syringe. The cartridge contains two separate pastes that will be mixed in the syringe.

4. Spatulas. Each will be used to mix a specific type of material.

5. Amalgamator. This machine shakes a capsule or tip containing two materials to mix them.

6. d. Place in an amalgamator, select time and speed of shaking, and activate timer.

7. c. Place in automix syringe, affix tip, and squeeze handle.

8. a. Eject directly onto area of interest.

9. b. Place equal lengths of the materials on a pad.

10. a. Obtain correct scoop, liquid measure, spatula and flexible bowl.

▼ Chapter 5 ▼

1. Pumice or quartz

2. Pumice and/or tin oxide

3. Diamond polishing paste or quartz

4. Pumice

5. Quartz (sand)

6. Use medium or fine grit abrasive in a water or oil lubricant. Position it carefully. Begin polishing at cervical area and move toward occlusal or incisal. Use a constant dabbing motion to apply and reapply abrasive, and keep abrasive moving. Use low to medium speed and light to moderate pressure. Renew abrasive frequently.

7. Same as #6.

8. Begin polishing with the coarsest grit you will use, then proceed with progressively finer grits until you have completed the task.

9. Use rouge, low to medium speed and light to moderate pressure. Keep abrasive moving over crown. Renew abrasive frequently.

10. Use low to moderate speed. High speed heats and may destroy a substrate.

▼ Chapter 6 ▼

1. Sealants are used to prevent caries by isolating the tooth surface from environmental microorganisms and acids.

2. Both restored and sound teeth are susceptible to decay. Restored teeth are particularly vulnerable at the tooth-restoration interface, where microleakage can occur. Teeth fitted with fixed orthodontic appliances are vulnerable at the appliance-tooth interface, where the appliances trap and accumulate microorganisms and are difficult to keep clean.

3. Retention is improved by ensuring the tooth is correctly etched and dry, the unsupported enamel rods that exist after etching are not broken by touching the tooth surface with an explorer or other instrument, and the sealant material is placed and cured without moisture contamination.

4. Composite might be chosen because of its superior strength or its ability to bond to a composite restoration that is already in place. Glass ionomer might be chosen for a patient or area that is particularly susceptible to decay, where moisture control is difficult, or to bond to an adjacent glass ionomer restoration.

5. Mechanical interlocking of sealant material and enamel is created by painting the tooth surface with an etchant, which creates microscopic depressions on the tooth surface. The sealant material can then flow into the depressions, creating tiny interlocked "fingers" of enamel and material.

6. Select a tinted material.

7. Select a composite material. If acrylic is to be used, select a filled material. Whichever is used, ensure the most complete cure possible.

8. Seal the tooth-restoration interface with a glass ionomer or fluoride-containing sealant material. Glass ionomer would bond to the tooth and release fluoride into the surrounding tooth structure. Fluoride–containing acrylic would also release fluoride for a limited time.

9. As above, glass ionomer would be the material of choice to seal the tooth-appliance interface, but acrylic could be used.

10. Select a dual cure material. Light curing would provide immediate, but not necessarily complete, cure. Chemical curing would provide a more complete, but not immediate, cure. A dual cure material would provide for both actions, thereby making available the most satisfactory cure. If moisture control in the area is difficult, selecting a glass ionomer material would also help to ensure a more satisfactory cure.

▼ Chapter 7 ▼

1. a. Home
2. c. She will need to stop both smoking and drinking while bleaching.
3. b. Dentin hypersensitivity; trim tray short of margins.
4. d. Oxygen
5. c. Amalgam restorations bleach more rapidly. This statement is false because amalgam restorations do not bleach.
6. Take an alginate impression of the arch(es) to be bleached, pour the impression(s), and make a polymer bleaching tray on the resulting model(s.)
7. Quick start method
8. Speak about the possibility that she may be too young for bleaching because the enamel and pulp of the teeth may not be ready for it yet and the gingiva is not yet at its final level. Discuss the fact that the dentist will need to determine whether or not her teeth are ready.
9. The restoration will need to be replaced because esthetic restorations do not whiten. Your role will be to educate the patient about the need for replacing the restoration.
10. Choose the 15% concentration because the others are only for in-office use under the supervision of a dentist.

▼ Chapter 8 ▼

1. Work gently and confidently, and distract patient with conversation about pleasant topics as you work. Center tray over arch before compressing it over the teeth. If patient seems to be experiencing any difficulty, ask her to breathe deeply and lift one foot (or two, if need be!) above the chair.
2. Examine the mouth and estimate its size. Try in a tray that appears to be correct. It should fit loosely from front to back and side to side, cover the maxillary tuberosity or the retro-mandibular triangle as appropriate, extend almost to the mucobuccal fold and not be so large as to be uncomfortable to the patient.
3. Leave it in the mouth at least one minute beyond set. Hook your finger over the top of the set impression and gently pull straight down to

break the suction between the impression and the tissues. Remove the impression with a single continuous pull.
4. Rinse the impression under gently running water to remove any blood, saliva or debris. Gently shake any excess water out. Spray impression with disinfectant solution and seal it in a plastic bag for the time recommended by the disinfectant manufacturer.
5. Wear a mask. Let the alginate sit 2–3 seconds following fluffing, and recover the container immediately after proportioning the powder.
6. b. Slowly
7. a. Cool, dry; 12 months
8. d. Compressive strength
9. f. All of the above
10. b. Study models

▼ Chapter 9 ▼

1. *Rationale for yes:* Even if the impression used to pour a model were disinfected, it might still contain harmful microorganisms. *Rationale for no:* Impressions are disinfected, so it is unlikely that substantial numbers of harmful microorganisms would be present on the impression surface and survive on the model.

   Autoclaving would ruin a model. Models contain water. Water from the autoclave would also penetrate the model. These factors would cause it to swell, weaken, and crumble. As the cycle proceeded, water in the model would be converted to steam and lost. When the model dried, it would shrink. All semblance of accuracy would be lost.

   Immersion for any length of time would cause fluid to enter the model and the result would be swelling, weakening, and crumbling. Immersion for shorter periods of time (10–15 minutes) would likely not cause appreciable harm if the model were not going to be used for an indirect restoration.

   Spraying a model with disinfectant and sealing it in a plastic bag would likely provide disinfection without harm.
2. Neither. It is poor shear strength. If the model fell perfectly flat, it would not break.
3. Stone or die stone
4. Die stone
5. Prevent voids
6. Expand
7. Crystallization
8. 24 hours
9. a. Weaken
10. b. It has straight sides.

▼ Chapter 10 ▼

1. Resin bonding agent
2. Alternative 1: calcium hydroxide, varnish and a strong base such as zinc phosphate or zinc poly-carboxylate; Alternative 2: amalgam bonding agent alone or over calcium hydroxide
3. Alternative 1: glass ionomer; Alternative 2: etchant, primer and acrylic resin
4. Glass ionomer
5. Zinc phosphate, zinc polycarboxylate or glass ionomer
6. g. Primer
7. c. Zinc phosphate
8. b. Varnish
9. d. Acrylic resin
10. a. Glass ionomer
11. f. Zinc polycarboxylate
12. a. Glass ionomer
13. e. Zinc oxide and eugenol
14. e. Zinc oxide and eugenol
15. b. Varnish or e. Zinc oxide and eugenol

▼ Chapter 11 ▼

1. c. Glass ionomer
2. b. Flowable
3. c. Filler particle size and amount
4. b. Microfilled
5. a. Filler
6. e. All of the above
7. a. Both statements above are true
8. b. Strength; composite
9. a. Ejected from this syringe tip
10. b. Light cured
11. d. More filler creates a stronger material
12. Either c or e
13. Class II and IV restorations will likely be exposed to biting forces and will need the strength composite provides. Class IV restorations are also located in the anterior, and the translucency of composite presents a more natural appearance. Class V restorations are not subject to biting forces, may be anterior or posterior, and located on the labial or lingual. Appearance would be an issue for anterior labial restorations; composite would be the more likely choice there. Either material could be used for lingual or posterior restorations. Glass ionomer may also be the material of choice for any Class V preparation where it is difficult to control moisture.
14. Greater numbers of smaller, more regularly shaped filler particles can be packed into a given volume of resin. This in turn leaves smaller areas filled with resin between the particles. When composite is polished, resin wears away more rapidly than the harder particles. Polishing wear is more even when more of the surface is a single material. A surface that reflects light more evenly appears shinier to the human eye.
15. Itaconic acid attacks the reinforcing calcium fluoroaluminosilicate glass bead surfaces in glass ionomer. Decomposing surface molecules liberate calcium, fluorine, aluminum and sodium, which are then available to recombine into a hard polymer matrix with glass reinforcing particles and free fluoride scattered throughout.
16. Curing shrinkage occurs toward the light source as resins polymerize. It can be controlled by curing in layers and from several angles. Curing in layers allows the shrinkage of each layer to be incorporated into, and no longer stress, remaining layers. Curing from several angles varies the direction of shrinkage so that it is not concentrated in a particular area. Concentrated stress is more likely to cause bond fracture in the affected area.
17. Composite is formed of acrylic resin, which is colorless. Because it is colorless, it is translucent and can be tinted a variety of shades. Opaquers may also be added to decrease translucency. Glass ionomer contains zinc oxide particles, which are opaque. Glass ionomer can never be translucent but is able to be tinted a variety of shades.

▼ Chapter 12 ▼

1. Strength, ease of placement and cost are important considerations, but appearance matters less.
2. Zinc-containing alloy: plasticity of the mix
    Nonzinc alloy: dry environment during placement not achievable
    Low copper alloy: restoration will not be subjected to strong biting forces
    High copper alloy: restoration will be subjected to strong biting forces
3. Mercury dissolves the outer layers of the alloy particles. The ions in solution recombine to form a silver-based matrix with reinforcing particles scattered throughout.
4. Painting the cut dentin surface with varnish or bonding the restoration to the tooth.
5. Ensure there is adequate tooth structure remaining, build up the core if there is not, ensure an adequate thickness of amalgam is placed, avoid placing a base, and bond the restoration to the tooth surface.

6. d. Mixing by shaking
7. c. Healing time
8. a. Wet
9. b. Wet and dull
10. e. All of the above

▼ Chapter 13 ▼

1. Stock trays are purchased ready-made from the manufacturer. Custom trays are made to fit a specific patient.

2. Take an alginate impression. Pour a gypsum model. Select a material and construct the tray using the correct technique for that material. Trim, smooth and pierce the tray as indicated. Clean and disinfect the tray and replace it on the model.

3. A stock, custom or dual impression tray could be used. Which one is selected would be the operator's choice, although a custom tray would provide a better fit and a stock or dual impression tray would save time. Regardless of tray type, quadrant coverage would be adequate but not excessive.

4. A quadrant or sextant tray could be used, depending on the location of the prepared tooth. To ensure adequate but not excessive coverage, a quadrant tray should be used for a posterior preparation and a sextant tray for an anterior preparation.

5. You will need a flexible polymer sheet for vacuum or pressure forming a tray and must trim the resultant tray to extend only over the area to be bleached.

6. One bite tray will record how the two arches occlude.

7. You will need the beads, a scoop to measure them, the model, warm water to soften the beads, a sheet of wax to make the spacer, a lab knife or spatula to make holes for the stops and gather the softened beads together in one mass, and lubricant to paint on the spacer to make it easier to remove.

8. Make a spacer and stops on the model. Paint the spacer with lubricant. Soften the beads in warm water. Gather them, knead the mass to homogenous consistency, adapt the material to the model, form a handle, and smooth the tray edges. Remove the spacer, lightly readapt the tray to the model and allow the material to cure.

9. Holes in a custom tray relieve pressure during the impression procedure. They allow the material to flow through and mechanically interlock the tray and set material.

10. Stops are placed in a custom tray to prevent it from being seated too deeply during the impres-

sion procedure. They are made by cutting holes in the spacer and pushing tray material into the holes.

▼ Chapter 14 ▼

1. d. Both a and c. It is a suspension of particles in water and has a thermoplastic set. The accuracy, though good, is not on par with the newer rubber materials.

2. d. Is thixotropic

3. c. Light

4. b. Record anatomic detail well

5. e. Hydrocolloid

6. c. Vinyl

7. a. Squeeze out equal lengths

8. d. Its set is thermoplastic

9. a. Silicone

10. c. Vinyl, although there are polyether cartridges that can be mixed in a machine

▼ Chapter 15 ▼

1. c. The immediate need is to provide comfort and chewing ability to the patient. Any appearance change would be slight for some time. As long as the tooth was protected from the environment, decay would also take some time to develop. Not placing a temporary restoration would leave the prepared tooth extremely vulnerable to decay but would affect adjacent teeth only indirectly.

2. b. Composite is the usual material of choice for temporary veneers. Preformed alloys are not esthetic and would not be used. Acrylic is possible but more time-consuming.

3. d. A temporary restoration is cemented or bonded in place and either procedure, if done correctly, is adequate to protect the tooth as long as the cement or bonding agent remains intact. Margin discoloration is inherent in material sorption and the pigments to which a restoration is exposed. It does not depend on the expected longevity of the restoration.

4. d. Curing speed is unrelated to material contact with calcium. Curing heat may damage cells and curing shrinkage may lock the temporary restoration to the tooth.

5. a. An individualized mold that can be relined to construct a temporary restoration.

6. b. Doughy flash is trimmable. Drippy, flowable or stiff material cannot be molded or trimmed.

7. e. The margin, contacts and occlusion should all be checked.

8. a. Stainless steel provides the strength that may be necessary for relatively long-term use. Polycarbonate and acrylic wear readily and aluminum is more time-consuming to construct.

9. c. Acrylic can be used for either temporary crowns or bridges. Stainless steel, aluminum and polycarbonate are preformed shells that are used only for crowns.

10. e. Crimping pliers are necessary to fit the cervix of a preformed crown. A periodontal probe measures pocket depth and a vitalometer measures the response of a tooth pulp to an electrical stimulus. A lab engine with bur and an explorer may be useful when delivering a temporary crown, but are not necessary to its fitting.

▼ Chapter 16 ▼

1. This thin, opaque layer of porcelain is used to mask the metallic color of the underlying coping.

2. This temporary wax coping forms a pattern for casting a permanent metal one.

3. This platinum foil matrix is used to retain everything in position during construction of a fired porcelain restoration.

4. Firing porcelain is baking it at high temperatures to fuse the feldspar particles together.

5. An impression is taken and a stone die poured. A wax model is made on the die. The pattern is placed on a sprue, invested in a casting ring, and the filled ring set aside to allow the investment material to set. The invested pattern is heated to ignite and burn it, leaving a hole in the hardened investment that will serve as a mold for casting. The permanent material is forced into the mold through the sprue and allowed to cool.

6. Porcelain or ceramic material is applied to the metal substructure and fired to fuse the metal substructure and esthetic veneer together.

7. An intraoral camera is used to make a digital image of the prepared tooth. The image is stored in the computer and used to define and construct a three-dimensional image of the final restoration. The image is used to control a rotating abrasive disk to cut the restoration from a ceramic block. Final adjustment cuts are controlled by hand. The cut restoration is hand stained to match adjacent teeth.

8. The tooth is prepared and the preparation coated with a thin layer of separating lubricant. The inlay is formed in, but not bonded to, the preparation, and cured. It is removed from the preparation and cured further using heat at a higher temperature and for a longer period of time than could be used in the mouth, then cleaned and polished.

9. c. Porcelain

10. a. Increases its hardness and strength

11. d. Both a and c. Kaolin is opaque and becomes sticky when wet.

12. e. All of the above. High noble, gold-based alloys are used for crowns, bridges, and metal substructures. They are also used for inlays and onlays, but those options were not available in the question.

13. b. Toxicity of the metal in its pure state. The metals will be chemically combined in the finished restoration. The important consideration is biocompatibility of the finished restoration rather than of the metals in their pure states.

14. e. Both a and b. Silver whitens, hardens, increases tarnish and decreases the corrosion resistance of an alloy.

15. c. Margin integrity. The curing shrinkage of resin sometimes results in fracture of the bond holding the composite to the tooth. Fractured bonds leave open margins that are susceptible to microleakage and secondary decay.

▼ Chapter 17 ▼

1. Cements attach material two ways: (a) filling in defects on the tooth and material surface, and (b) bonding.

2. If the cement dissolves, the tooth-material interface opens, predisposing the underlying tooth preparation to secondary decay.

3. Polymer and combination cements bond. Glass ionomer and polycarboxylate bond chemically and resin bonds mechanically.

4. The operator makes an assessment of the characteristics of the cement and its record of success for similar applications in relation to the conditions in the patient's mouth and personal preference.

5. Z-O-E is too weak and soluble to be used for permanent cementation.

6. a. Premature set

7. b. Polymer

8. d. Resin

9. a. Brittle

10. d. Zinc phosphate and glass ionomer

11. c. Glass ionomer

12. b. Free acid is present

▼ Chapter 18 ▼

1. Osseointegration is bonding of an implant to bone. It requires 2–6 months to occur and depends on interaction between bioactive ceramic materials and living tissues.

2. A perimucosal seal is formed when gingival fibers encircle an implant and cells from the sulcus epithelium attach to its ceramic coating.

3. Titanium, a reactive metal, becomes passive when it reacts with surface oxygen to form a tough, adherent, nonreactive titanium oxide surface film.

4. Placement of a subperiosteal implant is accomplished by the following procedures: (1) surgery to prepare the bone and take an impression of it; (2) closure, healing, and fabrication of a metal implant frame; (3) reopening of the site and placement of the frame; (4) healing; (5) fabrication and placement of the prosthesis.

5. Placement of an endosteal implant is accomplished through the following procedures: (1) surgery to place the implant fixture and cover; (2) closure and lack of loading until osseointegration occurs; (3) reopening of the site and placement of the abutment and healing cap; (4) healing; (5) fabrication and placement of the prosthesis.

6. a. Calcium–phosphate ceramics

7. d. Titanium

8. d. Both a and c. An implant prosthesis is cemented or screwed in position.

9. c. Prevent implant scratching

10. b. At the titanium–ceramic interface

▼ Chapter 19 ▼

1. b. Cobalt-chromium alloy

2. e. All of the above

3. c. Horizontal; vertical

4. b. Shellac

5. a. Vertical dimension; jaw relationships

6. b. Thermosetting; shrink as they cure

7. d. Benzoyl peroxide

8. c. The statement is correct but the reason is not accurate.

9. d. Cobalt-chromium alloy and inert colored fibers

10. a. Hardens

11. Saddle

12. Clasp

13. Base

14. Flange

▼ Chapter 20 ▼

1. Different tasks, materials, timelines and goals underlie each type of procedure. Another major concern is whether any vital tissue remains and can be stimulated to cause formation of new hard or soft tissue.

2. Calcium hydroxide alone or mixed with parachlorophenol may be placed in an immature canal. If the material is left in place for several months to a year and covered with a temporary restoration, a damaged immature tooth can be stimulated to form an apex or to repair breaks in the cementum root cover.

3. Many endodontic procedures are completed because the pulp or periapical tissues are infected. Regardless of whether infection is present or not, when instruments are inserted into a pulp cavity, that normally sterile environment becomes contaminated with external microorganisms. Disinfectants help to control any resurgence of bacteria that are already present, and to discourage new infection.

4. Sealers are used to close the microspace between the tooth and the filling material to prevent fluids and microorganisms from entering the area.

5. If a sealer or filler shrinks excessively, a portion of the area will no longer be sealed. This permits microleakage, with its attendant problems of fluid, pigment, acid and bacteria entry.

6. Formocresol is a phenol derivative that is caustic to bits of bleeding tissue that stubbornly remain in the pulp canal following pulp extirpation. It also irritates any underlying vital pulp and the periapical tissues, which results in the formation of granulation tissue. Formocresol works by diffusion and volatization.

CASE STUDIES

Provide both the requested information and the rationale for your responses.

1. Your patient is a 13-year-old male who is new to the office. His medical history indicates he has received regular dental care since he was approximately 3 years old, has no known allergies or medical problems, does not mind receiving dental care and plays in three sports leagues in season: baseball, basketball and soccer. Clinical and radiographic examination reveal asymptomatic occlusal caries in teeth A and J. His only other remaining primary tooth is H. All of his permanent second molars are erupted and all of his erupted permanent teeth are sound.

   A. Suggest education that should be provided to the patient and his parents.
   B. What would be the likely treatment for teeth A and J?
   C. What treatment may be indicated for some of the permanent teeth?

2. Your patient is a 36-year-old male whose dental care has been completed in your employer's office for the past seven years. His medical history states that he has temporal lobe epilepsy that is well controlled by medication, and he was hospitalized for chest surgery during his preschool years, mental illness when he was a teenager and hernia repair and knee reconstruction as a young adult. Even now, he is quite frightened each time he must receive medical or dental care. He is here today for observation of healing progress following removal of tooth #30. In the mandible, tooth #31 is present and has a small buccal amalgam restoration; tooth #32 is missing. In the maxilla, tooth #1 is missing and teeth #2 and #3 are both present and sound.

   A. What are his options for replacement of tooth #30?
   B. Given his fear of receiving dental care and the replacement options available, which option would require that he undergo the fewest, least invasive procedures?
   C. Which options would be permanently fixed in the mouth and what would be the advantage of that characteristic?
   D. Which option would be removable and what would be the advantages and disadvantages of selecting that option?
   E. Which option would help to retain the normal bone height and contour in the area of the lost tooth and what would be the advantages and disadvantages of selecting that option?

3. Your patient is a 7-year-old girl who fell off her bicycle and fractured tooth #8. After clinical and radiographic examination the dentist determines that although the root is not complete and the fracture is at the junction of the middle and cervical thirds of the crown, the tooth can be saved. He recommends that the child receive immediate endodontic therapy followed by restorative care at an appropriate later time.

   A. What types of endodontic therapy could be used to treat this child and which one do you think the dentist would be likely to select?
   B. In addition to the appropriate endodontic instruments, what materials would the assistant need to prepare for this procedure?
   C. What items would be needed to prepare these materials?
   D. Why wouldn't an irrigating agent be used?
   E. Why would calcium hydroxide be used and how would it be prepared?

4. Your patient is a 54-year-old woman who presents with both extrinsic and intrinsic stain on her maxillary incisors. She has no health problems and takes better than average care of her teeth but is known to be allergic to eugenol. She works full time as a receptionist in an advertising agency, where she needs to look her best, and is unhappy with the staining. Clinically, she has slight gingival recession on the labial of tooth #8 and an old amalgam restoration that still has sound margins on the lingual of tooth #10.

   A. What procedure should be used to remove the extrinsic stains?
   B. What material would likely be chosen to complete this procedure?

251

C. What procedure could be used to remove the intrinsic stains?

D. What material would likely to be chosen to complete it?

E. Although all of the teeth may experience discomfort, which tooth may be particularly susceptible and what preventive measures could be employed to prevent that from happening?

5. The patient is a 35-year-old divorced male who is slightly overweight and is a heavy smoker. He works as an air courier and has a very irregular schedule. He has no visible caries but does have heavy lingual staining and proximal composite restorations in three of his maxillary incisors. He has taken sporadic care of his teeth but has a new girlfriend whom he wants to impress favorably. He has come in today to request that his teeth be bleached, as inexpensively and quickly as possible.

A. Is the patient an appropriate candidate for bleaching at this time?

B. What type of education about bleaching does he need to receive?

C. Once he becomes an appropriate candidate, what bleaching regimen would be most appropriate?

D. In view of his composite restorations, what problems could occur as a result of the bleaching process and what precautions could be taken to prevent them from happening?

E. How long would he need to wait after completing bleaching before he could replace the restorations if he chose to do so?

6. Your patient is a 43-year-old female with no known medical problems or allergies. She has three children and no dental coverage. She is afraid of dentists and last visited the office four years ago for a toothache. The aching tooth was removed and has not been replaced. She is here today because tooth #12 is sensitive to cold. The dentist determines it has extensive proximal caries but can be saved, and after consulting with the patient prepares the tooth for a direct restoration.

A. What materials could be selected for a direct restoration in this area?

B. What are the advantages and disadvantages of each type?

C. If the major criteria are cost and ease of placement, what material will be selected?

D. If the major criterion is esthetics, what material will be selected?

E. Assuming the material ultimately selected is composite, what intermediary materials are likely to be used in this deep restoration?

7. Your 27-year-old patient has porcelain veneers on teeth #7–#10, and composite restorations on all four first molars. Her other teeth are sound.

The dentist has asked you to polish all of her teeth and then give her a fluoride treatment.

A. What grit of abrasive should you select for polishing?

B. What type of fluoride should you select?

C. Which material is more vulnerable to damage from use of the wrong abrasive grit or type of fluoride?

D. How are each of the components of the composite material susceptible to damage?

E. What type of damage could result from use of the incorrect type of fluoride on the veneers?

8. Your 38-year-old patient will have orthodontic bands attached to his maxillary first molars with zinc phosphate cement this afternoon. Once the bands are in place, you will seal each band–tooth interface.

A. What other technique and materials could be used to bond these brackets to the tooth?

B. Select one of the materials and state why you chose it.

C. Describe how this material would be prepared.

D. How would you clean up following its use?

E. Why is it an advantage to seal the band–interface area if a metal oxide cement is used?

9. Your patient is an 82-year-old male smoker who lives alone and has no dental coverage. His last visit to the dentist was 21 years ago. He has several carious lesions but is only concerned about the lower left side, which "hurts." The dentist determines that tooth #18 is the problem and recommends a direct restoration. The patient agrees, "if I can pay for it a little at a time." Following consultation and cavity preparation, the dentist is concerned that the tooth may not quiet down easily and asks that you place a temporary restoration and reappoint the patient in 5–7 weeks for additional observation.

A. Why might a temporary restoration be helpful in this case?

B. What kind of material should be prepared for use as a temporary restorative?

C. How is this material prepared?

D. Is it legal in your state for you to place a temporary direct restoration?

E. If the tooth eventually quiets down, is it legal in your state for you to place a permanent direct restoration?

10. Your patient is a 61-year-old female non-smoker who repeatedly clenches her teeth. She takes excellent care of her teeth but has developed a shallow Class V lesion partly on the crown and partly on the root of all of her lower premolars. The dentist had characterized these as abfraction lesions that you know are due to chewing forces bending the teeth and possibly breaking the brittle tooth at the gumline. There is no

decay but these areas are catching food and that is causing gingival irritation in the area. The dentist had previously placed composite restorations in these areas but they keep popping out due to the bending and resultant breaking of the mechanical bond with the tooth. The patient would like to know if there might be a better option to fill these lesions.

A. What material might be better for the patient than composite for restoration of these teeth?

B. Will etching and mechanical bonding be needed prior to placement of this material?

C. Following preliminary set, what material could be placed over this restorative material to allow it to set completely before it is exposed to air and oral fluids?

D. Once this restorative material is set, how likely is it to dissolve in oral fluids?

11. Your patient is an 18-year-old female with no medical problems. Clinical and radiographic examination reveals no caries, periodontal disease or orthodontic problems. She does, however, have noticeable, discolored pitting on the labial of teeth #7 and #9 that is visible when she talks or smiles.

A. What could be done to correct this problem?

B. What types of materials could be used?

C. Which type appears more natural?

D. If the more natural, more expensive material is selected to correct the problem, what procedures will need to be completed and what materials will be used to do so?

E. If the less natural, less expensive material is chosen, what procedures will need to be completed and what materials will be used to do so?

12. Your 47-year-old patient is having a crown made for tooth #3. He has no known allergies but is a bruxer and has a particularly strong bite.

A. What materials would provide the occlusal strength needed plus the esthetic facial appearance the patient prefers for this crown?

B. How many appointments would normally be needed to construct and deliver it?

C. What type of luting or bonding agent would provide the strength necessary to attach this crown permanently to the tooth?

D. If the patient has to wait for the crown to be made and delivered, how could his facial appearance and oral function be maintained in the interim?

E. Once the crown has been attached to the tooth, how likely is the luting or bonding agent to dissolve in oral fluids?

F. How would allied dental personnel check to learn whether the luting or bonding agent had in fact dissolved?

13. Your 25-year-old patient was diagnosed with AIDS last year. He is undergoing aggressive treatment and progressing well. Last week the dentist placed a Class V composite restoration on the facial of tooth #20. The patient has returned complaining of redness, soreness and formation of small blisters on the soft tissue adjacent to the new restoration.

A. Do you think the patient has made the right choice in returning to his dentist or that he should have called his physician for an appointment?

B. What do you think the problem may be?

C. Suggest a way that your belief about the cause of the problem could be tested and what you would expect to see if it were correct.

14. Your 52-year-old patient has an old Class V amalgam restoration on tooth #29. For the past few months, the tooth has been bothered when she drinks acid colas or iced or hot drinks. The dentist has determined there is no decay, fracture, crack, infection or gingival recession present, has gone into the next operatory to give a local anesthetic injection, and has asked that while she is gone you educate the patient regarding why she may be experiencing this problem.

A. What is the likely reason for the problem?

B. How will you explain this to her?

15. Your 78-year-old male patient is present for a routine examination. He has been a conscientious dental patient throughout his life and has noticed that there is a small open area surrounding an amalgam restoration that was placed some years ago on one of his lower right teeth. This restoration was not bonded in place. Clinical and radiographic examination reveals there is no other hard or soft tissue problem in the area and the dentist determines that it is not necessary to replace the restoration.

A. What is the likely condition this gentleman has discovered?

B. How will you explain this to him?

C. How likely is this condition to persist indefinitely?

16. You will be taking impressions for study models.

A. What material should you use?

B. How should you select and fit the trays?

C. How should you evaluate whether your impressions are good or not?

D. How should you care for your impressions after they are taken?

E. What material should you use to pour them?

F. How will you know when the impressions and models are ready to be separated?

17. Your patient is having a ceramic crown made for tooth #21. Today is the initial appointment in the process. The dentist prefers alginate for preliminary impressions, vinyl polysiloxane for final impressions and bites, and acrylic for tem-

porary crowns. She also prefers to use a single phase material and dual impression technique whenever possible.

    A.   What materials will you need to get ready to use at this appointment? Which will not be needed?

    B.   What type of tray will you need to ready for use?

    C.   How will you care for the finished impression before it is poured?

    D.   If you are asked to pour the impression, what material will you use?

    E.   If you are asked to ready the impression for transport to a dental laboratory, how will you prepare it?

18.   You have been designated the hazard control coordinator for your office.

    A.   What kinds of hazards need to be controlled in a dental office?

    B.   What agencies can you contact for help in understanding the regulations that apply to hazard control in the dental environment?

    C.   What types of written policies and procedures do you need to put in place to control chemical hazards in compliance with OSHA standards?

    D.   What types of training are required?

    E.   What is an MSDS file and how is it utilized to help control hazards?

    F.   Why do waste disposal procedures matter?

19.   You have been asked to train a new employee in your office. She has no dental experience and will be learning both by observing you work and by specific short instruction sessions you will hold with her.

    A.   What will you teach her about storing materials?

    B.   How can she tell which spatula needs to be used for mixing which material?

    C.   How can she know which scoop is used to measure which powder?

    D.   How can she know whether to use a glass slab or a paper pad for mixing?

    E.   How can she know if the cement she is mixing is ready for use?

    F.   How can she know if the impression material she is mixing is ready for use?

20.   Your 5-year-old patient presented with severe decay in all of his molars. Today the dentist has prepared teeth A and B for crowns and asked you to fit and place them.

    A.   What kind of crowns should you select?

    B.   How would you fit these crowns?

    C.   What kind of material could be used to attach the crowns to the teeth?

    D.   Describe to the mother how long the child will need to use the crowns.

21.   Your healthy 16-year-old patient presented on an emergency basis. Tooth #23 was avulsed (knocked out) when she fell during gym class on the metal pipe edging a circular trampoline. The dentist reimplanted the tooth and now the task is to stabilize it in position.

    A.   What will be placed to stabilize the tooth?

    B.   What types of material can be used to make it?

    C.   Although the young woman's parents gave permission for the treatment, they were upset at the time and are now somewhat unsure of what was done and how it will be beneficial to their daughter. What will you tell the parents when you again describe the treatment she received and why it was done?

    D.   The parents are also concerned that the treatment may ultimately be unsuccessful. Explain to them what other options exist for restoring form and function in the area if this treatment fails.

22.   You are removing stain from the teeth of a 31-year-old male patient who is a smoker. You do not seem to be making much headway in removing the tobacco stain on the maxillary lingual surfaces.

    A.   Suggest some possible causes for your lack of success.

    B.   Describe the measures you could take to improve your success rate without harming the teeth.

23.   One of the hygienists is extremely busy and has asked you to get a sealant set-up ready for her next patient, a 9-year-old girl who will be having her four first molars sealed. The office policy is to polish the surfaces to be sealed, to use unfilled, acrylic sealant material that does not contain fluoride, and to provide a fluoride treatment following the sealant procedure.

    A.   What will you need to get ready?

    B.   What would need to be added to the set-up if the sealant material were a filled type?

    C.   What will need to be done if the finished sealant is slightly high?

    D.   What will you tell the child and the parent when you give them post-operative directions?

    E.   How could you check the curing light before use to be sure it was working correctly?

24.   One of the assistants is extremely busy and has asked you to make a custom quadrant bead tray so that it will be ready for a final impression later in the afternoon.

    A.   What technique will you use to make the tray?

    B.   What do you need to have on hand to complete the task?

    C.   How does this type of tray harden?

D. What do you need to do to the finished tray to assure the impression does not remain in the mouth when the tray is removed?

E. How far ahead of the appointment does this step need to be taken?

25. Your 65-year-old female patient is considering having an endosseous implant to replace tooth #13, which was extracted. She has talked with the dentist and office manager about the procedure but is having difficulty making up her mind. Today she brought a friend with her to help with the decision. You have been asked to provide explanations to the friend, who has not heard the previous discussions.

A. Explain to the patient and her friend what an endosseous implant is.

B. Describe how an endosseous implant becomes a single unit with the bone.

C. Explain the procedures that will need to be completed to prepare the implant site, and place the implant and prosthesis.

D. Explain why an implant is preferable to a partial denture or conventional bridge.

E. Describe the oral hygiene measures the patient will need to follow if an implant is placed.

RATIONALES FOR CASE STUDIES

▼ Case Study 1 ▼

A. The patient and his parents should be educated to the importance of using an athletic mouthguard when playing sports and to placing sealants on sound permanent teeth that have pits and fissures.

B. If there are no permanent successors to teeth A and J, direct restorations would likely be placed in order for the patient to use them as long as possible. Since the patient is 13 years old, if the permanent successors are present and reasonably near eruption, the primary molars would probably not be treated.

C. Sealants may be indicated for the permanent molars and premolars that have erupted. If deep pits exist on other teeth, such as the lingual surfaces of the maxillary anteriors, sealants may be indicated for them as well.

▼ Case Study 2 ▼

A. Tooth #30 could be replaced with an implant, a fixed bridge or a partial denture.

B. Construction of a partial denture would be least invasive and require only an impression plus fitting and delivery procedures.

C. A conventional bridge or implant would be permanently fixed in the mouth. The advantage of a fixed replacement is that it feels more like a natural tooth.

D. The partial denture would be removable. It would be less expensive, the procedures to construct it would be less invasive, it would be easier to keep clean and it would maintain the form and function of the dental arch. It would place force on the adjacent teeth, while making them more difficult to clean, fail to maintain the height of the alveolar bone and appear less natural.

E. An implant would maintain normal arch form and function, normal bone height and contour, avoid placing destructive forces on adjacent teeth, and appear and feel more natural. It would also be more expensive than a removable denture, require a longer time and more invasive

procedures to construct, and meticulous oral hygiene procedures.

▼ Case Study 3 ▼

A. Available endodontic therapies include pulp capping, pulpotomy, pulpectomy and apexification. It is likely the dentist would choose apexification because of the child's age and the fact that the root is not yet fully formed.

B. Calcium hydroxide and zinc oxide and eugenol temporary restorative material would be needed.

C. A small mixing pad, spatula and an instrument to carry the material to the mouth would be needed to place calcium hydroxide. Similar items would be needed to place zinc oxide and eugenol powder and liquid. If the Z.O.E. were in a preloaded capsule, the capsule, a triturator and an instrument to place the material would be required.

D. An irrigating agent is used to flush away debris and tissue fluid, and to provide lubrication for instruments entering the canal. Because the tooth is vital, it is probably not infected and does not contain debris. This means irrigation and disinfection are likely contraindicated.

E. Calcium hydroxide is used to stimulate production of dentin, cementum and a root apex, and would be would be mixed on a paper pad with a ball-pointed instrument or small spatula.

▼ Case Study 4 ▼

A. Polishing with an abrasive would remove the extrinsic stains.

B. Pumice slurry or a prepared prophylaxis paste is the usual choice for polishing tooth surfaces with an abrasive.

C. The instrinsic stains should be able to be removed with external beaching.

D. Hydrogen or carbamide peroxide is the usual material of choice for external bleaching procedures.

E. Tooth #8 is particularly susceptible to discomfort because of the recession. To prevent this problem, the bleaching tray may be cut back slightly or the exposed area may be covered with a thin layer of acrylic bonding agent. If discomfort occurs, the number of hours of bleaching per day may be reduced or fluoride may be used in the bleaching tray in alternation with the bleaching agent.

▼ Case Study 5 ▼

A. No, he is not. The teeth should be cleaned of external deposits and stain and his oral hygiene habits should be regular and effective before the bleaching process begins. He also needs to refrain from smoking during the bleaching process and preferably beyond that. His ability and willingness to do that needs to be ascertained.

B. He needs to know about the need to gain control of his oral hygiene and smoking habits before beginning bleaching. He needs to know that his teeth will need to be cleaned before starting. He needs to know about the possibility that increased contrast between his composite restorations and newly-lightened teeth will make the restorations appear darker following bleaching, and he should know there may be a need to touch up the bleached teeth periodically.

C. A quick-start method would provide the immediate change he has requested and would also be more practical, given his erratic schedule.

D. As noted, the restorations may appear darker following bleaching. There may also be leakage of the bleaching material into the microspaces between the teeth and restorations if composite bonds to the teeth have broken, and that may cause discomfort. Microleakage can be prevented by placing a clear acrylic seal over the tooth-restoration interface, although this is rarely done, and then only after discomfort actually occurs. It is more common to combat discomfort by substituting fluoride for bleach in the bleaching tray.

E. The new, lighter color obtained from bleaching requires approximately two weeks to stabilize. Additionally, bond strengths of composite to teeth may be decreased if the restorations are replaced sooner.

▼ Case Study 6 ▼

A. Composite or amalgam could be used for a direct restoration in this tooth. Glass ionomer is not indicated when chewing forces are present.

B. Composite is esthetic, translucent, strong and can be bonded to the tooth surface. It is technique-sensitive and requires placement in a dry field. Amalgam is not esthetic but is relatively strong, inexpensive and easy to place.

C. Amalgam may be the material of choice if cost and ease of placement are the major criteria for selection and esthetics are not important.

D. Composite is the material of choice if esthetic appearance is the major criteria for selection and a dry field can be obtained.

E. An etchant, dentin primer and acrylic bonding agent will be used either in combination applications or separately.

▼ Case Study 7 ▼

A. You should select fine or very fine grit abrasives for the veneers and fine or medium grit abrasives for the composite restorations and natural teeth.

B. Sodium fluoride should be used.

C. Composite is more likely to be roughened by larger abrasive particles. Porcelain is a hard material but can be scratched by very hard abrasives.

D. Glass can be etched by acidic flourides, and the plastic is easily abraded.

E. Acidic fluorides can etch them, roughening the surface.

▼ Case Study 8 ▼

A. Glass ionomer or another polymer cement could be used to bond brackets directly to the teeth, although whether this is advisable or not would depend on what the orthodontist planned to accomplish.

B. Glass ionomer is a frequent choice. It flows well, forms a thin film beneath the bracket, does not require etching and bonding and leaches fluoride into the surrounding tooth surface.

C. Glass ionomer cement is available as a powder and liquid, and in a preloaded capsule or tip. The powder and liquid are mixed on a paper pad; a preloaded capsule or tip is shaken for the prescribed time in a triturator.

D. Glass ionomer is easily removed before set with a 2 × 2 gauze. Once set, it can be scrubbed off using soap and water or run through the ultrasonic cleaner. Usually only the spatula or placement instrument tip needs to be cleaned because glass ionomer is hand mixed on a paper pad.

E. Sealing the interface area helps to prevent the decalcification that may accompany orthodontic appliance placement. Bands catch food readily and can be very difficult to clean. Sealing the interface creates a smooth surface that is not hospitable to plaque attachment, makes cleaning easier and if done with a glass ionomer sealant, provides a temporary source of topical fluoride for the immediate area.

▼ Case Study 9 ▼

A. A temporary restoration provides for maintenance of tooth comfort, form and function, and contains eugenol, an irritant that stimulates the pulp to form new dentin. This new dentin serves as an insulating bridge that protects the pulp from chemical and thermal injury.

B. Temporary direct restorations in vital teeth are made with reinforced zinc oxide and eugenol.

C. Temporary restorative material is available as a powder and liquid and in a preloaded capsule. One scoop of powder and one drop of liquid are placed on a paper pad, the powder is divided into 2–4 large increments, and each increment is spatulated into the liquid separately. Mixing time is less critical than for many other materials and time may be taken to assure the powder particles are well crushed into the liquid. Preloaded capsules are placed in a triturator and shaken for the manufacturer's recommended time.

D. Those duties that can be delegated to allied dental personnel are specific to each state. Many states allow allied dental personnel to place temporary direct restorations. It is important to know specifically what is and is not permitted in the jurisdiction in which you practice.

E. Again, duty delegation is state specific. Few states permit allied dental personnel to place permanent direct restorations. Be sure you know what is and is not permitted in your practice jurisdiction.

▼ Case Study 10 ▼

A. Glass ionomer would be a strong contender for the material of choice because it is esthetic, bonds chemically to the tooth and because it is more flexible than composite so will be less likely to pop out of the tooth.

B. No. Glass ionomer bonds chemically to the tooth.

C. Bonding agent or glass ionomer varnish (also termed glaze) could be placed over the new restoration to protect it during the first 24 hours while it is setting.

D. Once polymer materials are set, they are virtually insoluble in oral fluids. The problem with glass ionomer is wear, not dissolution. There is no occlusal wear on a Class V restoration, but tooth brushing will likely abrade the material over time.

▼ Case Study 11 ▼

A. Depending on the severity of the pitting, veneers or crowns could be used to correct the problem. Veneers are the more likely choice as they require removal of less hard tissue.

B. Veneers could be made of either porcelain (ceramic) or composite (an acrylic family material). Ceramic is the more natural-appearing choice and composite ("bonding") is the simpler, less-expensive choice. Newer composites are, however, quite lifelike and often represent a viable choice. Crowns could also be made of either all porcelain (jacket crowns) or porcelain fused to metal.

C. Because glass materials can have coloring agents and opacifiers placed in the material before it is processed, thereby making a nearly infinite number of shades and opacities available, and because glass materials are covered with a clear smooth glaze, they are the most natural-appearing. Composite does, however, contain a large percentage of translucent fillers, can be tinted a nearly infinite number of shades and can appear exceedingly lifelike.

D. Porcelain veneers require removal of a thin portion of enamel, and the taking of a highly accurate impression. This impression is sent to the lab, where a die is poured with a gypsum stone. Porcelain frits are mixed and vibrated onto the die until the correct shape is obtained. The veneer is then fired (baked at high temperature) and may be returned to the patient for try-in. A final layer is added and the veneer is again fired to form a smooth glaze over the surface. Porcelain crowns require removal of more tooth structure during tooth preparation but are formed in the same manner as veneers. Composite temporary veneers are ordinarily placed while the patient is waiting for the ceramic veneers to be completed.

E. Teeth are prepared for composite veneers in similar manner to the way they are prepared for ceramic ones. Composite veneers are placed directly on the tooth, however, so the tooth can be prepared and the restoration placed at a single appointment. The prepared tooth is etched, an acrylic bonding material is placed, and the composite bonded to it.

▼ Case Study 12 ▼

A. Ceramic fused to metal would provide both strength and esthetics. Gold or base metal alloy alone would not be esthetic and ceramic alone might not be strong enough.

B. Ceramic fused to metal crown fabrication normally requires two appointments—one for preparing the tooth, taking the impression and placing the temporary crown, and one to fit, cement and finish the finished crown, and teach the patient how to care for it.

C. Any of the permanent cements could be used. Zinc phosphate cement is a relatively strong metal oxide cement that has a long track record of success in cementing metal castings to the tooth surface. Glass ionomer cement can be used and will bond chemically to the tooth. Resin cement can also serve as a relatively strong bonding agent between the tooth and metal.

D. Tooth comfort, form and function would be maintained through placement of a temporary acrylic crown.

E. Zinc phosphate cement is known to dissolve in oral fluids over time. Composite and other polymer cements are virtually insoluble once set but wear if the margin is accessible to abrasion.

F. The margins of the crown would need to be carefully checked with an explorer at each examination appointment. Areas where cement has dissolved or chipped away, or the bond is no longer present, can be felt with a fine explorer tip.

▼ Case Study 13 ▼

A. The patient has likely made a correct choice in returning to the dentist for observation.

B. Since the signs and symptoms exhibited are classic indicators of local soft tissue irritation, and since they appeared so soon after the placement of a new restoration, it is likely the bothersome area is a local reaction to composite material. Whenever adverse tissue response is involved, however, the dentist must consider a broad range of clinical causes. Infection, injury, allergy, and medication are some of the factors that would likely be considered for this young patient with AIDS.

C. The restoration could be removed and replaced with one of another material. If the signs and symptoms then subside, it is likely the source of the problem has been correctly identified.

▼ Case Study 14 ▼

A. The patient may be experiencing pain resulting from bond fracture and the resulting sensitivity due to microleakage.

B. Heat and cold cause the tooth and the amalgam to expand and contract, but at different rates. This pulls on the interface between the tooth and the restoration, causing it to break down. Now, a tiny space exists between the tooth and the restoration. Acids or fluids can seep into this area, get underneath the restoration, travel toward the pulp (a soft tissue in the middle of the tooth) and cause sensitivity.

▼ Case Study 15 ▼

A. It is likely ditching is present around the amalgam restorations.

B. When a metal restoration is placed, there is a tiny space between it and the tooth. Because this restoration is metal it is susceptible to corrosion, metal fatigue and fracture. Tiny corrosion bits have fractured off the edges of this restoration, leaving an open ditch around it instead of a tiny space. This can be a good thing, because the corrosion bits fall into and eventually fill the space, sealing the cut part of the tooth against entrance of cavity-causing germs and undesirable matter dissolved in the saliva. This takes awhile, though, so decay can start next to the restoration. The dentist believes the best thing to do here is to let the restoration continue its self-sealing course.

C. It is theoretically possible for the ditching condition to persist indefinitely, if the ditch is filled before decay gains a foothold and the adjacent tooth structure remains strong. What more frequently happens, however, is that the decay process outpaces the self-sealing process and secondary decay ultimately appears underneath the restoration. This generally takes some time, so some dentists believe it is safe to "watch" the restoration for awhile and replace it when there is a clear need. Other dentists believe it is best to replace a ditched amalgam as soon as it appears because it will eventually need to be replaced anyway. Still other dentists believe it is best to bond the amalgam restoration to the tooth in the first place, thereby sealing the microspace and not depending on the amalgam to be self-sealing.

▼ Case Study 16 ▼

A. Alginate is usually used to take impressions for study models.

B. First, observe the patient's mouth for arch size and form, and the presence of any lesions, tori, bone irregularities or a very high palatal vault. Then select a tray that appears to be the approximate size and shape needed and try it in the mouth. It should be inserted gently, loosely cover the arch from front to back and side to side, include the mandibular retromolar pads or maxillary tuberosities and be deep enough to record the mucobuccal fold. If it is slightly short in length or height, utility wax can be used to add to the dimensions slightly. If is too narrow or more than slightly short, a larger tray should be selected and tried in.

C. The mandibular impression should record the retromolar pads, the lingual ridge, the mucobuccal fold, and all of the teeth, and should not exhibit voids, tears or drag areas. The maxillary impression should record the maxillary tuberosities, palatal vault, mucobuccal fold and all of the teeth, and again should not exhibit voids, tears or drag areas.

D. The impressions should be rinsed in gently running water to remove any blood, saliva or debris; the fluids gently shaken out; the entire impression sprayed with disinfectant; the impression sealed in a plastic bag; the bag labeled with the patient's name, the date and the time; and the impression left in the sealed bag for the disinfectant manufacturer's recommended time.

E. Alginate impressions are poured with one of the gypsum materials. Which one is selected depends on the use to which the model will be put and the dentist's policy on the material to be used. Plaster is strong enough to use for study models and looks quite elegant. Some dentists prefer that study model impressions be poured in stone, which is stronger and less likely to discolor, chip or fracture.

F. Impressions and models can be separated when the model is no longer warm to the touch.

▼ Case Study 17 ▼

A. You will need single phase vinyl polysiloxane to take an impression of the area of interest, the opposing area, and a bite registration. You will also need the brand of acrylic material the dentist prefers to make a temporary crown. Alginate is not needed in the dual impression technique; it is used in the conventional technique when a preliminary impression must be taken to enable a model to be poured and a custom tray made or to make a model of the opposing arch to use as a guide to the proper occlusal form.

B. You will need to prepare a quadrant dual impression tray.

C. The impression should be rinsed of blood, saliva and debris, then disinfected by immersion in disinfectant solution for the manufacturer's recommended time, or sprayed with disinfectant and placed in a labeled plastic bag and sealed for the recommended time. Vinyl polysiloxane impressions should not be poured for 2–6 hours following disinfection to allow any gases formed in the setting process to dissipate.

D. Final impressions are poured with gypsum. Because this impression will be used to make a crown, die stone should be used to provide adequate strength, accuracy, and abrasion resistance.

E. The impression should be rinsed, placed in disinfectant solution in a sealed plastic bag and labeled with the patient's name, the dentist's name and the date. A prescription should be prepared for the laboratory that provides directions for how the dentist wants the crown constructed; this prescription may be prepared by the assistant, hygienist or dentist, but must be signed by the dentist. Unless the lab stops at the office to pick up cases on a routine basis, the lab or shipping company should be contacted for case pick-up.

▼ Case Study 18 ▼

A. Physical hazards, infectious materials, the possibility of fire, and chemical hazards need to be controlled in a dental facility. Radiation should also be controlled, but is outside the scope of this text.

B. OSHA, the Occupational Safety and Health Administration, can be contacted for help with hazard control regulations. The CDC, the federal Centers for Disease Control and Prevention, can be contacted for advice in controlling infectious hazards. The EPA, the federal Environmental Protection Agency, can be contacted for advice concerning hazardous chemical disposal. The ADA, the American Dental Association, and OSAP, the Organization for Sterilization and Asepsis Procedures, are private agencies that provide substantial advice concerning dental facility hazard control policies and procedures. Additionally, state or regional counterparts of the agencies named above offer similar advice to dental facilities located in their geographic jurisdictions.

C. The following need to be written and accessible:

Identification by name and task all individuals exposed to chemical hazards
Labeling of hazardous chemicals
Policies concerning procedures for the use, storage and disposal of hazardous and infectious materials
Comprehensive chemical inventory
An MSDS file
Documentation of employee training

D. Training must be provided to new hires, to all affected employees when a new chemical is introduced and when procedures are changed, and at least annually to continuing employees.

E. An MSDS (Material Safety Data Sheet) file is a compendium of comprehensive chemical information sheets for all chemicals used in the dental facility. If a spill or leak occurs, information concerning what to do is then readily available from the MSDS sheet. The manufacturer is responsible for providing MSDS to purchasers of its chemicals. The dental facility is responsible for assuring that an MSDS is on file for each chemical used and all of the MSDS in its file are current. These two regulations aim to assure that the available information is always current.

F. Waste disposal can affect the quality of our air, water and soil, and result in damage to people, ecosystems and animals. Dentists who disregard EPA or OSHA regulations are also subject to fines, an unproductive use of money.

▼ Case Study 19 ▼

A. Materials should be stored where it is cool and dry and the light is not strong. New materials should be placed in the rear of the storage area so that the oldest materials are used first. (FIFO: First in, first out)

B. Common sense is her best guide. Small spatulas are used for mixing small amounts of material, large spatulas, for larger amounts. Other distinguishing characteristics for the large spatulas are: tapered blade sides for impression material, straight blade sides for model materials and convex blade sides for alginate.

C. Each scoop is unique to its material. For this reason, store each scoop with the powder it is used to proportion, and always return it to that position after it is used and cleaned.

D. Virtually all powder and liquid materials are mixed on a paper pad. The exceptions are zinc phosphate cement, which is always mixed on a cool, dry glass slab; plus alginate and gypsum, which are mixed in a flexible rubber bowl.

E. Check the label to see if it is a polymer cement. All polymer cements are ready for use when they are homogenous in color and consistency, and still have a glossy surface. If it is not a polymer, it will be a metal oxide cement. This type should also be homogenous in color and consistency. If a metal oxide cement is to be used for luting, it should flow off the end of the spatula, not drip off or stick to it. If it is to be used for basing or a temporary restoration, it should be able to be rolled into a small ball.

F. All properly mixed impression materials should be homogenous in color and consistency. In addition, alginate should be creamy and the rubber base materials should have a glossy surface.

▼ Case Study 20 ▼

A. Stainless steel crowns would be used.
B. Stainless steel crowns are fitted by cutting and crimping the cervix of the preformed shell with scissors and pliers.
C. Cement is used as a luting agent.
D. The child will need to use these crowns until the permanent premolars erupt.

▼ Case Study 21 ▼

A. A periodontal splint will be placed.
B. The splint can be made with wire, or specially constructed cloth strips and a polymer.
C. The dentist replaced the tooth in its socket, then placed a splint to hold it in position while the area heals. Position is maintained by attaching the splint to the tooth that was put back in place plus its neighbors, which are still firmly anchored in their sockets.
D. Should the reimplantation not be successful, there are other ways to replace the tooth — an implant, a bridge or a partial denture. An implant is a substitute tooth root that is anchored in the bone and topped with a replacement tooth. A bridge is a replacement tooth that is attached to nearby teeth. A partial denture is a partial plate. In this case, the partial would have only one replacement tooth, as all the other teeth are intact. These may never need to be considered, though, if the re-implantation treatment is successful.

▼ Case Study 22 ▼

A. Possible causes include using too fine an abrasive grit (the abrasive might not be hard enough or coarse enough to remove the stain), using too high a polishing speed (this could fling the abrasive off the tooth), not renewing the abrasive frequently enough (so the particles are too small and round to be effective, or simply no longer present), not adapting your hand position so the abrasive can reach the tooth, or applying the abrasive with too much pressure or without adequate moisture (either of these would prevent the abrasive from moving freely over the tooth surface).

B. You could follow the principles of effective abrasive use: use an appropriate grit (medium for natural teeth in this case), moderate speed and pressure, keep the area moist, move your hand so the abrasive both contacts and moves over the tooth surface, apply abrasive with a dabbing motion and renew the abrasive frequently.

▼ Case Study 23 ▼

A. You would need to obtain plain pumice slurry, prophylaxis angle and cup, acid etch material, sealant material, a curing light, a mirror, explorer, fluoride gel, an appropriately sized fluoride tray, dental floss and items to maintain a dry field.

B. Articulating paper and a scaler or bur would need to be added to remove any high spots if a filled material were used. High spots on sealants made with unfilled material work themselves out through occlusion; those on sealants made with filled material need to be removed by a dental professional.

C. Nothing will need to be done because the sealant material is unfilled. You would, however, want to advise the parent and child that the sealant would need a few days to wear in to the usual bite position.

D. Your daughter has had a fluoride treatment so she should not eat or drink for 30 minutes. I've checked and the sealant seems to be very securely attached. However, if it should come off, call the office so it can be reapplied. How long a sealant lasts in the mouth depends on many factors that differ from person to person. We'll be checking it each time your daughter comes in for an examination, and it is likely that some years in the future it may need to be reapplied. Sealants do wear away over time.

E. A light meter is used to check curing light efficiency. The light tip is placed on a small circle on the device and turned on. A needle on the device immediately rises to the level of the light's photo output. The actual output is compared to the manufacturer's recommended output to assure the light is still working efficiently. A light that does not reach recommended levels may not cure materials effectively and should not be used until it is repaired.

▼ Case Study 24 ▼

A. You will soften the beads in warm water and shape them over a model by hand.

B. You will need a model of the patient's mouth, wax to make a spacer, a knife or sharp instrument to prepare the wax for making the stops, a lubricant to enable easy separation of the tray and spacer, scissors to cut away any excess material, and warm water.

C. Cooling hardens this thermoplastic material.

D. The finished tray should be painted with a rubber base adhesive and the adhesive should be allowed to dry before the impression material is placed in it. The adhesive will hold the set impression material to the tray.

E. Adhesive painting and drying require 10–15 minutes, but can be done ahead of time without affecting the performance of the adhesive.

▼ Case Study 25 ▼

A. An implant is an artificial tooth root that is anchored in the bone and will be connected to a replacement for the tooth that was removed.

B. The surface of the implant is biologically active and attracts bone to form on it. Given enough time the implant and bone fuse into a solid unit, a phenomenon termed osseointegration.

C. Once a decision is made to proceed with the implant, several appointments over several months time will be required to complete it. First, surgery is required to prepare the bone and place the artificial root and its cover into it. The site is left alone for 2–6 months to allow the implant and bone to become a single unit. Once this has happened, the site is reopened, and the cover is removed and replaced with a connector that extends into the mouth. A healing cap is used to cover the connector while the gum tissue heals. When this has happened, the healing cap is removed, a precisely fitted cylinder is placed over the implant, an impression is taken, a replacement tooth is made, and the replacement tooth is attached to the implant. Overall, it can take 6–9 months to complete the process.

D. An implant is preferred for tooth replacement because it appears and feels natural, maintains facial contour and dental arch form and function, results in less bone loss, and remains fixed in position. It can be cleaned in ways similar to a natural tooth. Replacement with a conventional bridge or partial denture results in more bone loss, therefore a less natural facial contour and arch form. Partial dentures and bridges also require that adjacent teeth be cut down to receive the replacement tooth, place more forces on adjacent teeth and make them more difficult to clean. A partial denture appears and feels less natural. It can be removed for cleaning but tends to collect stain and deposits unless scrupulously cleaned on a regular basis.

E. The patient with an implant just like one with natural teeth needs frequent, thorough, conscientious professional examination and prophylaxis, and an individualized home care plan. The plan should be conscientiously followed.

Crossword Puzzles

Why Dental Materials?

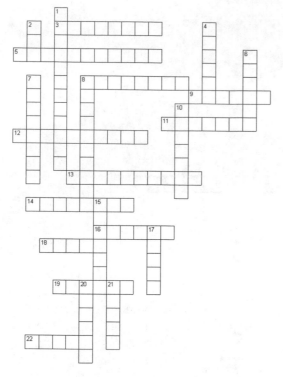

1. bridge that has a pontic at either or both ends
2. working cast of one tooth
4. single fixed indirect restoration that replaces one or more teeth
6. type of restoration that is formed in the mouth
7. restoration used to connect a pontic to a neighboring tooth
8. type of implant that is anchored within the bone
10. removable replacement for all the teeth in an arch
15. replacement for the root of a tooth that has been lost
17. indirect restoration similar to a filling but made outside the mouth
20. device used to redistrubute mechanical forces
21. indirect restoration that includes the cusps of a chewing surface

Across

3. material that attaches two solids together
5. a tooth repair
8. appearing natural
9. esthetic restoration of a facial surface to improve its appearance
11. thin plastic coating over areas that are vulnerable to tooth decay
12. mold of a patient's oral structures
13. flexible plastic cover that fits over the teeth and absorbs and distributes traumatic forces
14. material used to cut, shape, or polish teeth

16. each replacement tooth in a bridge
18. duplicate of oral structures
19. type of impression tray made specifically to fit one patient very well
22. indirect restoration that replaces all the surfaces of a natural tooth crown

Vocabulary 1

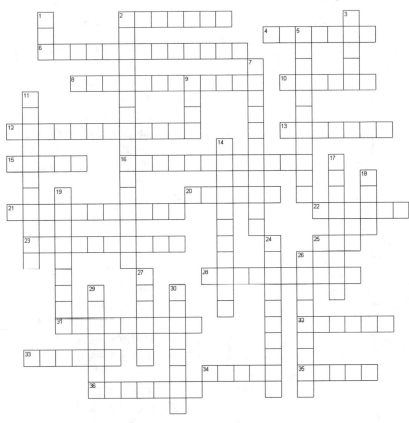

Down

1. hardened
2. characteristic of affecting an oral tissue benignly
3. lightness or darkness (shade) of a color
5. property of absorbing some light and permitting some to pass through
7. allergic response to a foreign substance
9. polymer set
11. material that flows in response to pressure
14. property of permitting all light to pass through
17. type of solid that has a regular arrangement of internal atoms
18. ability to move to conform to the shape of a container
19. type of solid that may flow after set
24. device for selecting the shade of a material to be used
26. resistance to flow
27. material composed of relatively rapid-moving atoms
29. material composed of a chain of repeating units
30. type of bonding in which tooth and material share surface electrons or a weak electrical current

Across

2. attaching a material to a tooth surface so the two are continuous with one another
4. type of light that should be used for shade selection
6. set in which material softens when heated and hardens when cooled
8. tooth property often termed sparkle
10. this tooth tissue is translucent
12. entrance of fluids and dissolved substances into the space between a tooth and a material
13. polymer that sets following mixing with another chemical plus application of light
15. reflected light waves that are visible
16. is a chemical set reversible or irreversible?
20. this tooth tissue is opaque
21. type of solid that does not conduct electricity well
22. should a shade be selected before or after a tooth preparation procedure is completed?
23. exaggerated local response of skin or mucous membrane to a material
25. color name
28. type of bonding in which material and tooth are interlocked
31. polymer that sets when mixed with another material
32. property of absorbing all light
33. vividness (saturation) of a color
34. material composed of relatively slow-moving atoms
35. poisonous
36. arrangement of atoms in the type of solid that has consistent melting and solidifying temperatures

Vocabulary 2

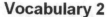

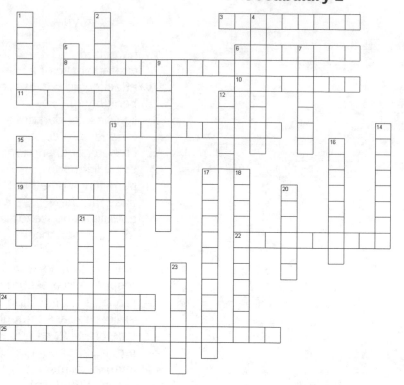

Down

1. amount of force applied
2. force placed on a material
4. pitting and disintegration of a metal from exposure to electrochemical forces
5. cutting (pushing and pulling) load
7. metal discoloration from exposure to electrochemical forces
9. this type of material flows well over the surface of a wet solid
12. open area surrounding a restoration
13. the breaking up of a solid
14. another word for absorption
15. process of a liquid's covering the surface of a solid
16. resistance to stress
17. resistance of a metal to compressive stress
18. pushing load
20. when a material is heated its size will usually do this
21. temporary deformation followed by relaxation
23. twisting load

Across

3. resistance of a metal to tensile stress
6. breakage
8. this type of material does NOT flow well over the surface of a wet solid
10. when a material is cooled its size will usually do this
11. internal rearrangement of atoms to adjust to stress
13. change in shape resulting from the effects of strain
19. pulling load

22. return to original state before stress was applied
24. ability of a substance to dissolve in a liquid
25. resistance to wear (2 words)

Using Materials Safely

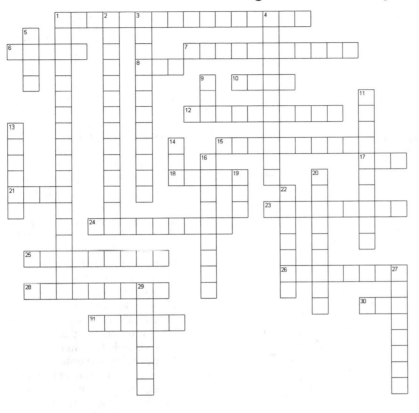

Down

1. letters or symbols in the white diamond indicate any ___ that must be taken
2. day that indicates when a chemical should no longer be used
3. this type of waste may be discarded in a closed, unlabeled, leakproof bag
4. how soon must a chemical in a secondary container be used in order for a secondary label not to be required?
5. may or must employees with actual or potential exposure to hazardous chemicals have access to the employer's written safety program?
9. equipment worn to protect a dental health worker from chemical and microbial harm
11. contaminated materials may transfer this type of microorganisms to a patient or dental health worker
13. the number in the ___ diamond of a hazardous material label indicates the risk of chemical reactivity
14. federal agency that must grant approval before a dental material can be marketed
16. suggestion of an appropriate method for complying with a law or regulation
19. federal agency that is charged with protecting the natural environment
20. term that describes the period during which a chemical is at appropriate strength
22. an MSDS must be in this language, but may contain other languages as well
27. this must be provided to employees with actual or potential exposure to hazardous chemicals when they are hired and when new hazards are introduced
29. type of chemical exposure that occurs from repeated contact with a small amount of a chemical over a long period of time

Across

1. the ADA seal of acceptance indicates a dental material is ___
6. a special mask may need to be worn to protect a dental worker from this form of a chemical
7. the OSHA Hazard Communication Standard aims to provide the worker with this
8. fire risk is indicated in this color diamond
10. manufacturer or importer's sheet that provides comprehensive information about a chemical
12. directive from an official agency that must be followed
15. the most important aspect of infection control is ___ of the need for and practice of rigorous infection control procedures
17. influential federal agency that issues guidelines for safe dental practice
18. type of chemical exposure that occurs from contact with a large amount of a chemical in a short time
21. federal agency charged with protecting dental personnel from chemical harm
23. comprehensive listing of chemicals used in a facility
24. this type of waste is either biologically or chemically hazardous
25. the number in the blue diamond of a hazardous material label indicates its ___ risk
26. this should be readily available to clean up a chemical spill
28. to do this, it is necessary to wear thick, protective utility gloves
30. dental organization that operates a voluntary acceptance program for dental materials
31. needles and instruments with sharp edges are termed ___

Using Materials Sensibly

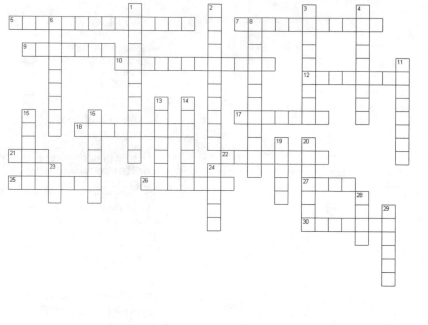

Down

1. mixing motion in which the liquid is brought to the powder and compressed into it
2. are polymers usually hydrophilic or hydrophobic?
3. disposable multi-dose, two-compartment containers of unmixed material
4. area of the mouth in which metal alloys are most likely to be used
6. mixing motion that consists of sweeping back and forth across a surface
8. small machine that cuts models to esthetic proportions
11. moving a submerged spatula tip in circles
13. instrument used to mix materials together
14. two tubes of paste are proportioned by extruding equal ____ of the materials
15. mixing motion in which the spatula is moved in circles
16. plastic is this type of material
19. this is used to cure many polymer materials
20. squares of this material are softened and adapted to working casts using a vacuum or pressure former
23. unit dose of material that will be applied directly into the mouth with a small applicator gun
24. mixture of metals
28. true or false: metal restorations are safe
29. pick up a mixed mass of material with a spatula

Across

5. small machine that uses pressurized air to soften and adapt plastic materials to working casts
7. small machine that shakes materials to mix them
9. type of glass used when esthetics is important but biting forces are a factor
10. small machine that uses a vacuum to soften and adapt plastic materials to working casts
12. type of restorations made with glass materials
17. mixing motion that consists of stropping and lifting spatula slightly when changing direction
18. type of glass used where esthetics is critical and biting forces are low
21. this material is softened in warm water or over a low flame
22. type of bowl in which mixing is done
25. disposable multi-dose container of premixed material
26. small cylinder of pre-measured materials separated by a thin membrane
27. reusable mixing surface
30. long, thin tube through which material is expelled onto the area of interest

Abrasives

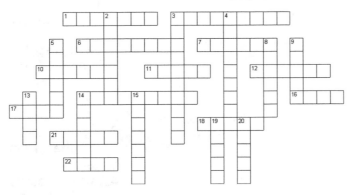

Down

2. connector for attaching a disk or wheel to a handpiece or angle
3. how often should an abrasive in use be renewed?
4. softer material over which an abrasive is rubbed
5. type of abrasive that should not be used on natural teeth
8. thin abrasive paste
9. thin piece of plastic or metal with abrasive on one side
13. this speed is counterproductive when using abrasives
14. a gray powder utility abrasive that is used for finishing and polishing natural and artificial surfaces
15. as abrasives are used, they become this size
19. an area of abrasive use should be kept _____ to dissipate heat
20. reddish-brown abrasive used in the laboratory for polishing gold

Across

1. hard natural or synthetic abrasive that generates much heat when cutting natural teeth
3. cutting and smoothing
6. mild white powder abrasive used for polishing enamel and metals
7. material residue of abrasive use
10. should an abrasive be harder or softer than the substrate on which it is used?
11. as abrasives are used the particles become this shape
12. sand abrasive supplied on disks and strips
14. smoothing a surface to create a shine
16. this tooth tissue can be injured when excessive heat is generated during abrasive use
17. type of abrasive that produces a shine
18. another name for corundum
21. mixture of abrasive and binder pressed into a thin shape and mounted on a mandrel
22. by-product of abrasive use

Dental Sealants

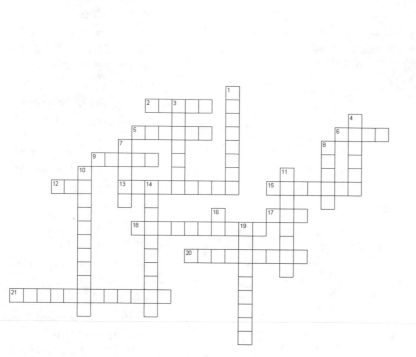

1. a high spot on a sealant made with this type of material will adjust itself through normal use
3. type of polymer used for the vast majority of sealants
4. when glass ionomer sealant material is used, completing this placement step thoroughly is not essential
7. true or false: a tooth prepared to receive a sealant should be smooth
8. this type of pumice is used for polishing so as not to interfere with bonding
10. as polymers, would you expect sealant materials to be hydrophilic or hydrophobic?
11. filler in a sealant increases this property of the material
14. this type of sealant material does not need to be mixed
16. yes or no: sealants need to be applied only once
19. sealants work by using this technique to prevent microorganisms and acids from reaching the tooth surface

Across

2. material used as a filler to increase the strength of some sealant materials
5. this part of a polymer is very weak
6. true or false: a fluoride treatment is not always provided after a sealant is placed
9. a properly etched tooth surface should be the color of this material
12. should the tooth surface be wet or dry during sealant placement?
13. this type of sealant material requires mixing of two materials
15. this technique is used to create multiple depressions on the tooth surface to facilitate mechanical interlocking
17. yes or no: sealants are cost-effective
18. this type of acid is most often used for etching
20. this sealant material is the same polymer as acrylic, but is much more heavily filled
21. type of sealant polymer that bonds chemically to the tooth and leaches fluoride

Tooth Whiteners

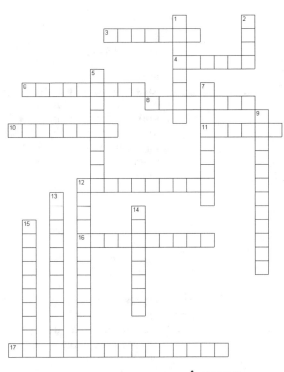

Down

1. material added to carbamide peroxide to increase the viscosity of whitening gels
2. true or false: whitening is generally successful in removing colors associated with aging
5. type of peroxide that combines oxygen with nitrogen
7. category of chemicals used for both internal and external bleaching
9. this type of restoration occasionally turns orange following bleaching
12. bleaching materials can travel through these to irritate the pulp in young teeth with large pulps
13. removal of staining from use of this antibiotic while teeth are forming is problematic
14. type of bleaching completed at home by patients, sometimes under professional supervision
15. method of carrying whitening gel to the teeth in home whitening systems

Across

3. this type of restoration may appear darker following bleaching
4. except for whitening strips, the patient brushes (before or after) the bleach is applied
6. because there is no data on how bleaching affects women with this condition, bleaching is not indicated for them
8. it takes about this long for a new tooth color to stabilize and residual peroxide to clear following bleaching
10. type of bleaching that is reserved to the dentist
11. active ingredient in tooth whiteners
12. this whitening product has a low concentration of peroxide and is designed for daily use
16. this is the most common soft tissue side effect from bleaching teeth
17. this is the most common dental side effect of bleaching teeth

Alginate

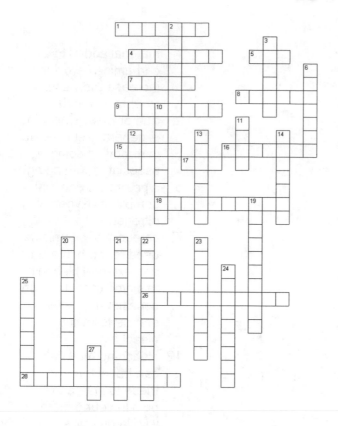

Down

2. this type of alginate requires a short time to set
3. blood and saliva ___ the set of gypsum materials used to pour impressions
6. should an alginate impression be sprayed or immersed in disinfectant
10. loss of water to the environment followed by shrinking of an alginate impression
11. alginate should be stored where it is dark and this temperature
12. the liquid state of alginate material
13. alginate is an (elastic or inelastic) impression material
14. relaxed patients who are treated gently are less apt to experience this problem
19. alginate is used to make this item
20. the term for water trapped between the fibrils in set alginate
21. alginate has this type of set
22. mounting finished models on an artificial jaw joint in correct relationship to each other
23. how do accelerators and retarders working at the same time affect the setting time?
24. what is the ultimate fate of an impression?
25. what type of tray is used to carry alginate paste to the mouth?
27. the patient's head should be tipped in this direction for taking a mandibular impression?

Across

1. this is done to alginate material before it is proportioned
4. a set alginate impression should be removed from the mouth with one motion because it has little of this type of strength
5. the semisolid state of alginate material
7. true or false: alginate takes impressions that record detail exceptionally accurately
8. to shorten the setting time when using alginate, use this temperature of water
9. alginate materials should be protected from exposure to this during storage
15. item poured from an alginate impression to make a duplicate of the oral anatomy
16. in what direction should the patient's head be tipped for a maxillary impression
17. this type of material is often used to record occlusal relationships when alginate impressions are taken
18. gain of water from the environment followed by swelling of an alginate impression
26. a set alginate imprssion ahould always be placed on a flat surface tray side down because it has little of this type of strength
28. alginate is this type of material

Model and Die Materials

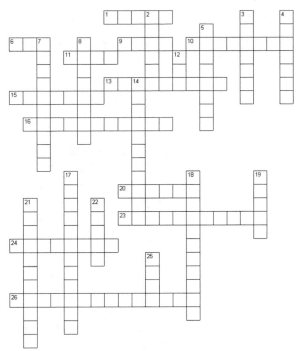

Down

2. number of milliliters of water needed for mixing 100 grams of stone
3. type of gypsum with most irregular powder particles
4. portion of the powder particle where setting reaction takes place
5. most dense, most abrasion resistant type of set gypsum
7. setting process which gives off heat
8. speed to use when pouring models
12. what actually fills an "empty" (unpoured) impression
14. powder form of gypsum
17. set of directions from a dentist to the laboratory technician for constructing a restoration
18. a commonly used accelerator for gypsum set
19. gypsum material used for all types of working casts except dies
21. water needed for mixing and pouring a gypsym model, but not for setting
22. duplicate of oral structures
25. usual color of dental stone

Across

1. usual color of plaster material
6. replica of one tooth
9. area of air in the gypsum mix
10. small motor with a flat top attached; used for bringing trapped air bubbles to the surface of a mix
11. temperature of poured gypsum when initial set has been reached
13. set mass form of gypsum
15. approximate amount of time following pouring that a gypsum model is fully set
16. type of structure which forms set gypsum
20. usual color of die stone powder
23. effect of adding water to the hemihydrate form of a gypsum material
24. chemical that slows the setting reaction
26. type of rock mined and processed to make gypsum

Intermediary Materials

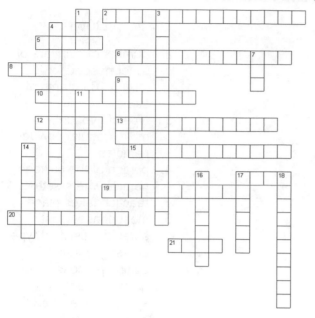

Down

1. material used for temporary restorations
3. water-based liner that has a basic pH and dissolves easily in oral fluids
4. process currently believed to cause pulpal sensitivity
7. calcium hydroxide can be used under these types of restorative materials
9. type of varnish that interferes with bonding and inhibits resin set
11. tenacious coat of ground hydroxyapatite crystals and protein that forms as dentin is cut
14. contemporary method of sealing cut dentin tubules to eliminate microleakage
16. material conventionally used to seal cut dentin tubules
17. material painted on cut dentin to soften and wet it
18. correct consistency of material that will be used as a base or temporary restoration

Across

2. combination cement that is mixed quickly like a polymer and has the reinforced strength of zinc oxide
5. thin layer of material applied to a cavity preparation to change its surface chemistry, irritate the pulp or serve as a bonding agent
6. highly acidic cement that may damage the pulp unless it is first protected with calcium hydroxide
8. is the compressive strength of Z.O.E. good or poor?
10. lining material that can set in the presence of moisture, bonds to the tooth and leaches fluoride
12. accelerator for zinc oxide and eugenol materials
13. popular polymer bonding agent
15. surface layer of a polymer; it does not harden as long as it is on the surface
17. intermediary materials are used to protect this tissue
19. part dentin, part hardened polymer layer that serves to anchor an esthetic direct restoration
20. type of varnish that can be used under all types of direct restorative materials
21. insulating coat placed on a cavity preparation floor

Esthetic Direct Restoration Materials

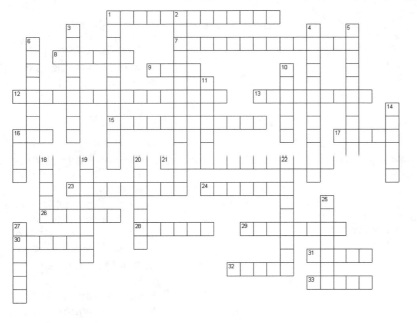

Down

1. charged chemicals that react with resin atoms to begin polymer hardening
2. unbound chemical in set glass ionomer that can diffuse into surrounding tooth tissue
3. material in a composite that responds to a chemical or light activator
4. esthetic material of choice where moisture control is difficult and biting forces are minimal to absent
5. type of bond created between composite and the tooth surface
6. blend of approximately equal amounts of composite and glass ionomer
10. composite material that contains both large and small size filler particles
11. this may be placed over a composite margin to preserve its integrity
14. curing light efficiency should be monitored by allied dental personnel at least this often
16. this type of cure seeks the speed of a light cure and the thoroughness of a chemical cure
18. composite reinforcing particles may be made of this translucent material
19. low viscosity composite material
20. a type of polymer used in composite restorative material
22. this undesirable process occurs as composite is curing
25. ion on the tooth surface with which glass ionomer bonds
27. opaque composite materials are used to simulate this tissue

Across

1. this process can result in staining of composite restorations
7. another type of polymer used in composite restorative material
8. composite and acrylic resin are similar but composite has much more of this type of material
9. true or false: etching is required for bonding composite to the tooth
12. blend of a greater amount of glass ionomer and a lesser amount of composite
13. this material may be used during composite finishing to ensure debris does not stain the new restoration
15. shaping and reinforcement of little remaining tooth structure to create adequate support for a restoration
16. type of environment required for composite set: wet or dry
17. particle size chosen for strength
21. this type of personal protective attire must be worn when using a curing light
23. esthetic direct restorative that can be used for all types of cavity preparations
24. all esthetic direct restoratives are this type of material
26. linking agent that prevents the loss of composite surface filler particles as the restoration wears
28. two paste composite systems will require this action
29. very high viscosity composite material that can be condensed into a cavity preparation
30. translucent composite materials are used to simulate this tissue
31. one paste composite systems will be cured using this tool
32. true or false: etching is required for bonding glass ionomer to the tooth
33. particle size which polishes best

Non-esthetic Direct Restoration Materials

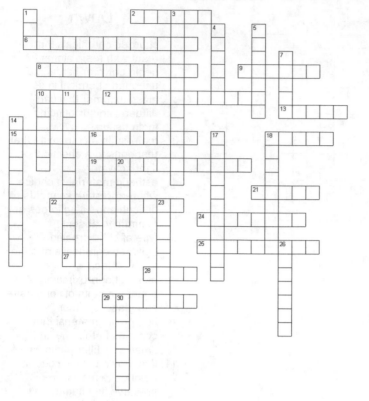

Down

1. metal oxide and oil of cloves cement used for temporary direct restorations
3. the reinforcer in set amalgam
4. correctly mixed amalgam should make this sound when being pushed into the carrier
5. type of alloy that contains a mixture of irregular filings and round droplets
7. wearing a mask protects against this form of mercury
10. some operators choose to use amalgam bonding agent as a ___ rather than to bond with it
11. cause of tooth pain when dentin tubules have been cut
14. surgical removal of the apical portion of a tooth root
16. poor support under an amalgam restoraiton may cause this to fracture
17. mixing of alloy and mercury
18. type of alloy comprised of round droplets
20. size of condenser needed for pushing spherical alloy particles into position
23. visible space around an amalgam restoration margin
26. material conventionally used to seal cut dentin tubules
30. metal in amalgam that is hazardous when it is free

Across

2. metal in amalgam alloy that reduces tarnish and corrosion, and increases restoration strength
6. mercury that is needed for amalgam preparation and handling but not for its set
8. mercury from dental unit waste lines contributes to pollution of these environmental features
9. physical state of mercury at room temperature
10. indicate whether set amalgam is dangerous or safe
12. the operator who bonds an amalgam restoration to the tooth is trying to prevent this
13. preloaded capsules of alloy and mercury are categorized by amount as one, two or three ___ sizes
15. means by which Z.O.E. temporary restorative material acts on the tooth
18. correctly mixed amalgam should appear like this
19. set amalgam characteristic that causes some operators to choose not to bond amalgam to the tooth
21. flow after set
22. type of restoration that is placed from the root end of a tooth following an apicoectomy
24. type of alloy comprised of irregular filings
25. what mercury does to alloy particles when the two materials are mixed
27. repeated expansion and contraction of an amalgam restoration may cause this to fracture
28. metal in amalgam alloy that may contribute to delayed, excessive expansion
29. metal alloy used for direct restorations

Impression Trays

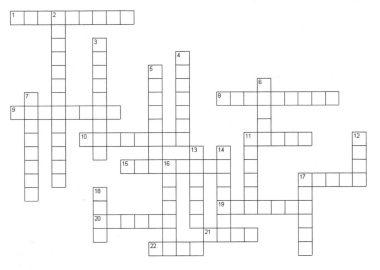

Down

2. type of set exhibited by polystyrene custom tray bead material
3. material painted on a spacer to facilitate its later removal
4. type of material used to make custom trays and athletic mouthguards
5. before being used for a rubber base impression, a custom tray must be painted with this material
6. materials with three types of polymer cure are available to make custom trays: cooling, mixing and
7. _____ tray that covers half an arch
11. wax placed over the model when constructing a custom tray to leave room for the impression material
12. tray that takes an impression of both arches at the same time
13. tray made specifically to fit an individual patient
14. tray that covers the arch from canine to canine
16. copolymer added to custom tray material to stiffen it
17. this type of adaptation is used to pull softened material over a model to make a custom tray
18. tray used to record occlusal relationships

Across

1. another name for a quadrant tray
8. dimensional property of polymers that is of concern when making a custom tray
9. tray that covers an entire arch
10. another name for a sextant tray
11. tray purchased ready-made from the manufacturer
15. this type of adaptation is used to push softened material over a model to form a custom tray
17. copolymer added to mouthguard and bleaching tray material to make it more flexible
19. material rolled similar to pie crust to make a custom tray
20. another name for a dual impression tray
21. small projection of custom tray material into the space on the tissue side of a custom tray
22. acrylic custom trays are not made in the mouth because so much of this is produced during setting

Final Impression Materials

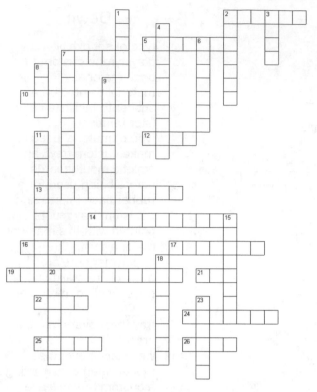

Down

1. most accurate rubber base material
2. light body rubber base material is ejected from this type of applicator
3. rubber base viscosity is described using this term
4. consistency and color of rubber base material desired at end mixing process
6. one link in a polymer chain
7. an impression made of this material sorbs fluids and should not be immersed for long disinfection times
8. this characteristic of impression materials enables them to record tissue detail accurately
9. this property of an impression material is necessary for the impression not to be damaged on removal
11. thixotropic rubber base materials that provide both flow and bulk to the finished impression
15. this rubber base material begins the setting reaction of rubber base materials
18. type of rubber base material that shrinks excessively as it cures
20. rubber base materials of this viscosity are used alone in a tray
23. this property of the finished impression is provided by light body material

Across

2. dimensions recorded by an impression material must remain ____ for the restoration to fit the patient correctly
5. all of the rubber bases are this type of material
7. extra heavy body rubber base material
10. type of material which smells bad and stains clothing
12. this property of the finished impression is provided by heavier body material
13. hazardous catalyst found in polysulfide material
14. are rubber base materials hydrophilic or hydrophobic?
16. disposable, two-compartment multi-dose container of rubber base and catalyst materials
17. two pastes of rubber base material are proportioned in equal ____
19. type of set exhibited by reversible hydrocolloid material
21. types of impressions and different types of impression-taking techniques for which vinyl material is used
22. another name for reversible hydrocolloid
24. an impression made with mercaptan material will most likely be used to make this item
25. type of material in which the polymer particles of reversible hydrocolloid are suspended
26. layer of light body material placed in an indentation to record accurate detail in the area of interest

Materials for Temporary Coverage

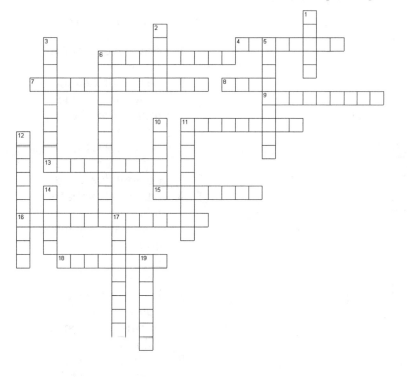

Down

1. material that can be used to cool a polymer material while a temporary restoration is being formed on a tooth
2. thin, quickly made polymer form used to place acrylic material over the prepared tooth or model
3. materials for temporary coverage all liberate heat on setting, so are described as ___
5. type of cement used to lute temporary coverage to a tooth
6. type of material used to make preformed esthetic shell crowns
10. instrument used to crimp cervix of stainless steel crown so it will fit the tooth
11. type of crown for temporary use
12. item in which a temporary material can be placed to carry it to the tooth
14. excess material
17. dimensional concern associated with polymer curing
19. resin material used for temporary crowns and bridges

Across

4. anterior temporary restorations must be made of this type of material
6. temporary restorations perform this function for prepared teeth
7. purpose of using a cotton roll or bite stick when cementing a temporary restoration
8. this tissue can be injured if setting acrylic is left on the tooth too long
9. the height of this must be checked and adjusted if indicated after a temporary restoration has been placed
11. permanent material used to make veneers
13. polymer material used for temporary veneers
15. posterior temporary restorations must exhibit this property to resist biting forces
16. type of preformed crown used in posterior pediatric applications
18. these contacts must be checked and adjusted as indicated after a temporary restoration has been cemented

Materials for Permanent Indirect Restorations

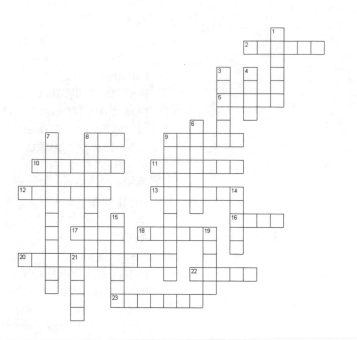

Down

1. clay used to make ceramic
3. portion of indirect restorations which must be thoroughly checked to assure the bond to the tooth has not broken or the cement dissolved
4. type of alloy that is more subject to fracture, tarnish and corrosion
6. porcelain restorations may crack or craze because they are ___
7. porcelain simulates enamel well because it exhibits this property
8. team member who customarily fabricates indirect restorations
9. property of resin that makes it less prone to fracture
14. thin, smooth surface coating on a porcelain restoration
15. glass material used for veneers, crowns, inlays and onlays
19. combination of metals used for all types of indirect restorations and for substructures that will be veneered
21. selective polishing is or is not appropriate for metal indirect restorations

Across

2. ceramic appears less natural because it is ___
5. acrylic material used for inlays, ceramic repairs and cementing when translucence is desired
8. number of appointments ordinarily required for a metal alloy or resin inlay restoration
9. baking glass material at a high temperature
10. the technique of making ceramic restorations by milling them to shape
11. team member who designs indirect restorations
12. pouring or injecting liquefied glass into a mold
13. grinding a block of ceramic into shape
16. type of fluoride which may damage ceramic restoration surfaces
17. grit of abrasive that should be used on all types of indirect restorations
18. mineral used to make ceramic
20. material used to seal an open margin on a metal indirect restoration
22. type of metal that is relatively inert and resists tarnish and corrosion well
23. porcelain restorations may be easily ___ if scaled with a heavy hand

Cements

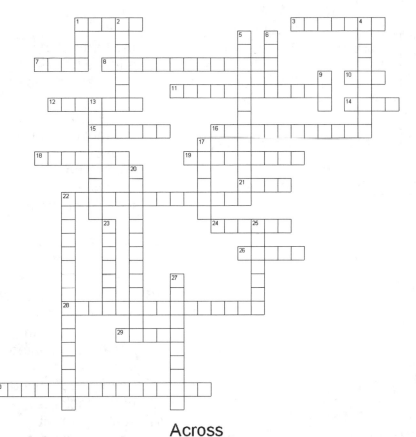

Down

1. to cement; to attach two solid materials together using a cement
2. oil of cloves
4. because Z.O.E. is weak, it should be used only for this type of luting
5. these materials work by interlocking with the tooth or sharing electrons with it
6. polymer cement that bonds mechanically to the tooth surface
9. the type of environment required for cement placement and setting
13. are polymer cements soluble or insoluble over time in oral fluids?
17. which is proportioned first for a cement mix: powder or liquid?
20. metal oxide cement that remains sufficiently acid to damage pulp tissue unless the tooth is protected with a basic liner
22. type of pad that should be used to mix cements
23. should polymer cements be mixed quickly or slowly?
25. are metal oxide cements soluble or insoluble over time in oral fluids?
27. type of acid used in zinc phosphate cement liquid

Across

1. cement used as a protective sealer coating on cut dentin tubules under a restoration
3. family of intermediary materials used as bases, liners, and luting agents
7. would you incorporate more or less powder in a cement mix for greater strength?
8. this inexpensive metal oxide cement is used primarily to cement ___ or orthodontic bands
10. metal oxide cement that is used for temporary applications
11. polymer cement that bonds chemically to the tooth and leaches fluoride into surrounding tooth structure
12. does the pH of zinc polycarboxylate cement rise rapidly or slowly?
14. cement used as a protective floor layer under a restoration
15. should metal oxide cements be mixed quickly or slowly?
16. unique property of resin cement
18. Z.O.E. cement is not used under this type of restorations because it retards their set

19. glass ionomer cannot be used to cement jacket crowns made of this material because it expands as it sets
21. this type of film thickness is preferable when cementing
22. luting agents work by ___ on the surfaces of the two materials involved
24. the surface of a polymer cement should have this appearance when it is ready to use
26. this should be done to separate powder particles before they are proportioned
28. combination cement that is mixed like a polymer but has the strength of a reinforced metal oxide
29. this should be done to liquids to prevent them from evaporating
30. basic liner used to protect tooth pulp from acid cement

Materials for Dental Implants

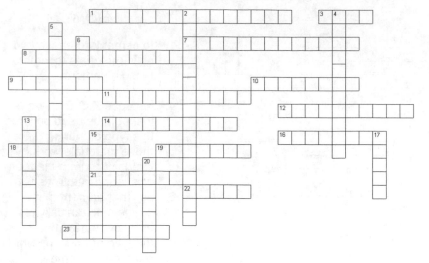

Down

2. the forming of surface bonds between an implant and bone
4. these procedures are most likely to cause implant scratching
5. replacement restoration attached to an implant
6. plaque and calculus do or do not form on implants
13. serious problem that may occur at the ceramic-titanium interface of coated implants
15. metal usually used to make implants
17. scalers or probes used on implants should be made of this material
20. tooth replacement that is anchored in or on the bone

Across

1. the attachment of sulcus epithelium cells to an implant
3. connector between a subperiosteal implant frame and a prosthesis
7. implant placed on the bone under the periosteum
8. non-harmful, sometimes beneficial, interaction between a material and tissue
9. substructure of an endosseous implant
10. porous ceramic bone substitute that promotes osseointegration
11. full or partial denture supported by implants or retained tooth roots
12. cover placed on an implant following osseointegration to allow formation of a perimucosal seal and esthetic gingival shaping
14. type of implant that is anchored in the bone
16. cover for implant when the impression for a prosthesis for an endosseous implant is being taken
18. characteristic describing non-reactivity of an implant surface film with the surrounding environment
19. surface problem that may occur from rough treatment of an implant
21. connector between an implant fixture and a prosthesis
22. non-reactive
23. item placed between epithelium and the implant-bone complex to prevent interference with osseointegration

Denture Materials

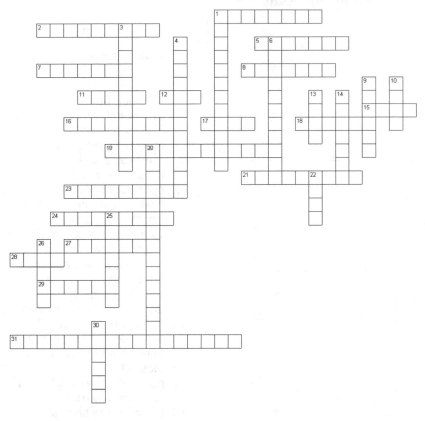

Across

1. material that may pit cobalt-chromium or gold alloy frameworks
2. supporting skeleton of a denture
5. material used for denture bases, saddles and teeth
7. type of denture that replaces some of the teeth and associated structures in one arch
8. removable replacement of some or all of the teeth and associated structures in one arch
11. container for holding materials in position while a denture being constructed
12. connector between parts of a denture framework
15. portion of denture that mimics the soft tissue and fits over the alveolar ridge
16. polymer used to improve the fit of a denture or provide a more resilient surface
17. shape of artificial denture teeth
18. portion of denture base that extends vertically toward the mucobuccal fold
19. fluid sorption into a denture may result in this problem
21. encircling border located at the deepest part of the denture flange
23. type of denture constructed prior to surgery and delivered at the final surgical appointment
24. temporary denture base
27. one of the materials used to make a baseplate
28. soft metal sometimes used for denture frameworks, especially in the palate
29. portion of a partial denture that overlies the soft tissue and supports the teeth
31. distance between the patient's nose tip and chin center when teeth are present

Down

1. type of denture constructed after surgery and tissue healing are complete
3. arch-shaped block of wax attached to base plate to maintain vertical dimension
4. type of acrylic used in dentures
6. polymer used to promote healing of irritated tissue under a denture
9. materials inserted into a denture base to simulate blood vessels
10. horizontal extension near a partial denture clasp that provides vertical support
13. type of denture that replaces all the teeth and associated structures in one arch
14. liquid methacrylic acid material
20. metal alloy used for denture frameworks
22. this catalyst causes the most complete cure of denture material
25. powder that consists of set, ground methyl methacrylate
26. retainer; partial denture extension that partly encircles an abutment tooth
30. a baseplate plus the artificial teeth that will be used in a denture

Endodontic Materials

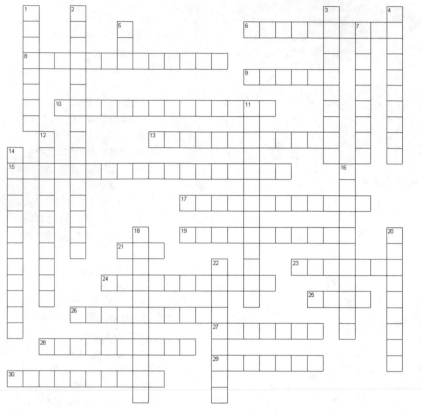

Down

1. phenol-based medicament that works by volatization and diffusion but is less irritating than formocresol
2. irrigating solution that releases oxygen and bubbles to loosen debris
3. device used to dry an open root canal
4. type of materials used to remove pulp tissue and fill the resulting space
5. material used for temporary coverage of endodontic materials
7. irrigating agents are applied using this process
11. procedure used to stimulate formation of an apex on an immature tooth
12. removal of all pulp from a non-vital tooth
14. a sealer functions to prevent this process
16. type of sealer that may be used to prevent material loss or lessen post-operative pain
18. irrigating agents provide this for subsequent instrumentation of the cavity
20. removal of only the coronal pulp from a vital tooth
22. device used to isolate a tooth during pulp therapy procedures

Across

6. flushing of debris and tissue fluid from a pulp cavity
8. sterile salt and water solution used for irrigation
9. agent used to fill the microspace between the tooth and filling material
10. instrument used to spin sealer into a tooth
13. irrigating agents may also have this function
15. occasional unintended, adverse consequence of placing calcium hydroxide in a pulp cavity
17. sterile solution that flushes microorganisms away but does not reduce their numbers appreciably
19. natural thermoplastic polymer used to fill root canal spaces
21. device used to access the pulp by cutting the tooth
23. essential oil that is used as a pulp irritant and mild antiseptic
24. formaldehyde and cresol solution sometimes used to cauterize small, bleeding tissue tags
25. irrigating agent that dissolves debris and tooth shavings, disinfects the cavity, and coats its surface
26. agent used to sterilize or disinfect the cavity
27. a patient may have this reaction to placement of a eugenol sealer
28. removal of all pulp from a vital tooth
29. eugenol sealer does or does not set completely
30. type of sealer that may shrink excessively

Why Dental Materials? (p. 266)

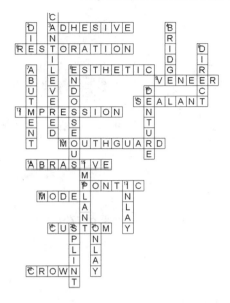

Vocabulary 1 (p. 267)

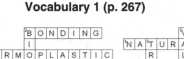
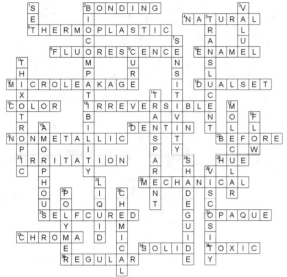

Vocabulary 2 (p. 268)

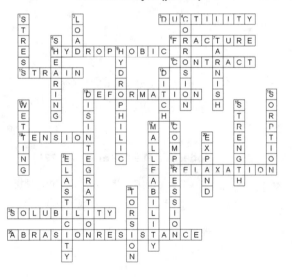

Using Materials Safely (p. 269)

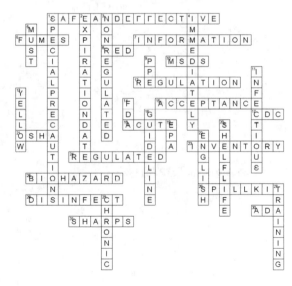

Using Materials Sensibly (p. 270)

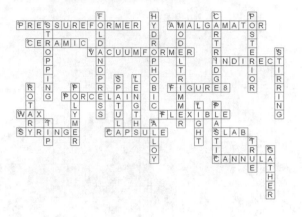

Abrasives (p. 271)

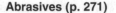
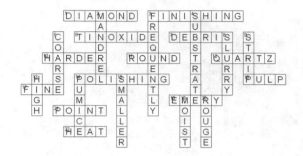

Dental Sealants (p. 272)

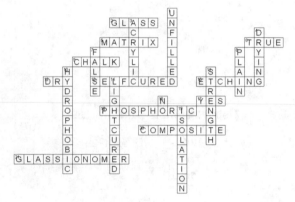

Tooth Whiteners (p. 273)

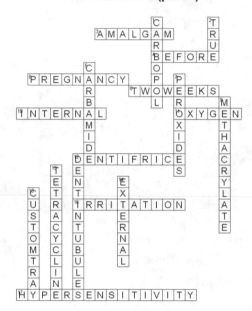

Alginate (p. 274)

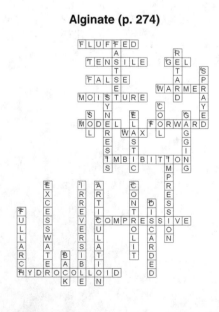

Model and Die Materials (p. 275)

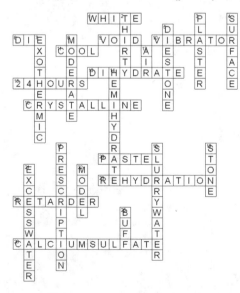

Intermediary Materials (p. 276)

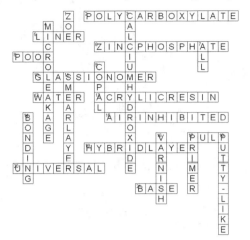

Esthetic Direct Restoration Materials (p. 277)

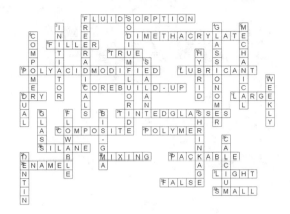

Non-esthetic Direct Restoration Materials (p. 278)

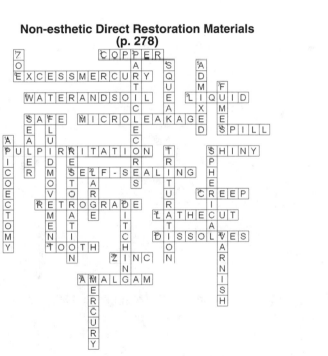

Impression Trays (p. 279)

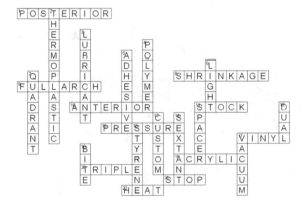

Final Impression Materials (p. 280)

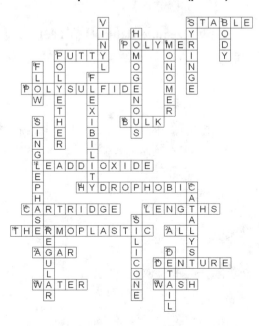

Materials for Temporary Coverage (p. 281)

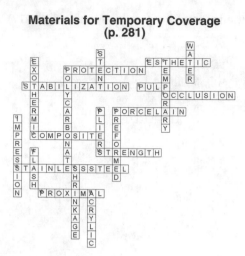

Materials for Permanent Indirect Restorations (p. 282)

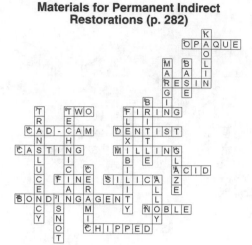

Cements (p. 283)

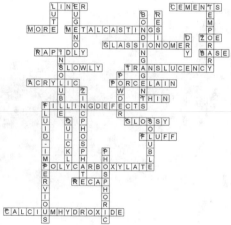

Materials for Dental Implants (p. 284)

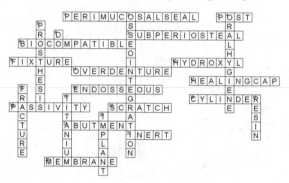

Denture Materials (p. 285)

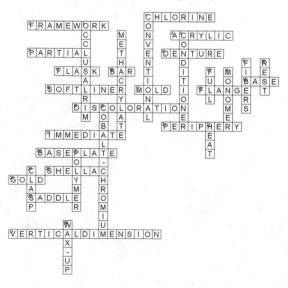

Endodontic Materials (p. 286)

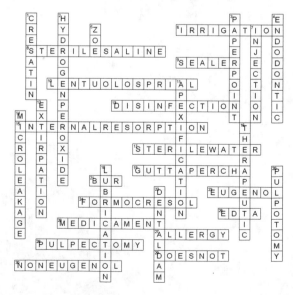

Competency Evaluations

Evaluation of Competence for Chapter 1: Items Made with Dental Materials

Student's Name: _____ Date: _____

Directions to evaluator: Show the student a model or picture of the indicated item and ask for its name and use(s). Place a check mark in the appropriate column when a criterion is NOT met. Leave other areas blank. This will direct the student's attention to any area that may still need work, while clearly indicating those areas that have been mastered.

Student identifies:	Name	Use(s)	Instructor Comment
Direct restoration			
Indirect restoration			
Esthetic material			
Nonesthetic material			
Veneer			
Inlay			
Onlay			
Crown			
Conventional bridge			
Cantilevered bridge			
Abutment			
Pontic			
Unit, including the number in the bridge displayed			
Full denture			
Partial denture			
Overdenture			
Implant			
Model			
Impression			
Custom tray			
Mouthguard			
Occlusal splint			
Periodontal splint			
Sealant			
Wax			
Abrasive powder			

Competence assessment: To be judged competent, the student will correctly identify at least 24 (_____) and will correctly indicate at least one use for 22 (_____) of the 26 items displayed. [Competence = 26−2 (-_____) names and 26−4 (-_____) uses.]

_____
Instructor's Signature/Date

Evaluation of Competence for Chapter 2:
The Vocabulary of Dental Materials

Student's Name: _____ Date: _____

Directions to evaluator: Ask the student to define each word or phrase listed below and to describe how what it signifies is related to the patient's oral health and appearance, or the successful use of a material in the mouth. Place a check mark in the appropriate column when a criterion is NOT met. Leave other areas blank. This will direct the student's attention to any area that may still need work, while clearly indicating those areas that have been mastered.

Term	Definition	Relationship to Health, Appearance or Material Use	Instructor Comment
Biocompatibility			
Irritation			
Sensitivity			
Toxicity			
Microleakage			
Varnish			
Bonding (both mechanical and chemical)			
Hue of a material			
Value of a material			
Chroma of a material			
Shade guide and selection			
Translucent			
Opaque			
Fluorescence			
Solid			
Liquid			
Polymer			
Monomer			
Material flow			
Material viscosity			
Thixotropic material			
Thermoset material			
Thermoplastic material			
Light cured polymer material			
Heat cured polymer material			
Dual cured polymer material			
Compressive load/strength			
Tensile load/strength			
Torsion/resistance to torsion			

Stress/strain			
Deformation/relaxation/elasticity			
Thermal expansion/contraction			
Abrasion resistance			
Tarnish/corrosion			
Hydrophobic/hydrophilic/wetting			
Sorption/solubility			
Material disintegration			

Competence assessment: To be judged competent, the student will correctly define at least 34 (_____) of the terms and phrases, and will correctly describe the relationship of the process signified by the term or phrase of at least 32 (_____) of the 74 definitions and relationships requested. [Competence = 37−3 (-_____) definitions and 37−5 (-_____) uses.]

_____
Instructor's Signature/Date

Evaluation of Competence for Chapter 3:
Using Materials Safely

Student's Name: _____ Date: _____

Directions to evaluator: Ask the student to describe each process or concept listed below, including how each relates to patient and dental personnel safety. Place a check mark in the appropriate column when a criterion is NOT met. Leave other areas blank. This will direct the student's attention to any area that may still need work, while clearly indicating those areas that have been mastered.

Process or Concept	Explanation	Relationship to Safety	Comments
FDA approval program			
ADA acceptance program			
Harm from a chemical			
Chemical integrity			
Chemical exposure			
Agency regulations and guidelines for chemical use in dentistry			
Hazard Communication Standard			
Eye and fire safety regulations			
Spill clean-up			
Mercury characteristics and clean-up			
Waste disposal procedures			
Infection control			

Competence Assessment: To be judged competent, the student will correctly explain 10 of the 12 (_____ of 12) concepts and processes, and describe the relationship of 10 of the 12 (_____ of 12) processes and concepts to patient and personnel safety. (Competence = 20 of 24 criteria met.)

_____
Instructor's Signature/Date

Evaluation of Competence for Chapter 4:
Using Materials Sensibly

Student's Name: _____   Date: _____

Directions to evaluator: Ask the student to state the properties of each type of material listed below and how they relate to its selection or rejection for use in an individual patient or a particular area of the mouth. Place a check mark in the appropriate column when a criterion is NOT met. Leave other areas blank. This will direct the student's attention to any area that may still need work, while clearly indicating those areas that have been mastered.

Type of Material	Properties	Relationship to Selection	Instructor Comment
Metal alloy			
Glass			
Plastic			

Competence assessment: To be judged competent, the student will correctly name at least 5 properties of each of the 3 materials listed and describe at least 3 relationships of the material to selection for use in an individual patient or area. (Competence = 5 × 3 properties and 3 × 3 relationships.)

_____
Instructor's Signature/Date

Laboratory Component: Cross Task Equipment and Skills

Student's Name: _____   Date: _____

Directions to evaluator: Show the student a model or picture of the indicated item and ask for its name and use. Place a check mark in the appropriate column when a criterion is NOT met. Leave other areas blank. This will direct the student's attention to any area that may still need work, while clearly indicating those areas that have been mastered.

Small Equipment Item	Name	Use	Instructor Comment
Flexible bowl			
Non-flexible bowl			
Paper pad			
Glass slab			
Alginate spatula			
Impression spatula			
Cement spatula			
Vacuum former			
Pressure former			
Model trimmer			
Curing light			
Light box			

Competence assessment: To be judged competent, the student will correctly identify at least 10 (_____) and indicate at least one use for 9 (_____) of the 12 items displayed. [Competence = 12−2 (-_____) items and 12−3 (-_____) uses.]

Directions to evaluator: Show the student a sample or a picture of the indicated item type. Ask him/her to name the type of packaging and describe the method by which it would be prepared for use. Place a check mark in the appropriate column when a criterion is NOT met. Leave other areas blank.

Packaging	Type	Preparation Method	Instructor Comment
Powder and liquid			
Two tubes of paste			
Polymer sheet			
Capsule			
Unit dose tip			
Multidose syringe			
Cannula			
Cartridge			

Competence assessment: To be judged competent, the student will correctly identify and indicate the preparation method for at least 7 (_____) of the 8 items displayed. [Competence = 8−1 (-_____) items and 8−1 (-_____) preparation methods.]

Directions to evaluator: Ask the student to demonstrate each preparation technique. Place a check mark in the appropriate column when a criterion is NOT met. Leave other areas blank.

Preparation Technique	Executed Correctly	Instructor Comment
Rotary mixing		
Fold and press mixing		
Stropping		
Figure 8 mixing		
Stirring		
Mixing and gathering a powder and liquid		
Mixing and gathering two pastes		

Competence assessment: To be judged competent, the student will demonstrate correct preparation technique for 6 (_____) of the 7 methods listed. [Competence = 7−1 (-_____) techniques.]

_____

Instructor's Signature/Date

Evaluation of Competence for Chapter 5: Abrasives

Student's Name: _____ Date: _____

Directions to evaluator: Ask the student to identify a sample or picture of the indicated item and state its usual use. Place a check mark in the appropriate column when a criterion is NOT met. Leave other areas blank. This will direct the student's attention to any area that may still need work, while clearly indicating those areas that have been mastered.

Student identifies:	Name	Use	Instructor Comment
Pumice			
Tin oxide			
Quartz			
Emery			
Aluminum oxide			
Diamond chips			
Rouge			
Disk or wheel			
Stone or point			
Mandrel			
Strip			
Powder			
Slurry			
Cake			

Competence assessment: To be judged competent, the student will correctly identify at least 12 (_____) and state the usual use of at least 10 (_____) of the 14 items displayed. [Competence = 14−2 (-_____) names and 14−4 (-_____) uses.]

Directions to evaluator: Ask the student to describe how each characteristic of abrasive particle selection and use listed below affects cutting efficiency. Place a check mark in the appropriate column when a criterion is NOT met. Leave other areas blank.

Abrasive Characteristic	Effect	Instructor Comment
Particle size		
Particle smoothness		
Particle hardness		
Application speed		
Application pressure		

Competence assessment: To be judged competent, the student will correctly describe the effect of at least 4 (_____) of the 5 characteristics on abrasive cutting efficiency. [Competence = 5−1 (-_____) effects.]

Directions to evaluator: Ask the student to describe how each process listed below is accomplished. Place a check mark in the appropriate column when a criterion is NOT met. Leave other areas blank.

Process	Description	Instructor Comment
Abrasion		
Selection of an abrasive to use		
Selection of a grit to use		
Preparation of an abrasive slurry		
Cutting and contouring		
Polishing		
Prevention of hard and soft tissue damage when using an abrasive		
Retention of an abrasive on a substrate		
Maintaining the cutting ability of an abrasive		

Competence assessment: To be judged competent, the student will correctly describe how to accomplish at least 7 (_____) of the 9 processes listed. [Competence = 9−2 (-_____) processes.]

_____

Instructor's Signature/Date

Evaluation of Competence for Chapter 6: Sealants

Student's Name: _____ Date: _____

Directions to evaluator: Show the student a sealant on a patient, or a model or picture of a sealant. Ask the student to provide its name and uses, then describe sealant materials as listed below. Place a check mark in the appropriate column when a criterion is NOT met. Leave other areas blank. This will direct the student's attention to any area that may still need work, while clearly indicating those areas that have been mastered.

Student identifies:	Name	Instructor Comment
Sealant		
Uses (3)		
Materials (3) of which made		
Category into which all of these materials fall		
Mechanism of sealant action		

Competence assessment: To be judged competent, the student will correctly complete at least 4 (____) of the 5 items. [Competence = 5−1 (-____) identifications.]

Directions to evaluator: Ask the student to describe each of the sealant materials as listed below. Place a check mark in the appropriate column when a criterion is NOT met.

Student describes acrylic resin sealant material:	Description	Instructor Comment
Components		
Activation and curing		
Properties		
Relationship of each property to the clinical use and longevity of acrylic sealants		

Student describes composite sealant material:	Description	Instructor Comment
Components		
Activation and curing		
Properties as compared to acrylic		
Relationship of differences in acrylic and composite properties to their clinical use and longevity		

Student describes glass ionomer sealant material:	Description	Instructor Comment
Components		
Activation and curing		
Properties		
Relationship of each property to the clinical use and longevity of glass ionomer sealants		

Competence assessment: To be judged competent, the student will correctly complete at least 9 (_____) of the 12 items. [Competence = 12−3 (-_____) descriptions.]

Directions to evaluator: Ask the student to describe each process listed below. Place a check mark in the appropriate column when a criterion is NOT met.

Student describes means of controlling pertinent clinical factors:	Description	Instructor Comment
Isolation of the area to be sealed		
Ease of material placement		
Sealant visibility		
Sealant retention		
Sealant wear		

Competence assessment: To be judged competent, the student will correctly complete at least 4 (_____) of the 5 items. [Competence = 5−4 (-_____) descriptions.]

Laboratory Component: Sealant Placement

Directions to evaluator: Following demonstration and practice, ask the student to place a sealant. Place a check mark in the appropriate column when a criterion is NOT met. Leave other areas blank. This will direct the student's attention to any area that may still need work, while clearly indicating those areas that have been mastered.

Student correctly completes the following steps:	Description	Instructor Comment
Education of the patient		
Cleaning of the area to be sealed		
Etching/flushing		
Inspection for correct etching		
Thorough isolation of the area		
Material application and curing		
Inspection for adequate retention and adequate but not excessive extension and occlusal height		
Provision of a fluoride treatment		
Provision of post-operative directions		
Safe, efficient operation of handpiece and curing light		
Adherence to infection control protocol		

Competence assessment: To be judged competent, the student will correctly complete at least 10 (_____) of the 11 steps. [Competence = 11−1 (-_____) steps.]

_____

Instructor's Signature/Date

Evaluation of Competence for Chapter 7: Tooth Whiteners

Student's Name: _____   Date: _____

Directions to evaluator: Show the student selections of samples or pictures of whitening products. Ask the student to describe the materials as listed below. Place a check mark in the appropriate column when a criterion is NOT met. Leave other areas blank. This will direct the student's attention to any area that may still need work, while clearly indicating those areas that have been mastered.

Student identifies or describes	Identification or Description	Instructor Comment
Type of material		
Its use and mechanism of action		
Components of whitening gels		
Contribution of each component to the whole		
Product types displayed		
Application regimen for each type		
Efficacy of bleaching		
Safety of bleaching		
Longevity of results		

Competence assessment: To be judged competent, the student will correctly complete at least 7 (_____) of the 9 items. [Competence = 9−2 (-_____) identifications.]

Directions to evaluator: Ask the student to describe each of the processes listed below. Place a check mark in the appropriate column when a criterion is NOT met.

Student describes the following processes and their relationship to whitening success	Description	Relationship	Instructor Comment
Preparation for bleaching			
Evaluation of patient for appropriateness of bleaching treatment			

Competence assessment: To be judged competent, the student will correctly complete both (_____) of the items. [Competence = 2−0 (-_____) descriptions.]

Directions to evaluator: Ask the student to describe the means of preventing or controlling each bleaching-related problem listed below. Place a check mark in the appropriate column when a criterion is NOT met.

Student describes means of preventing or controlling the following bleaching-related problems	Means	Instructor Comment
Dentinal hypersensitivity		
Gingival irritation		
Temporary white spots		
Color change in methacrylate restoration		
Temporary response, then reversion to original color		
Tooth color does not lighten		
Cervical third of tooth appears darker		
Esthetic restoration does not respond to bleaching		
Amalgam restoration appears darker		

Competence assessment: To be judged competent, the student will correctly describe at least 7 (_____) of the 9 means. [Competence = 9−7 (-_____) descriptions.]

Laboratory Component: Construction of a Bleaching Tray

Directions to evaluator: Following demonstration and practice, ask the student to construct a custom bleaching tray. Place a check mark in the appropriate column when a criterion is NOT met. Leave other areas blank. This will direct the student's attention to any area that may still need work, while clearly indicating those areas that have been mastered.

Student correctly completes the following steps	Step	Instructor Comment
Preparation of model		
Selection and placement of tray material		
Safe, efficient operation of the vacuum or pressure former		
Adherence to lab infection control and cleanup protocols		

Tray constructed can be used	Criterion	Instructor Comment
Reservoirs on teeth to be bleached, if requested		
Trimmed to appropriate height		
Edges rounded and smooth		
Fits over and covers teeth of interest		
Is not open in the cervical area		
Has no bubbles, burns, holes or sag areas		

Competence assessment: To be judged competent, the student will correctly complete all (_____) of the 10 steps and criteria. [Competence = 10−0 (-_____) steps and criteria.]

_____
Instructor's Signature/Date

Evaluation of Competence for Chapter 8: Alginate

Student's Name: _____ Date: _____

Directions to evaluator: Show the student samples or pictures of alginate products. Ask the student to describe the material as listed below. Place a check mark in the appropriate column when a criterion is NOT met. Leave other areas blank. This will direct the student's attention to any area that may still need work, while clearly indicating those areas that have been mastered.

Student identifies the material	Identification	Instructor Comment
Name		
Type		
Components		
Contribution of each component to the whole		
Product types displayed		
Mechanism of action at the procedural level		
Mechanism of action at the chemical level		
Advantages/disadvantages		
Safety		
Used to pour alginate impressions		

Competence assessment: To be judged competent, the student will correctly identify at least 7 (_____) of the 10 items. [Competence = 10−3 (-_____) identifications.]

Directions to evaluator: Ask the student to describe each of the processes listed below. Place a check mark in the appropriate column when a criterion is NOT met.

Student describes the following processes	Description	Instructor Comment
Selection of alginate material		
Proper storage of alginate		
Maintenance of operator safety during alginate use		
Selection of a tray for an alginate impression		
Material preparation		
Prevention of patient gagging		
Prevention of impression tearing		
Care of a finished alginate impression		

Competence assessment: To be judged competent, the student will correctly complete 7 (_____) of the 8 processes. [Competence = 8−1 (-_____) descriptions.]

_____
Instructor's Signature/Date

Laboratory Component: Evaluation of Alginate Impressions

Directions to evaluator: Following demonstration and practice, ask the student to select appropriate trays, then take maxillary and mandibular alginate impressions and a wax bite. Circle any unmet criterion. This will direct the student's attention to any area that may still need work, while clearly indicating those areas that have been mastered.

Mandibular Impression	Maxillary Impression	Bite	Self-Evaluation
Includes: All of lingual border All of mucobuccal fold All teeth The gingival tissue The alveolar mucosa Both retromolar pads Exhibits no: Voids Drag areas	Includes: All of palate All of mucobuccal fold All teeth The gingival tissue The alveolar mucosa Both maxillary tuberosities Exhibits no: Voids Drag areas	Includes: Complete occlusal or incisal surface of each tooth that is present and in occlusion Centered arches Rounded posterior corners Exhibits no: Areas of bite-through Tears Slides (unless patient has one) Double impressions	Presents specific information Recognizes areas done well Recognizes areas done poorly Provides specific remedies for each problem encountered Satisfactory = no more than 1 deviation
			General Educated patient Prevented any incipient gagging Followed labeling, infection control and disinfection protocols Stored impression properly during disinfection
Satisfactory = no more than 2 mild or moderate, or 0 major deviations	Satisfactory = no more than 2 mild or moderate, or 0 major deviations	Satisfactory = no more than 1 mild deviation	Satisfactory = no more than 1 deviation

Comments: _____

Grading: Place an X over the word *satisfactory* if any major criterion (maxillary impression, mandibular impression, bite, self-evaluation and general) is unacceptable. If 5 of 5 major criteria are met, grade = 95 (____); 4 of 5, grade = 85 (____); 3 of 5, grade = 75 (____); 2 of 5, grade = 55 (____), and 0 of 5, grade = 50 (____).

_____
Instructor's Signature/Date

Evaluation of Competence for Chapter 9: Model and Die Materials

Student's Name: _____ Date: _____

Directions to evaluator: Show the student samples or pictures of gypsum models and gypsum, metal and epoxy dies. Ask the student to describe them as listed below. Place a check mark in the appropriate column when a criterion is NOT met. Leave other areas blank. This will direct the student's attention to any area that may still need work, while clearly indicating those areas that have been mastered.

Student identifies	Identification	Instructor Comment
Name of the item		
Material of which it is made		
Uses of gypsum, metal and epoxy dies		
Materials in the gypsum family		
Properties of each of the gypsum materials		
Why the properties of the three gypsums differ		
Uses of each type of gypsum		
Mechanism of gypsum action at the procedural level		
Components of gypsum materials		
Contribution of each component to the whole		
Responsibilities of team members in the construction of gypsum models		

Competence assessment: To be judged competent, the student will correctly identify at least 9 (_____) of the 11 items. [Competence = 11−2 (-_____) identifications.]

Directions to evaluator: Ask the student to describe each of the processes listed below. Place a check mark in the appropriate column when a criterion is NOT met.

Student describes the following processes	Description	Instructor Comment
Proper storage of gypsum materials		
Selection of gypsum material for a specific task		
Maintenance of operator safety during gypsum use		
Use of a laboratory prescription		
Obtaining proper material flow		
Mixing gypsum materials		
Pouring gypsum materials		
Crystallization/exothermic setting		

Syneresis		
Imbibition		
Handling of gypsum models after set		
Development of maximum material strength		

Competence assessment: To be judged competent, the student will correctly complete 10 (_____) of the 12 processes. [Competence = 12−2 (-_____) descriptions.]

_____

Instructor's Signature/Date

Laboratory Component: Evaluation of Gypsum Models

Directions to evaluator: Following demonstration and practice, ask the student to pour maxillary and mandibular alginate impressions. Circle any unmet criterion. This will direct the student's attention to any area that may still need work, while clearly indicating those areas that have been mastered.

Anatomic Portions Include	Bases	Trimming	Self-Evaluation
Mandibular: All of the tissue details present in the impression	Mandibular: Extends 1/2" – 1 1/2" beyond arch Thickness is 1/2" – 1 1/2"	General: Operated machine correctly Operated machine safely Cleaned machine and area at end of trimming session	Presents specific information Recognizes areas done well Recognizes areas done poorly Provides specific remedies for each problem encountered
Maxillary: All of the tissue details present in the impression	Maxillary Extends 1/2" – 1 1/2" beyond arch Thickness is 1/2" – 1 1/2"	Achieved acceptable result: Posterior cuts Posterior side cuts Anterior side cuts Maxillary midline cuts Mandibular anterior rounding	Satisfactory = no more than 1 deviation
Both arches exhibit no: Voids Drag areas Fractures Areas of excess stone Surface roughness Color streaks Mold	Both arches exhibit no: Voids Drag areas Areas of excess stone Surface roughness Color streaks Fractures Mold		General
			Worked efficiently Followed infection control protocol Labeled and stored model properly
Satisfactory = no more than 2 mild or 0 major deviations	Satisfactory = no more than 2 mild or 0 major deviations	Satisfactory = no more than 3 mild or 2 moderate deviations	Satisfactory = 0 deviations

Comments:

Grading: Place an X over the word *satisfactory* if any major criterion (anatomic portions, bases, trimming, self-evaluation, and general) is unacceptable. If 5 of 5 major criteria are met, grade = 95; 4 of 5, grade = 85; 3 of 5, grade = 75; 2 of 5, grade = 55; and 0 of 5, grade = 50.

Instructor's Signature/Date

Evaluation of Competence for Chapter 10:
Intermediary Materials

Student's Name: _____ Date: _____

Directions to evaluator: Show the student samples or pictures of the various intermediary materials. Ask the student to describe them as listed below. Place a check mark in the appropriate column when a criterion is NOT met. Leave other areas blank. This will direct the student's attention to any area that may still need work, while clearly indicating those areas that have been mastered.

Student defines and states the use(s) of	Identification	Use(s)	Instructor Comment
Intermediary materials			
Base			
Varnish			
Liner			
Calcium hydroxide			
Zinc oxide and eugenol			
Zinc phosphate			
Zinc polycarboxylate			
Glass ionomer			
Primer			
Acrylic resin			

Competence assessment: To be judged competent, the student will correctly identify at least 9 (_____) of the 11 identifications and 8 of 11 uses. [Competence = 22−5 (-_____) identifications and uses.]

Directions to evaluator: Ask the student to describe each of the processes listed below. Place a check mark in the appropriate column when a criterion is NOT met.

Student describes the following processes	Description	Instructor Comment
Pulp protection through the use of intermediary materials		
Pulp protection through selection of a base and/or varnish		
Pulp protection through selection of bonding materials		
Dentin bonding		

Competence assessment: To be judged competent, the student will correctly describe 3 (_____) of the 4 processes. [Competence = 4−1 (-_____) descriptions.]

Directions to evaluator: Ask the student to describe the properties of each material listed below, then indicate how each relates to the health of the tooth. Place a check mark in the appropriate column when a criterion is NOT met.

Material	Properties	Relationship	Instructor Comment
Copal varnish			
Universal varnish			
Calcium hydroxide			
Zinc oxide and eugenol			
Zinc phosphate			
Zinc polycarboxylate			
Glass ionomer			
Dentin primer			
Acrylic resin bonding agent			

Competence assessment: To be judged competent, the student will correctly describe 7 (_____) of the 9 property sets and 7 (_____) of the 9 relationship sets. [Competence = 18−4 (-_____) descriptions.]

Laboratory Component: Preparation and Transfer of Intermediary Materials

Directions to evaluator: Following demonstration and practice, ask the student to prepare, transfer and clean up after use of each of the materials listed below. Place a check mark in the appropriate column when a criterion is NOT met.

Material	Preparation	Transfer	Cleanup	Instructor Comment
Copal varnish				
Universal varnish				
Calcium hydroxide				
Zinc oxide and eugenol base				
Zinc phosphate base				
Zinc polycarboxylate base				
Glass ionomer base				
Glass ionomer liner				
Dentin primer				
Acrylic resin bonding agent				

Competence assessment: To be judged competent, the student will correctly prepare, transfer and clean up following use of 9 (_____) of the 10 materials. [Competence = 30−3 (-_____) tasks correctly completed.]

_____
Instructor's Signature/Date

Evaluation of Competence for Chapter 11:
Direct Esthetic Restorative Materials

Student's Name: _____   Date: _____

Directions to evaluator: Ask the student to define and state the use(s) of each material listed below. Place a check mark in the appropriate column when a criterion is NOT met. Leave other areas blank. This will direct the student's attention to any area that may still need work, while clearly indicating those areas that have been mastered.

Student defines and states the use(s) of	Definition	Use(s)	Instructor Comment
Direct esthetic restorative material			
Composite			
Glass ionomer			
Blended direct esthetic restorative material			
Compomer			
Polyacid modified glass ionomer			
Core buildup			

Competence assessment: To be judged competent, the student will correctly identify at least 5 (_____) each of the 7 definitions and uses. [Competence = 14−4 (-_____) identifications and uses.]

Directions to evaluator: Ask the student to describe the composition and setting reaction of each material listed below. Place a check mark in the appropriate column when a criterion is NOT met.

Student describes the composition and setting reaction of:	Composition	Setting Reaction	Instructor Comment
Composite			
Glass ionomer			

Directions to evaluator: Ask the student to describe the properties of each material listed below and describe how each affects its clinical selection and the success of a restoration made from it. Place a check mark in the appropriate column when a criterion is NOT met.

Student describes the properties and their relationship to selection of that material for a specific use and the clinical success of a restoration made with	Properties	Relationship	Instructor Comment
Composite			
Glass ionomer			

Competence assessment: To be judged competent, the student will correctly describe the composition and setting reaction of both (_____) of the materials and both sets of properties and relationships. [Competence = 4−0 (-_____) descriptions.]

Laboratory Component: Preparation and Transfer of Direct Esthetic Restorative Materials

Directions to evaluator: Following demonstration and practice, ask the student to prepare, transfer, and clean up after use of each of the materials listed below. Place a check mark in the appropriate column when a criterion is NOT met. Leave other areas blank. This will direct the student's attention to any area that may still need work, while clearly indicating those areas that have been mastered.

Material*	Preparation	Transfer	Cleanup	Instructor Comment
Acid etchant				
Conventional composite				
Flowable composite				
Packable composite				
Self-cure direct esthetic material				
Light cure direct esthetic material				
Dual cure direct esthetic material				
Esthetic restorative material packaged in a syringe				
Esthetic restorative material packaged in a capsule				
Esthetic restorative material packaged in a unit dose tip				
Esthetic restorative material that must be expelled through a cannula				
Esthetic restorative material packaged as powder and liquid				

*Preparation, transfer and cleanup of one material may demonstrate competence in more than one category, as, for example, when a light-cured, flowable composite packaged in a syringe and expelled through a cannula is prepared, transferred and the area cleaned after use, or a light-cured glass ionomer packaged in a capsule is prepared, transferred and the area cleaned after use.

Competence assessment: To be judged competent, the student will correctly prepare, transfer and clean up following use of 11 (_____) of the 12 materials. [Competence = 36−3 (-_____) actions.]

_____
Instructor's Signature/Date

Evaluation of Competence for Chapter 12: Nonesthetic Direct Restorative Materials

Student's Name: _____   Date: _____

Directions to evaluator: Show the student samples or pictures of nonesthetic direct restorations. Ask the student to describe each material as listed below. Place a check mark in the appropriate column when a criterion is NOT met. Leave other areas blank. This will direct the student's attention to any area that may still need work, while clearly indicating those areas that have been mastered.

Student discusses dental amalgam	Discussion	Instructor Comment
Identifies restoration made with this material		
Alloy types and their composition		
Alloy selection		
Uses		
Preparation		
Characteristics when correctly prepared		
Placement		
Setting reaction		
Safe use and disposal procedures		
Prevention of restoration and tooth fracture when amalgam is used		
Microleakage when amalgam is used		
Restoration self-sealing		
Restoration ditching		

Competence assessment: To be judged competent, the student will correctly discuss at least 10 (_____) of the 13 listed concepts. [Competence = 13 − 3 (-_____) discussions.]

Student discusses reinforced zinc oxide and eugenol	Discussion	Instructor Comment
Identifies restoration made with this material		
Uses		
Mechanisms of action on the tooth		
Preparation		
Clinical concerns when Z.O.E. is used		
Longevity		

Competence assessment: To be judged competent, the student will correctly discuss 5 (_____) of the 6 listed concepts. [Competence = 6 − 1 (-_____) descriptions.]

_____
Instructor's Signature/Date

Laboratory Component: Preparation and Transfer of Dental Amalgam

Directions to evaluator: Following demonstration and practice, ask the student to prepare, pick up, transfer and clean after use of amalgam in the situations listed below. Place a check mark in the appropriate column when a criterion is NOT met. This will direct the student's attention to any area that may still need work, while clearly indicating those areas that have been mastered.

Amalgam Placement Task	One-spill Mix	Two-spill Mix	Three-spill Mix	Instructor Comment
Place matrix and wedge, if indicated				
Select as requested				
Triturate				
Pick up from squeeze cloth or amalgam well				
Transfer carrier				
Transfer appropriate condenser				
Repeat as needed				
Transfer instruments (explorer, carver, burnisher) as needed to complete placement				
Remove matrix and wedge, if necessary				
Transfer articulating paper, floss, wet cotton pellet as needed				
Remove stray bits of amalgam with high-volume evacuator				
Practice safe handling and scrap storage procedures				
Work efficiently				

Competence assessment: To be judged competent, the student will correctly meet 36 (_____) of the 39 criteria. [Competence = 39−3 (-_____) criteria.]

_____
Instructor's Signature/Date

Laboratory Component: Placement of Z-O-E Temporary Restoration

Directions to evaluator: Following demonstration and practice, ask the student to prepare material for and place a zinc oxide and eugenol restoration, then clean up after use of the material in the situations listed below. Place a check mark in the appropriate column when a criterion is NOT met. This will direct the student's attention to any area that may still need work, while clearly indicating those areas that have been mastered.

Student places Z-O-E temporary restoration	Step	Instructor Comment
Educates patient		
Selects powder and liquid OR preloaded capsule		
Mixes material to stiff, putty-like consistency OR triturates preloaded material		
Places in cavity		
Has patient bite material into occlusion OR carves to anatomy		
Removes remaining excess material		
Checks proximal anatomy and occlusal height		
Provides postoperative directions		
Cleans after use		
Follows infection control protocol		

Student achieves acceptable result	Criterion	Instructor Comment
Cavity completely filled		
Smooth surface		
Margins flush with tooth preparation		
Restored surface(s) replicate usual tooth anatomy		
No overhangs		
No occlusal high spots		
Restoration completed in reasonable amount of time		

Competence assessment: To be judged competent, the student will correctly meet 9 (_____) of the 10 steps and 6 of the 7 criteria for an acceptable restoration. [Competence = 10−1 (-_____) steps and 7−1 (-_____) criteria.]

_____
Instructor's Signature/Date

Evaluation of Competence for Chapter 13:
Impression trays

Student's Name: _____ Date: _____

Directions to evaluator: Provide the student with samples or pictures of trays and equipment and materials used to make them, then request that he/she select the one you name and indicate its use(s). Place a check mark in the appropriate column when a criterion is NOT met. Leave other areas blank. This will direct the student's attention to any area that may still need work, while clearly indicating those areas that have been mastered.

Student selects	Selection	Use(s)	Instructor Comment
Stock tray			
Custom tray			
Full arch tray			
Quadrant (posterior) tray			
Sextant (anterior) tray			
Dual impression tray			
Bite tray			
Polyvinyl sheet			
Polystyrene beads			
Self-cured resin monomer and polymer			
Vacuum former			
Pressure former			
Compound heater (or similar)			
Light box			
Rolling pin and board			

Competence assessment: To be judged competent, the student will correctly identify 13 (_____) of the 15 items displayed, and will correctly indicate at least one use for 15 (_____) of the 15 items displayed. (Competence = 15−2 (-_____) tray identifications and 15−0 (-_____) uses.)

_____
Instructor's Signature/Date

320   Competency Evaluations

Laboratory Component: Construction of Custom Trays

Directions to evaluator: Following demonstration and practice, ask the student to construct a bleaching tray, mouthguard, and custom final impression tray using your choice of the techniques listed below. Evaluate the adequacy of the completed tray. Place a check mark in the appropriate column when a criterion is NOT met. Leave other areas blank. This will direct the student's attention to any area that may still need work, while clearly indicating those areas that have been mastered.

Criterion	Quadrant Tray Using Polystyrene Beads	Bleaching Tray Using Vacuum or Pressure Former	Mouthguard Using Vacuum or Pressure Former	Full Arch Tray Using Light Box or Self-cure Resin
Fits over and covers teeth of interest				
Does not impinge on soft tissue				
Even spacing between tray and teeth		XXX	XXX	
Space adequate to hold impression material or, for a bleaching tray, bleaching gel			XXX	
Edges gently rounded and smooth				
Handle is securely attached		XXX	XXX	
Handle has sufficient bulk to hold easily		XXX	XXX	
Handle does not interfere with lips or teeth		XXX	XXX	
Stops placed away from teeth of interest		XXX	XXX	
Sufficient number of stops placed for size of tray		XXX	XXX	
Tray perforated for retention, if requested		XXX	XXX	
Tray cleaned of wax, loose plastic and air barrier coating				
Tray disinfected and placed on model				
Safe procedures followed				
Area cleaned following tray construction				

Competence assessment: To be judged competent, the student will meet 13 (____) of the 15 criteria for an acceptable custom tray, 8 (____) of 8 criteria for an acceptable bleaching tray, and 7 (____) of 7 criteria for an acceptable mouthguard. [Competence = ____ - ____ criteria met for technique demonstrated.]

_____
Instructor's Signature/Date

321

Evaluation of Competence for Chapter 14:
Final Impression Materials

Student's Name: _____ Date: _____

Directions to evaluator: Ask the student to describe each material, concept and technique listed below. Place a check mark in the appropriate column when a criterion is NOT met. Leave other areas blank. This will direct the student's attention to any area that may still need work, while clearly indicating those areas that have been mastered.

Student describes	Description	Instructor Comment
Definition and use of a final impression		
How a final impression material works in the mouth		
Properties of rubber base materials in general		
Properties of hydrocolloid material		
Comparison of rubber base and hydrocolloid final impression materials		
Differences among polysulfide, polyether, silicone and polyvinyl siloxane rubber base materials		
The body of a material		
Heavy, regular, and light body materials		
Single phase material		
Relationship of material viscosity to its selection for use		
Syringe technique		
Tray technique		
Putty-wash technique		
Direct placement technique		
Operation of a hydrocolloid conditioner		
Use of a water-cooled tray		
Disinfection of final impressions		

Competence assessment: To be judged competent, the student will correctly describe 13 (_____) of the 17 materials, concepts and techniques listed. [Competence = 17−5 (-_____) descriptions.]

_____

Instructor's Signature/Date

Laboratory Component: Preparation of Rubber Base Final Impression Materials

Directions to evaluator: Following demonstration and practice, ask the student to prepare and transfer rubber base final impression materials using your choice of the techniques listed below. Place a check mark in the appropriate column when a criterion is NOT met. Leave other areas blank. This will direct the student's attention to any area that may still need work, while clearly indicating those areas that have been mastered.

Criterion	Syringe Technique: Hand (H) or Automix (A)	Tray Technique: Hand (H) or Automix (A)	Putty-wash Technique: Hand (H) or Automix (A)	Direct Placement Technique: Automix	Machine Mixing Technique
Paints tray with adhesive and allows to dry, if needed				XXX	
Selects appropriate material(s) to use					
Proportions correctly	H	H	H	XXX	XXX
Combines base and catalyst correctly	H	H	H	XXX	XXX
Ensures all material is incorporated	H	H	H	XXX	XXX
Mixes to homogenous color and consistency	H	H	H	XXX	XXX
Gathers material into one mass	H	H	H	XXX	XXX
Loads evenly into tray or syringe				XXX	
Transfers correctly		XXX		XXX	XXX
Repeats when using second material of different viscosity					
Loads cartridge without difficulty	A	A	A		XXX
Affixes mixing tip and ensures air in tip is expelled and material is mixing properly	A	A	A		XXX
Affixes direct placement tip, if requested	A	XXX	A		XXX
Disinfects impression					

Cleans area and equipment following use			
Works neatly, safely			
Follows infection control protocol			
Total number of criteria to be met			
90% of total criteria =			

Competence assessment: To be judged competent, the student will meet 90% of the criteria for the technique and steps selected. The number of criteria to be met will differ depending on the total number of techniques and steps requested.

_____

Instructor's Signature/Date

Laboratory Component: Preparation and Use of Hydrocolloid

Directions to evaluator: Following demonstration and practice, ask the student to prepare and transfer hydrocolloid final impression material using the syringe technique. Place a check mark in the appropriate column when a criterion is NOT met. Leave other areas blank. This will direct the student's attention to any area that may still need work, while clearly indicating those areas that have been mastered.

Task to be completed	Task Completed Correctly	Instructor Comment
Select appropriate tray and syringe		
Select appropriate tray and syringe materials		
Liquefy materials in boiling compartment		
Transfer to storage compartment		
5 minutes before use, load tray (and syringe if not loaded prior to liquefying materials), attach water tubes to tray and transfer both tray and syringe to tempering compartment		
Transfer tempered syringe material to operator		
Scrape water-logged surface off tray material		
Receive syringe and transfer tray		
Activate circulation of cool water in tray		
Receive and disinfect impression		
Operate machine correctly		
Work neatly, safely and efficiently		
Clean area and equipment following use		

Competence assessment: To be judged competent, the student will correctly complete 12 (_____) of the 13 steps listed. [Competence = 13−1 (-_____) steps.]

_____
Instructor's Signature/Date

Evaluation of Competence for Chapter 15: Temporary Coverage

Student's Name: _____ Date: _____

Directions to evaluator: Ask the student to complete each task listed below. Place a check mark in the appropriate column when a criterion is NOT met. Leave other areas blank. This will direct the student's attention to any area that may still need work, while clearly indicating those areas that have been mastered.

Task to be completed	Description	Instructor Comment
Define temporary coverage		
State the uses of temporary coverage		
Describe why temporary coverage is necessary		
List the materials used for temporary coverage		
Discuss esthetics, ease of use, durability and cost in relation to temporary coverage		
Summarize the characteristics and uses of acrylic resin, composite and preformed crown temporary materials		
Given a description of a specific situation, select a material for temporary coverage		
Describe construction of a temporary restoration using a stent		
Describe construction of a block temporary		
Describe construction of a temporary restoration using an impression as a mold		
Describe construction of a temporary restoration using a preformed polymer crown		
Describe construction of a temporary restoration using a preformed stainless steel crown		

Competence assessment: To be judged competent, the student will correctly describe 9 (_____) of the 12 materials, concepts and techniques listed. [Competence = 12−3 (-_____) descriptions.]

_____
Instructor's Signature/Date

Laboratory Component: Construction and Cementation of a Temporary Restoration

Directions to evaluator: Following demonstration and practice, ask the student to construct and cement a temporary restoration using your choice of construction techniques. Then evaluate the adequacy of the restoration. Place a check mark in the appropriate column when a criterion is NOT met. Leave other areas blank. This will direct the student's attention to any area that may still need work, while clearly indicating those areas that have been mastered.

Criterion	Met	Instructor Comment
Created correct incisal overlap and overjet, if restoration is in anterior 　Recreates contact of natural tooth		
Created correct interproximal contacts 　At correct height to meet contacts of adjacent teeth 　Not overextended cervicoincisally/occlusally		
Created correct anatomic form 　Is neither too large nor too small for the space 　　to be filled 　Replicates contours of the natural crown 　Embrasures and interproximal areas are present		
Adapted restoration correctly 　Seats fully on preparation 　Covers entire preparation 　Does not rock 　Margin is not overextended 　Margin is flush with tooth preparation		
Finished surface well 　Smooth 　Has no voids 　Polished to a high lustre		
Cemented correctly 　Margin completely cemented 　No voids in cement line 　All excess cement removed 　Crown is not high		
Professional work habits exhibited during process 　Worked neatly, safely and efficiently 　Followed infection control protocol 　Self-evaluation acceptable		

Competence assessment: To be judged competent, the student will meet 6 (_____) of the 7 criteria. [Competence = 7−1 (-_____) criteria met.]

_____
Instructor's Signature/Date

Evaluation of Competence for Chapter 16:
Materials for Permanent Indirect Restorations

Student's Name: _____ Date: _____

Directions to evaluator: Ask the student to complete the indicated task. Place a check mark in the appropriate column when a criterion is NOT met. Leave other areas blank. This will direct the student's attention to any area that may still need work, while clearly indicating those areas that have been mastered.

Task to be Completed	Task Completed Correctly	Instructor Comment
Define a permanent indirect restoration		
List the materials used for construction of temporary restorations		
State the usual uses for each type of material		
Provide brief descriptions of the processes used to construct fired porcelain, cast ceramic, CAD-CAM, metal alloy and resin indirect restorations		
Describe margin and surface considerations and examination procedures for all types of indirect restorations		
Describe polishing considerations and care for ceramic, metal alloy, and resin restorations		
Describe fluoride treatment considerations and care for ceramic restorations		
Describe repair of fractured ceramic restorations		
Describe appointment scheduling for the various types of indirect restorations		

Competence assessment: To be judged competent, the student will complete 6 (_____) of the 9 tasks correctly. [Competence = 9−3 (-_____) tasks completed correctly.]

_____
Instructor's Signature/Date

Evaluation of Competence for Chapter 17:
Cements

Student's Name: _____ Date: _____

Directions to evaluator: Ask the student to complete each listed task. Place a check mark in the appropriate column when a criterion is NOT met. Leave other areas blank. This will direct the student's attention to any area that may still need work, while clearly indicating those areas that have been mastered.

Task to be Completed	Task Completed Correctly	Instructor Comment
Define and state the use of a luting cement		
Describe how joints are formed between teeth and material		
Differentiate metal oxide and polymer cements		
List metal oxide cements and state at least one use of each		
List polymer cements and state at least one use of each		
Discuss film thickness; cement acidity, strength and solubility; and development of secondary decay in relation to the use of cements		
Discuss the general principles of mixing any type of cement powder and liquid		
Discuss the principles of mixing powder and liquid that apply only to polymer cements		
Discuss the principles of mixing powder and liquid that apply only to zinc oxide cements		
Indicate how to tell when a cement is the proper consistency for luting		
Describe how to prepare a metal item for cementation		
State the type of environment necessary for cementation and why it is necessary		

Competence assessment: To be judged competent, the student will correctly complete at least 9 (_____) of the 12 tasks. [Competence = 12−3 (-_____) identifications and uses.]

_____
Instructor's Signature/Date

Directions to evaluator: Ask the student to describe the properties of each material listed below, then indicate how they relate to the health of the tooth. Place a check mark in the appropriate column when a criterion is NOT met.

Material	Properties	Relationship	Instructor Comment
Zinc phosphate cement			
Zinc oxide and eugenol cement			
Glass ionomer cement			
Resin cement			
Zinc polycarboxylate			

Competence assessment: To be judged competent, the student will correctly describe 4 (____) of the 5 property sets and 4 (____) of the 5 relationships. [Competence = 5−4 (-____) property sets and 5-4 (-____) relationships.]

Laboratory Component: Preparation and Transfer of Cements

Directions to evaluator: Following demonstration and practice, ask the student to prepare, test for correct preparation, transfer, and clean after use of, each of the materials listed below. Place a check mark in the appropriate column when a criterion is NOT met. This will direct the student's attention to any area that may still need work, while clearly indicating those areas that have been mastered.

Material	Preparation	Test for Correct Preparation	Transfer	Cleanup
Zinc phosphate luting cement				
Z-O-E luting cement				
Glass ionomer luting cement				
Resin luting cement				
Zinc polycarboxylate luting cement				

Comments _____

_____

_____

Competence assessment: To be judged competent, the student will correctly complete 18 (____) of the 20 tasks. [Competence = 20−2 (-____) descriptions.]

_____
Instructor's Signature/Date

Evaluation of Competence for Chapter 18: Materials for Dental Implants

Student's Name: _____ Date: _____

Directions to evaluator: Ask the student to complete the indicated task. Place a check mark in the appropriate column when a criterion is NOT met. Leave other areas blank. This will direct the student's attention to any area that may still need work, while clearly indicating those areas that have been mastered.

Task to be Completed	Task Completed Correctly	Instructor Comment
Define and state the use of a dental implant		
Given pictures of the two basic types of implants, identify each type and its components		
List the materials used to construct dental implants and the contributions of each to the whole		
Describe osseointegration		
Describe formation of a perimucosal seal		
Describe how an implant contributes to occlusal function		
Briefly describe the procedures for placing endosseous and subperiosteal implants		
Discuss mobility, microbial invasion, mechanical overload and scratching of the implant surface as they relate to implant function		
Describe means of examining and caring for implants that will maintain their surface integrity		

Competence assessment: To be judged competent, the student will correctly complete at least 8 (_____) of the 9 indicated tasks. [Competence = 9−1 (-_____) tasks correctly completed.]

_____
Instructor's Signature/Date

Evaluation of Competence for Chapter 19: Denture Materials

Student's Name: _____ Date: _____

Directions to evaluator: Ask the student to complete the indicated task. Place a check mark in the appropriate column when a criterion is NOT met. Leave other areas blank. This will direct the student's attention to any area that may still need work, while clearly indicating those areas that have been mastered.

Ask the student to	Task Completed Correctly	Instructor Comment
Define and differentiate conventional, immediate, full, partial and overdentures		
Given samples or pictures of full and partial dentures, name and state the purpose of each component		
Discuss the contributions dentures make to daily living		
Summarize the procedures for construction of a full denture		
Summarize the procedures for construction of a partial denture		
Discuss appointment scheduling for full and partial denture construction, delivery and follow-up care		
List the materials that may be used to construct denture bases and saddles; teeth; metal frameworks, connectors, clasps and rests; baseplates and occlusal rims; state why the dentist may select each one		
Describe the composition, reaction and characteristics of denture acrylic		
Discuss esthetics, tissue irritation, fracture, dimensional stability, material stability, discoloration, distortion and wear as they relate to the clinical success and longevity of a denture		
Discuss cobalt–chromium alloy in relation to the demands placed on a denture in the oral cavity		

Competence assessment: To be judged competent, the student will correctly complete at least 8 (____) of the 10 indicated tasks. [Competence = 10−2 (-____) tasks correctly completed.]

_____
Instructor's Signature/Date

Evaluation of Competence for Chapter 20: Endodontic Materials

Student's Name: _____ Date: _____

Directions to evaluator: Ask the student to complete the indicated task. Place a check mark in the appropriate column when a criterion is NOT met. Leave other areas blank. This will direct the student's attention to any area that may still need work, while clearly indicating those areas that have been mastered.

Ask the student to:	Task Completed Correctly	Instructor Comment
Define each of the following procedures: pulp extirpation, pulpectomy, pulpotomy, and apexification		
Differentiate pulp irrigating agents, medicaments, sealers and fillers on the basis of general function		
List and state the action(s) of each material used as an irrigating agent		
List and state the action(s) of at least four of the materials used as medicaments		
List and state the actions of each of the three types of sealers		

Competence assessment: To be judged competent, the student will correctly complete at least 4 (_____) of the 5 indicated tasks. [Competence = 5−1 (-_____) tasks correctly completed.]

_____
Instructor's Signature/Date

INDEX

liquids, 23
  mixing, 53
  mixing techniques, 55
  packaging materials, 52
load, 25–27

M

Maryland bridge, 6, 6f
Material Safety Data Sheets, 38
materials used in dentistry, 14. See also specific materials
  abrasion resistance, 28
  choosing, 30
  color selection. (see color)
  electrochemical forces, 28
  flow of, 24–25
  hydrophilic, 29, 30
  hydrophobic, 30
  intermediary. (see intermediary materials)
  load abilities, 25–26
  malleability, 27
  moisture, assessing when choosing materials, 29–30
  setting abilities, 25
  solidity, 23–24
  strength, 26–27
  thermal expansion and contraction, 27–28
  transparency of, 27–28
mechanical bonding, 19
mercury
  -alloy ratio, 144
  OSHA regulations, 39–41
  precautions when using, 143
  usage, 39
metacresylacetate (Crestatin), 233
metal alloy
  amalgam. (see amalgam)
  clinical considerations, 188–189
  composition, 187
  description, 45
  electoplating on final impressions, 99
  fabrication, 187–188
  high copper, 143
  materials, specific choices, 188
  noble, 187
  particles, shape of, 144
  properties, 187
  types, 187
  usage, 45
  use, 187–188
  zinc, 143
microleakage, 18–19
model trimmers, 48
models
  abrasion resistance, 107
  accuracy of finished product, 107

chemical level, 98–100
  constructing, 98
  definition, 98
  fractures, preventing, 107–108
  materials used, 98
  procedure, 98
  strength, 107
  study type, 8
  usage, 8, 98
  wetness of, 107–108
moisture, impact on dental materials, 29–30
monomers, 24
mouthguards, 11
  athletic, 155
  material selection, 155
MSDS. See Material Safety Data Sheets

N

National Transportation and Safety Board, 38
nickel, 188

O

occlusal registration, 8
Occupational Safety and Health Administration. See OSHA
onlay, 5
opacity, 130
Organization for Safety and Asepsis Procesures, 38
OSHA
  eye and fire safety, 39
  Hazard Communication Standard, 38–39
  mercury. (see mercury)
  regulations, 37–38
  spills and leaks, 39
osseointegration, of implants, 207, 208–209
overdenture, 6, 7

P

pads, 47
palladium, 188
paste
  blending, 52–53, 55
  two tubes, use of, 52–53
personal safety. See also OSHA
  chemicals, protection from, 36
  composites, when using, 135
  exposure to chemicals, 36–37
  hazard control, 36
plastics. See also polymers
  description, 46
  usage in dentistry, 46
platinum, 188
polymers. See also plastics
  as crown, 177
  cement, 195, 196

definition, 24
esthetics, use in situations where important, 46
heat cured, 25
light cured, 25, 158
polystyrene bead trays, 158
pontic, 6
porcelain
    as non-metallic solid, 23
    characteristics, 183
    clinical concerns, 186
    contraction, 45
    dentures, 220–221
    fracture repairs, 186–187
    restorations, making, 183–185, 186
    usage in dentistry, 45
    vs ceramic, 186
powders
    mixing, 52
    mixing techniques, 55
    packaging materials, 52
    preparation techniques, 55
pressure formers, 48
pressure forming (of trays), 157
processing waxes, 13
pumice, 69

Q

quartz, 69

R

regulatory agencies. See OSHA; safety
relaxation, 26
restorations. See also crown; inlay; onlay
    direct, 4
    indirect, 4–5
    overview, 4
    single tooth, 5
    temporary. (see temporary restoration)
reversible hydrocolloid, 169–170
rouge, 70

S

saddle, 6
safety. See also OSHA
    ADA Acceptance program. (see American Dental Association)
    FDA approval process, 35
    personal. (see personal safety)
    private resources of assessing, 35–36
    regulatory agencies, 37–38
sargenti paste, 234
sealants
    action, mechanism of, 74
    caries resistance, 76
    composition, 74

description, 12, 74
efficacy, 78
evaluation, 77
isolation, adequate, 74–75
materials used, 74
placement, 75, 77
resin, acrylic, 74
retention, 75
surface preparation, 76–77
usage, 12, 74
visibility, 75
wear, 75
sealers, 232–233
secondary impression. See final impression
setting, of dental materials, 25
shade selection. See color
sheets, 53
silver, 188
slabs, 47
sodium hypocholrite, 231
solids, 23–24
solubility, 30
sorption, 30
spatulas, 47–48
splints
    occlusal, 11–12
    periodontal, 12
    usage, 11
sterile saline solution, 229
strain, 26
strength
    malleability, 27
    overview, 26–27
    types of, 26
syringes, 55

T

temporary restorations
    acrylic resin, 174–175
    clinical concerns, 174
    composite use, 177
    definition, 174
    for broken or missing tooth, 175–176
    for mostly intact tooth, 176–177
    materials used, 174, 175t
    preformed crowns, 177
    rationale for use, 174
    usage, 174
thermoplastic set, 25
tin oxide, 69
tips, 53
tooth whiteners. See whiteners
toxicity, 18
transparency of dental materials, 22
trays, for impressions, 10, 91
    custom, procedures for, 155, 156

trays, for impressions (*con't*)
    for bleaching, 155
    for mouthguards, 155
    hand molding, 158
    light-cured polymer technique, 158
    materials used, 154
    perforated, 91
    polystyrene bead trays, 158
    pressure forming, 157
    rim lock, 91
    rolled acrylic dough technique, 159
    single arch, 154
    two arches, 154
    vacuum adaptaion, 156
trimming, 94
triturator, 118

V

vaccum formers, 48
vacuum adaptation, 156
varnish, 19
varnishes. See also specific materials and
    chemicals
    copal, 116
    materials used, 114
    overview, 115
    universal, 117
veneer, 5
viscosity, in composites, 129

W

waste disposal
    hazardous, 40–41
    overview, 41
    sharps, 41

water, sterile, 229
wetting, description of action, 29
whiteners
    action, mechanism of, 81
    application schedule, 84
    contraindications for, 82–84
    description, 81
    efficacy, 84
    gingival irritation, 85
    hypersensitivity to, 84
    indications for, 82
    materials used, 81
    preparation, 81, 82
    product types, 81
    trays for, 166
    troubleshooting, 84–85
    usage, 81

Z

zinc, 188
zinc oxide and eugenol (ZOE), 117, 118, 119,
    147–148, 198–200
    action, mechanism of, 147
    anatomy issues in placement, 148
    clinical concerns, 147
    containers, 147
    definition, 147
    procedure, 147
    pulp irritation, 147
    tooth response, assessing, 148
    usage, 147
zinc phosphate, 118–120, 197–198
zinc polycarboxylate, 120–121, 200–201